EXPERIMENTAL FOUNDATIONS
OF BEHAVIORAL MEDICINE:
CONDITIONING APPROACHES

EXPERIMENTAL FOUNDATIONS OF BEHAVIORAL MEDICINE: CONDITIONING APPROACHES

Edited by

Robert Ader
University of Rochester

Herbert Weiner
University of California

Andrew Baum
Uniformed Services University of Health Sciences

LEA LAWRENCE ERLBAUM ASSOCIATES, PUBLISHERS
1988   Hillsdale, New Jersey   Hove and London

Copyright © 1988 by Lawrence Erlbaum Associates, Inc.
All rights reserved. No part of this book may be reproduced in
any form, by photostat, microfilm, retrieval system, or any other
means, without the prior written permission of the publisher.

Lawrence Erlbaum Associates, Inc., Publishers
365 Broadway
Hillsdale, New Jersey 07642

Library of Congress Cataloging-in-Publication Data

Experimental foundations of behavioral medicine : conditioning
  approaches / edited by Robert Ader, Herbert Weiner, and Andrew Baum.
     p.   cm.
  Includes bibliographies and index.
  ISBN 0-8058-0139-1
  1. Medicine, Psychosomatic. 2. Conditioned response. I. Ader,
Robert. II. Weiner, Herbert. III. Baum, Andrew.
    [DNLM: 1. Behavioral Medicine. 2. Conditioning (Psychology) WB
100 E96]
RC49.E97   1988
616.08—dc19
DNLM/DLC   88-363
for Library of Congress   CIP

Printed in the United States of America
10 9 8 7 6 5 4 3 2 1

2. D. Felton
3. N. Cohen
4. F. Berkenbosch

4:00 - 6:00 p.m.
Room- Sunset Lounge
<u>Symposium B</u>
Biobehavioral Factors in Diabetes and Insulin Metabolism
1. B. Falkner
2. S. B. Johnson
3. A. La Greca

<u>EVENING</u>
7:00 p.m. Dinner - West Dining Room
8:00 - 9:30 p.m.
J. Dimsdale, Chair
8:00 - 8:30 p.m.
A. Leshner
Deputy Director, NIMH
NIMH Role in Behavioral Medicine
8:30 - 9:30 p.m.
R. Williams
The Trusting Heart

Prevention and Intervention In Health Research
1. M. Fletcher
2. M. Chesney
3. B. Andersen

4:00 - 6:00 p.m.
Room - Sunset Lounge
<u>Symposium B</u>
Obesity as Manifestation of Metabolic Defect
1. J. Hirsch
2. R. Keesey
3. R. Leibel

<u>EVENING</u>
7:00 p.m. Dinner - West Dining Room
8:00 - 9:30 p.m.
A. Shapiro, Chair
Presidential Address
N. Schneiderman
Biobehavioral Aspects of Hypertension

ACADEMY OF BEHAVIORAL MEDICINE RESEARCH
1989 PROGRAM
BEHAVIORAL ASPECTS OF DISEASE PROCESSES
Mohonk Mountain House
Lake Mohonk, New Paltz, New York

SUNDAY EVENING (June 11, 1989)
7:00 p.m. Dinner - West Dining Room
8:00 p.m. Opening Remarks - N. Schneiderman
8:10 - 9:30 p.m. Stress, Health and Aging - C. Eisdorfer

MONDAY (June 12)
9:00 a.m. - Noon - Plenary 1
Room - Council House
Psychosocial Stress and Immune Function
M. Stein, Chair
1. R. Glaser
2. J. Kiecolt-Glaser
3. A. Baum
4. A. Stone

3:30 - 6:00 p.m.
Room - Laurel Lounge
Symposium A
Basic Processes in Psychoneuroimmunology
1. R. Ader

TUESDAY (June 13)
9:00 a.m. - Noon - Plenary 2
Room - Council House
Biobehavioral Aspects of Diabetes and Metabolism
1. J. Skyler
2. D. Surwit
3. C. Bogardus
4. P. Cryer

3:00 - 4:00 p.m.
Business Meeting - Council House

4:00 - 6:00 p.m.
Room - Laurel Lounge
Symposium A

WEDNESDAY (June 14)
9:00 a.m. - Noon - Plenary 3
Room - Council House
Psychoimmunology and Disease
1. N. Klimas
2. S. Levy
3. S. Cohen

12:30 LUNCH

CONTENTS

CONTRIBUTORS ix

PREFACE xi

1

**LEARNED ASPECTS
OF CARDIOVASCULAR REGULATION** 1
  *Philip M. McCabe, Neil Schneiderman, Ray W. Winters,
  Christopher G. Gentile, Alan H. Teich*
Cardiovascular Concomitants of Operant Conditioning
  of Somatic Responses, 2
Direct Operant Conditioning
  of Cardiovascular Responses, 4
Behavioral Treatment of Hypertension, 7
Classical Conditioning, 8
Learned Modification of Elicited
  Cardiovascular Responses, 15
References, 18

2

PAVLOVIAN CONDITIONING OF ENDOCRINE RESPONSES 25
  Mark E. Stanton and Seymour Levine
Conditioned Endocrine Responses, 27

Dissociations of Conditioned Behavioral
and Endocrine Responses, 33
Properties of Endocrine Conditioning, 40
Summary and Conclusions, 43
Acknowledgments, 44
References, 45

3

THE PLACEBO EFFECT AS A CONDITIONED RESPONSE 47
Robert Ader
Behaviorally Conditioned Immunosuppression
and the Pharmacotherapy of Autoimmune
Disease in Animals, 49
A Conditioning Model of Pharmocotherapy, 56
Conclusions, 61
Acknowledgments, 63
References, 63

4

THE TREATMENT OF SCOLIOSIS BY CONTINUOUS AUTOMATED POSTURAL FEEDBACK 67
Barry Dworkin and Susan Dworkin
Introduction, 67
Method, 72
Results, 80
Discussion, 83
Conclusions, 84
References, 86

5

RELAXATION TRAINING IN ESSENTIAL HYPERTENSION 87
Prospects and Problems
W. Stewart Agras
Physiologic Effects, 88
Effects on Perception and Affect, 90
Behavior Changes, 91
Evidence for Efficacy in Essential Hypertension, 92
Evidence for Specificity of Effect, 100

Relaxation Training in the Management
  of Essential Hypertension, 105
Research Question, 106
References, 107

6

**THE SYNTHESIS OF MEDICAL AND BEHAVIORAL
SCIENCES WITH RESPECT TO BRONCHIAL ASTHMA**   111
  Thomas L. Creer
Definition of Asthma, 111
Conceptualizations of Asthma, 118
Psychological and Behavioral
  Interventions for Asthma, 127
Behavioral Contributions to the Management
  and Rehabilitation of Asthmatic Patients, 134
Application of Behavioral Techniques
  to Alter Patient Behaviors, 135
Summary, 152
References, 153

7

**STRESS, BEHAVIOR, AND GLUCOSE CONTROL
IN DIABETES MELLITUS**   159
  Richard S. Surwit
Diabetes and Stress, 160
Summary and Conclusions, 170
Acknowledgment, 171
References, 171

8

**A PROPOSAL FOR A CURRICULUM
IN BEHAVIORAL BIOLOGY AND MEDICINE
IN MEDICAL SCHOOLS**   175
  Herbert Weiner
The First Year, 177
The Second Year, 179
The Clinical Years, 181
References, 183

9

**TRAINING OF FAMILY PHYSICIANS
IN BEHAVIORAL MEDICINE**   185
Hiram B. Curry
Reference, 193

10

**TEACHING BEHAVIORAL CONCEPTS
IN CARDIOVASCULAR DISEASE WITH REMARKS
ON CHALLENGES TO MEDICAL EDUCATION**   195
Alvin P. Shapiro
Acknowledgment, 207
References, 207

AUTHOR INDEX   209

SUBJECT INDEX   219

CONTRIBUTORS

ROBERT ADER, PH.D.   Department of Psychiatry, School of Medicine and Dentistry, University of Rochester, 300 Crittenden Blvd., Rochester, NY 14642

W. STEWART AGRAS, M.D.   Department of Psychiatry, School of Medicine, Stanford University, Stanford, CA 94305

ANDREW BAUM, PH.D.   Department of Medical Psychology, USU School of Medicine, 4301 Jones Bridge Rd., Bethesda, MD 20814-4799

THOMAS L. CREER, PH.D.   Department of Psychology, Ohio University, Porter Hall, Athens, OH 45701

HIRAM B. CURRY, PH.D.   Professor and Chairman, Department of Family Medicine, Professor of Neurology, Medical University of South Carolina, Charleston, SC 29425

SUSAN DWORKIN, PH.D.   Department of Behavioral Sciences, School of Medicine, Milton S. Hershey Medical Center, Pennsylvania State University, Hershey, PA 17033

BARRY R. DWORKIN, PH.D.   Department of Behavioral Sciences, School of Medicine, Milton S. Hershey Medical Center, Pennsylvania State University, Hershey, PA 17033

CHRISTOPHER G. GENTILE Department of Psychology, Program in Behavioral Medicine, University of Miami, P.O. Box 248185, Coral Gables, FL 33124

SEYMOUR LEVINE, PH.D. Department of Psychiatry & Behavioral Science, Medical Center, Stanford University, Stanford, CA 94305

PHILIP M. McCABE Department of Psychology, Program in Behavioral Medicine, University of Miami, P.O. Box 248185, Coral Gables, FL 33124

NEIL SCHNEIDERMAN, PH.D. Department of Psychology, Program in Behavioral Medicine, University of Miami, P.O. Box 248185, Coral Gables, FL 33124

ALVIN P. SHAPIRO, M.D. Shadyside Hospital, 5230 Centre Ave., Pittsburgh, PA 15232

MARK E. STANTON, PH.D. Neurotoxicology Division (MD-74B), Health Effects Research Laboratory, U.S. Environmental Protection Agency, Research Triangle Park, NC 27711

RICHARD S. SURWIT, PH.D. Professor of Medical Psychology, Medical Center, Box 3842, Duke University, Durham, NC 27710

ALAN H. TEICH Department of Psychology, Program in Behavioral Medicine, University of Miami, P.O. Box 248185, Coral Gables, FL 33124

HERBERT WEINER, M.D. Neuropsychiatric Institute, Health Sciences Center, University of California, 760 Westwood Plaza, Los Angeles, CA 90024

RAY W. WINTERS Department of Psychology, Program in Behavioral Medicine, University of Miami, P.O. Box 248185, Coral Gables, FL 33124

PREFACE

As an interdisciplinary field of study, behavioral medicine has made a good case for itself in the clinic as well as the research laboratory. It may no longer be sufficient to document the role of behavioral factors in the development, progression, or recovery from disease or to illustrate the efficacy of behavioral strategies in the amelioration of symptoms of a wide range of physical disorders. We have, perhaps, reached the point at which to make another point, namely that the sophistication that characterizes the experimental analysis of behavioral processes can be used to achieve a more detailed and comprehensive understanding of the biobehavioral mechanisms underlying both the development and reduction of symptoms of disease.

From an experimental point of view, the apparently relevant strategies and interventions of the behaviorally oriented clinician are not new. By and large, they reflect and extrapolate from classic concerns of behavioral scientists. Primary among these is the issue of conditioning and learning. It would, of course, be an oversimplification to point to "learning" as *the* experimental foundation of behavioral medicine. Learning is, however, a fundamental process of adaptation to the physical and social environment and, implicitly or explicitly, extensions of classical and operant conditioning principles have provided the basis for many of the behavioral strategies of intervention designed to modify behavioral and physiological responses in clinically relevant ways. The principles and techniques are not new; what is new — and what we can credit to the behavioral medicine movement — is the application of these principles and techniques to the prevention of illness and to the alleviation of symptoms of disease.

From an experimental point of view, however, it sometimes appears that clinical practitioners, in applying behavioral modification techniques, have proceeded at a rate that far exceeds the experimental data upon which such interventions should be based. Based on the mostly clinical data that are available thus far, it is fair to say, perhaps, that behavioral interventions may sometimes be indicated, may sometimes by contraindicated, and that they are effective for some individuals in some clinical entities and are ineffective for other individuals and/or in other clinical entities. As empirically effective as some techniques have been for some individuals suffering from some physical disorders, the extent (and the limitations) of the role of behavioral and psychosocial factors in health and disease and the precise parameters for effective interventions are largely unknown. If this is so, who, then, will do the research, and who will be equipped to evaluate and apply this research? What constitutes the basic science foundations of behavioral medicine? And who will teach what substantive material to whom — and under what circumstances?

The focus of the meetings of the Academy of Behavioral Medicine Research held in Kiawah Island, SC in 1985 was on conditioning phenomena as one of the experimental foundations of behavioral medicine. The chapters included in the present volume are illustrative rather than exhaustive with respect to the relevance of conditioning to behavioral medicine and are representative but not a complete record of the proceedings of that meeting. As a point of departure for further discussion, the first group of chapters includes discussions of very basic conditioning effects in the regulation of physiological responses, the role of conditioning and learning in selected disease models, the precise application of conditioning principles, and speculative analyses of the potential of conditioning in the modification of clinically relevant responses. The final three chapters address some of the issues involved in teaching both the fundamentals and the applied components of behavioral medicine. We hope that this attempt to focus on basic research and, thus, education in behavioral medicine will prompt future meetings with a similar, if substantively different, emphasis.

The present volume represents only one outcome of the annual ABMR meetings and, for the success of this particular meeting, we would like to express our appreciation to those who gave such excellent presentations; to members of the Academy for their attention and spontaneous discussion; to Jerome E. Singer, the then outgoing Secretary-Treasurer of the Academy, and Peg Bang for their superb direction and organization of the meetings; and especially to the authors of the chapters that appear in this volume.

RA
HW
AB

1
LEARNED ASPECTS OF CARDIOVASCULAR REGULATION

Philip M. McCabe, Neil Schneiderman, Ray W. Winters,
Christopher G. Gentile, Alan H. Teich
University of Miami

The circulatory system distributes oxygen and other nutrients to bodily tissues, and returns carbon dioxide to the lungs and other products of metabolism to the kidneys. It also plays an important role in the regulation of body temperature and in the transport of hormones and other functional chemicals to target organs. The regulation of cardiovascular activity requires coordination of local, reflexive, and central nervous system (CNS) command activities.

Impulses initiated at intrinsic (e.g., visceral) or extrinsic (e.g., distance) receptors are relayed to the CNS, integrated within it at various levels of the neuraxis, and transmitted via efferents to the cardiovascular both negative feedback and positive feedforward processes, and by cellular and metabolic factors. Specific patterns of cardiovascular responses can therefore be associated with particular stimulus conditions as well as with species characteristics, metabolic demands, and the history of an organism with particular stimuli. Thus, cardiovascular responses to stimuli may vary as a function of novelty, habituation, or learning, as well as by tissue demands.

The procedure used to examine learned cardiovascular adjustments can be subsumed under the general rubrics of classical and instrumental conditioning. Classical, or Pavlovian, conditioning occurs when a neutral stimulus, termed the conditioned stimulus (CS), is paired with an unconditioned stimulus (US) that elicits cardiovascular responses in a reflexive fashion. The responses to the US are called unconditioned responses (URs). After repeated temporal pairings of the CS followed by the US, presentation of the CS alone acquires the ability to elicit anticipatory conditioned responses (CRs). Studies of cardiovascular classical conditioning have begun to provide important information about the manner in which the CNS integrates learned cardiovascular activity (for reviews, see Cohen & Randall, 1984; Schneiderman, in press).

Instrumental, or operant conditioning, occurs when the presentation or withdrawal of a specific stimulus (i.e., reinforcer or punisher) is made contingent upon an organism's specific response. Stimuli that increase the rate or magnitude of a specified response (e.g., food reward; shock termination) are defined as reinforcers. In contrast, stimuli that decrease response rate or magnitude (e.g., presentation of loud noise or shock) are termed punishers. In human operant conditioning studies in which feedback for making the specified response is the reinforcer, the procedure is known as biofeedback. Although instrumental and classical conditioning are both forms of associative learning, instrumental conditioning differs procedurally in that reinforcement (e.g., presentation of the US) is contingent upon the making of a response that is specified by the experimenter.

The relationship between instrumental conditioning and cardiovascular responses has been the focus of a great deal of research that can be categorized into two classes of studies. In the first category, the cardiovascular concomitants of situations in which a somatomotor act is reinforced (e.g., bar pressing to avoid shock) are measured. This strategy has been used extensively to study the role of stressful situations in the pathogenesis of hypertension. The second category of instrumental conditioning studies has examined specific cardiovascular responses as the operant (i.e., particular changes in cardiovascular activity are directly reinforced). The focus of these studies, typically referred to as biofeedback, has been to determine whether cardiovascular responses can be directly modified through operant learning.

The present paper shall examine: (a) the cardiovascular concomitants of operant conditioning of somatic responses, (b) the direct operant conditioning of cardiovascular responses, and (c) the classical conditioning of cardiovascular responses. The discussion concerning classical conditioning shall focus on the neural substrates of classically conditioned cardiovascular responses in rabbits. Finally, the consequences of pitting a CS against an *imperative* stimulus that elicits a cardiovascular response (i.e., one such as electric shock or exercise) will be discussed.

CARDIOVASCULAR CONCOMITANTS OF OPERANT CONDITIONING OF SOMATIC RESPONSES

Several animal studies have examined cardiovascular responses during shock-avoidance conditioning procedures. Exposure to continuous 2-hour shock avoidance in rhesus monkeys was found to lead to increases in cardiac output and arterial blood pressure (BP) in the early portion of the session (Forsyth, 1971). Over the course of the training session, however, cardiac output decreased from its maximal level, and total peripheral resistance increased due mainly to diminished muscle blood flow. Similar findings have been reported in dogs (Anderson &

Brady, 1973; Anderson & Tosheff, 1973; Anderson & Yingling, 1979; Lawler, Obrist, & Lawler, 1975), with the largest elevations in heart rate (HR) and cardiac output occurring early in the session, before shock avoidance has been mastered. During pre-avoidance periods in which the animal learned to anticipate the avoidance conditioning session, total peripheral resistance and BP progressively increased, while HR and cardiac output progressively decreased (Anderson & Brady, 1973; Anderson & Tosheff, 1973; Lawler et al., 1975). There have been a few reports where exposure to aversive instrumental conditioning has led to hypertension that extended beyond individual sessions. Prolonged exposure to shock-avoidance paradigms in rhesus (Forsyth, 1969) and squirrel monkeys (Benson, Herd, Morse, & Kelleher, 1969; Herd, Morse, Kelleher, & Jones, 1969) produced elevated BP during and after training sessions. Similar studies in squirrel monkeys have also demonstrated electrocardiographic (EKG) changes and myocardial damage after prolonged avoidance conditioning (Corley et al., 1979; Corley, Shiel, & Mauck, 1980).

In humans, Obrist and colleagues (Obrist et al., 1974; Obrist et al., 1978; Obrist, Light, McCubbin, & Hoffer, 1979) have used a signaled reaction-time task in which avoidance was made contingent on reaction-time performance. It was found that HR and carotid dp/dt increased following respone execution, and these cardiac changes could be abolished by a beta-adrengergic blockade. During the preparatory interval before the task, HR responses (both acceleration and deceleration) were under vagal control. When compared to other tasks (cold pressor, viewing an erotic film), the shock-avoidance reaction time task evoked the largest cardiac response, although all three tasks produced tonic elevations in HR (Obrist et al., 1979). Beta-adrenergic blockade resulted in a greater attenuation of HR during shock avoidance than during either the cold pressor or film.

Although large cardiovascular responses can be obtained during avoidance conditioning, these responses are generally transient and time-locked to the conditioning session. The data suggest that emotional stress alone does not lead to sustained hypertension. Several recent studies examining cardiovascular concomitants of aversive conditioning and its relationship to hypertension, however, have employed models that examine interactions among stress variables and other factors such as salt intake and/or genetic predisposition toward hypertension. These studies have been more successful in examining hypertensive processes.

The interactive approach has been used to study the Dahl salt-sensitive strain of rats that develop severe hypertension in response to excess salt ingestion. In one experiment, rats were required to press a lever to sustain themselves with food, but by doing so also exposed themselves periodically to electric shock (Friedman & Iwai, 1977). Rats exposed for six months to this approach-avoidance conflict while being fed a high-salt diet developed elevations of BP greater than those previously observed in conflict-exposed rats fed low-salt diets (Friedman & Iwai, 1976) and greater than those observed in unstressed rats given a high-sodium diet. Although these results suggest that the conflict paradigm exacerbated the hypertension, the data were confounded by the use of an operant conditioning procedure that resulted in severe food deprivation and weight loss.

Lawler and associates (Lawler, Barker, Hubbard, & Allen, 1980; Lawler, Barker, Hubbard, & Schaub, 1980b; Lawler, Barker, Hubbard, & Schaub, 1981) used a signaled conflict-avoidance paradigm to study the development of hypertension in the F1 offspring of a cross between Wistar-Kyoto and spontaneously hypertensive rats. Animals subjected to conflict ultimately developed tonic levels of systolic BP of about 185 mmHg, compared to maturation and cage restraint controls that had systolic BP of 150 mmHg and 165 mmHg, respectively. Although the results are interesting, a lack of control procedures separating the effects of conflict from physical (i.e., repeated shocks) and other behavioral (e.g., shock predictability) variables partially obscures the significance of the data. Nevertheless, the borderline hypertensive rat model described by Lawler would appear to represent a suitable model for studying the deveopment of hypertension in genetically predisposed individuals.

Anderson and colleagues have examined the effects of saline infusion and multiple daily avoidance sessions on BP in normotensive dogs (Anderson, Kearns, & Better, 1983). After two weeks of exposure to the salt-stress conditions, average 24-hour increases in BP over pre-treatment baselines were 23 mmHg in systolic and 11 mmHg in diastolic BP. In contrast, control animlas given two weeks of either saline infusion alone or avoidance conditioning alone showed negligible changes in BP. These results suggest that intermittent behavioral stress can interact with salt intake to increase BP chronically, however the mechanisms involved are not clear.

In an acute experiment, Grignolo, Koepke, and Obrist (1982) compared the cardiovascular and renal responses during signaled avoidance to responses elicited during treadmill exercise in dogs receiving concomitant infusion of saline. Both avoidance conditioning and exercise led to acute increases in HR and BP. Exercise also led to increased urine flow, sodium excretion, and glomerular filtration rate with no change in free water clearance. In contrast, avoidance conditioning induced decreases in urine flow and sodium excretion with no change in either filtration rate or free water clearance. Thus, the data suggest that changes in renal function during avoidance conditioning may play a role in chronic BP elevations.

DIRECT OPERANT CONDITIONING OF CARDIOVASCULAR RESPONSES

Since the first report that instrumental conditioning techniques could be used to modify HR in humans (Shearn, 1962), a great deal of research has explored the extent to which cardiovascular activity could be directly conditioned. By amplifying and displaying a physiological response in these experiments, the subject is able to detect small autonomic changes which then allows the individual to gain increased control over the response. To some learning theorists (e.g., Miller, 1969), an important issue in biofeedback research has been whether autonomic responses can be instrumentally conditioned without mediation via changes in respiration or somatomotor activity. Ordinarily, cardiovascular and somatomotor activity are closely coupled (Obrist, 1981; VanDercar, Feldstein, & Solomon, 1977), and thus conditioning of motor responses may lead to concomitant cardiovascular changes.

In an early series of animal operant conditioning studies by Miller and associates (DiCara & Miller, 1968; Miller, 1969), attempts were made to control somatomotor activity by paralyzing the animals with curare. Although initial studies reported substantial changes in cardiovascular responses as a function of conditioning, much of this work has been difficult to replicate and the issue remains clouded (Miller & Dworkin, 1974). In spite of these problems, from a clinical standpoint the issue of somatomotor mediation of operantly conditioned cardiovascular responses is not of major importance. As long as the desired cardiovascular response is obtained without major side effects due to the mediating factors, the problem of mediation is purely heuristic. Also, to the extent that the CNS normally integrates somatic and autonomic responses concomitantly, the question of independence of somatic versus autonomic regulation would appear to be an artificial distinction.

Another important issue in biofeedback research is the specificity of the desired response. This refers to the extent to which an operant procedure can modify a single response or pattern of response without affecting presumably related responses. For example, Shapiro and associates (Shapiro, Tursky, & Schwartz, 1970) were able to condition changes in systolic BP in humans without systematically influencing HR. If specific autonomically mediated activity can be selectively modified by instrumental conditioning procedures, it would be useful and clinically relevant to explore autonomic functions with these methods. Unfortunately, the issue of specificity is still somewhat equivocal and requires further exploration (Shapiro, 1977; Surwit, Williams, & Shapiro, 1982). Although the specificity of biofeedback training remains unresolved, basic research in this field typically focuses on modifying a single cardiovascular parameter. Therefore, the following sections will describe attempts to condition BP, HR, and vasomotor responses, independently.

Blood Pressure

Although most biofeedback research has been conducted with human subjects, an interesting series of programmatic studies has been carried out using restrained baboons (Goldstein, Ross, & Brady, 1977; Harris, 1980; Harris, Gilliam, Findley, & Brady, 1973; Harris & Turkkan, 1981a, b; Harris & Turkkan, 1982; Turkkan & Harris, 1981; Turkkan, Lukas, & Harris, 1982). In these experiments, in which food delivery and shock avoidance were contingent on specified increases in diastolic BP for 12 hours per day, sustained increases in both systolic and diastolic BP of up to 30-40 mmHg were maintained throughout the conditioning sessions. The HR was elevated at the start of each session but then gradually declined. During the ensuing 12-hour recovery period, HR continued to fall and BP returned to basal levels within 6-8 hours. During similar experiments in which BP increases were reinforced, selective alpha- and beta-adrenergic blockade attenuated the operantly condioned BP elevations. Plasma norepinephrine increased significantly during conditioning sessions, and increases in epinephrine approached significance. Plasma renin activity was not associated with the observed BP changes during training.

Most of the human studies dealing with operant control of BP use the noninvasive constant-cuff technique to obtain a relative beat-by-beat measure of BP, thereby providing immediate feedback to the subjects (Shapiro, Tursky, Gershson, & Stern, 1969). The results from these studies suggest that within the laboratory, normal individuals can produce increases in diastolic BP of up to 20 mmHg and decreases approximating 10 mmHg (Shapiro et al., 1970). Systolic BP changes can also be conditioned, but typically these responses are smaller (Shapiro et al., 1969). In addition, there is evidence that BP increases are easier to obtain than BP decreases (Surwit, Hager, & Feldman, 1977; Surwit et al., 1982).

Heart Rate

As was the case for BP, several studies using operant procedures in normal humans have reported average HR increases greater than 10 beats/minute (Blanchard, Young, Scott, & Haynes, 1974; Obrist et al., 1975; Wells, 1973). In one study, these differences were seen in only 6 out of 9 subjects, a point that emphasizes the importance of individual differences in biofeedback research (Wells, 1973). Heart rate decreases have been more difficult to obtain, with only a few reports of mean decreases greater than 5 beats/min (Sirota, Schwartz, & Shapiro, 1974, 1976).

An issue in biofeedback research is whether an individual can voluntarily control autonomic functions to some degree without feedback regarding the response system. Although this question is important to all cardiovacular responses, several studies dealing with this question have focused on HR (Bell & Schwartz, 1975; Bergman & Johnson, 1971, 1972; Davidson & Schwartz, 1976; Lang & Twentyman, 1974, 1976; Young & Blanchard, 1974). In subjects given instructions to control their HR, it has been reported that the addition of feedback did not significantly improve control (Bergman & Johnson, 1972). In contrast, it also has been demonstrated that increases in HR were largest in subjects given both feedback and instructions to control their HR (Bell & Schwartz, 1975; Davidson & Schwartz, 1976; Lang & Twentyman, 1974, 1976). The effects of instructions on HR decreases is not clear (Davidson & Schwartz, 1976; Young & Blanchard, 1974).

Vasomotor Activity

In an early study, Lisina (1965) trained subjects to increase forearm blood flow in order to avoid shock. Interestingly, subjects were only able to learn the response when they watched the polygraph tracing of their blood flow. It has been pointed out that this is rather crude feedback, and the subject could easily produce the responses through mediators such as respiratory maneuvers (Katkin & Murray, 1968). However, in a separate study, it was demonstrated that subjects could vasoconstrict the digits of the hand while skeletal motor activity was controlled (Synder & Noble, 1968). Thus, the data suggested that vasomotor activity can be instrumentally conditioned.

In animals there have been a few demonstrations of operant vasomotor control. In one study, dogs were trained to constrict their coronary vessels, decreasing coronary blood flow reliably (Ernst, Kordenat, Sandman, & Sandman, 1979). Anderson and Yingling (1979) were able to train dogs to elevate peripheral resistance (mean arterial pressure/blood flow in the ascending aorta) using shock avoidance as reinforcement. They attributed the increase in resistance to increased vasomotor tone because BP rose while cardiac output fell. Since peripheral resistance decreases as a concomitant of aversive classical conditioning, the rise in peripheral resistance produced by operant conditioning is attributable to the association of reinforcement to the cardiovascular response per se.

BEHAVIORAL TREATMENT OF HYPERTENSION

The behavioral treatment of hypertension has been undertaken using direct operant conditioning of BP (e.g., Kristt & Engel, 1975), biofeedback-assisted relaxation in conjunction with meditation (Benson, Rosner, Marzetta, & Klemchuck, 1974), or relaxation alone (Bali, 1979; Julius & Cottier, 1983). Although the results of several of these studies suggest that operant conditioning procedures may effectively reduce BP in hypertensives, a full-scale clinical trial to test this hypothesis has not been initiated.

Perhaps the best controlled of the studies attempted thus far was a randomized control study by Patel and North (1975). Half of the 34 enrolled patients were trained in biofeedback-assisted relaxation training involving the galvanic skin response and electromyogram; subjects were also instructed in relaxation procedures, which they practiced at home. The remaining half of the subjects rested on a couch, but were not given specific instructions or connected to the biofeedback equipment. Results indicated that systolic and diastolic BP decreased by 26 and 15 mmHg, respectively, in the experimental group as opposed to 9 and 4 mmHg, respectively, in the control group. Significant BP reductions were maintained at 12 months follow-up (Patel, 1975).

The above results are promising, but several caveats are in order. First, the role of learning as opposed to changes in life style or motivation have not been adequately assessed. Second, most studies that have not had high drop-out rates appear to have used a very small number of highly selected subjects that received considerable face-to-face attention. Third, the cost–benefit ratio of using conditioning as opposed to other modes of therapy has not been adquately addressed. Nevertheless, these findings suggest that learning procedures may be useful clinically under certain circumstances in the control of BP.

CLASSICAL CONDITIONING

Species (e.g., monkeys and pigeons) exhibiting increased somatomotor activity during a CS typically reveal an increase in HR (i.e., tachycardia) as the CR. In contrast, species exhibiting decreased somatomotor activity (e.g., rabbits, humans) reveal HR slowing (i.e., bradycardia) as the CR. The literature generally supports the notion that conditioned tachycardia, increases in cardiac output, and vasodilation in skeletal muscle occur when the CR includes movement; whereas, bradycardia is associated with an inhibition of somatomotor activity (e.g., Cohen & Obrist, 1975; Obrist & Webb, 1967; Schneiderman, 1970).

The directionality of the HR response appears to be more closely related to somatomotor activity than to the motivational properties of the US. In one study, for example, rabbits having access to lateral hypothalamic stimulation bar-pressed to receive stimulation and made approach responses to that side of a shuttle box in which stimulation occurred (Sideroff, Elster, & Schneiderman, 1972). In contrast, rabbits with access to medial hypothalamic stimulation did not bar-press for intracranial stimulation and made escape responses in the shuttle box. Pairing a tone CS with either lateral or medial hypothalamic stimulation as the US when the animals were loosely restrained elicited conditioned bradycardia as the CR. Thus, although medial and lateral hypothalamic stimulation had very different motivational properties, each provided an effective US for eliciting bradycardiac HR conditioning.

The HR CR in humans has also been studied as a function of different kinds of US (Wood & Obrist, 1968). A cognitive problem-solving task, slides of seminude women, and an exercise task were each used as the US. These stimuli differed in the constellation of URs that they elicited. Nevertheless, when a CS was paired separately with each US, the CR in each case consisted of bradycardia.

The neural substrates of learned cardiovascular adjustments are largely unknown but have begun to be studied programmatically in the baboon (e.g., Smith, Astley, Hohimer, & Stephenson, 1980), pigeon (Cohen & Randall, 1984), and rabbit (Schneiderman et al., 1986; Francis, Hernandez, & Powell, 1981). These efforts have begun to provide useful information about the manner in which the CNS integrates associative learning processes and cardiovascular performance.

Smith and his colleagues have used a procedure in the baboon in which the pairing of a visual or auditory CS with peripheral electric shock as the US is superimposed on a task in which the animal lever-presses for food (Smith et al., 1980; Smith, DeVito, & Astley, 1982). After a suitable number of CS-US pairings, presentation of the CS leads to a constellation of conditioned responses that includes lever-lift suppression, tachycardia, and increases in BP and terminal aortic blood flow. This integrated pattern of responses is termed the conditioned emotional response (CER).

Briefly, Smith and his collaborators have found that discrete bilateral hypothalamic lesions abolished the cardiovascular components of the CER without affecting the conditioned lever-pressing response or the cardiovascular concomitants of other behaviors (e.g., exercise). The finding that the lever-press CR was unaltered suggests that the loss of the cardiovascular CRs was not due to changes in motivation. In addition, the finding that the cardiovascular concomitants of behaviors such as exercise were unaltered suggests that the hypothalamic lesions interrupted a CNS pathway that may be fairly specific to learned cardiovascular responses.

Smith et al. (1980, 1982) also reported that electrical stimulation of the hypothalamic sites that subsequently interrupted conditioning when lesioned produced a constellation of responses similar to the cardiovascular CRs. Administration of horseradish peroxidase (HRP) to such sites produced retrograde labeling in a number of sites, including the septal region and amygdala.

Classical conditioning elicited by pairing a visual stimulus and peripheral shock in the pigeon elicits tachycardia as the CR (Cohen, 1982). Single-unit recording studies indicate that the primary contributor to the CR is an increase in sympathetic outflow, although a conditioned decrease in vagal tone is also involved. Lesion and histological studies suggest that the efferent pathway for the tachycardiac CR involves the avian amygdalar homologue, which projects through the posteromedial hypothalamus and maintains a ventromedial course through the rostral pons before passing through the ventrolateral medulla. The pathway then descends through the spinal cord before synapsing on sympathetic preganglionic neurons in the lateral horn. One of the more intriguing aspects of the studies conducted on HR conditioning in the pigeon is that they indicate that training-induced modifications of CS-evoked discharge occur in the sensory pathway at least as peripherally as the lateral geniculate nucleus (Cohen & Randall, 1984).

Whereas the pairing of a CS with peripheral shock in the monkey or pigeon leads to a tachycardic CR, similar pairings in humans or rabbits lead to a bradycardiac CR. In initial experiments exploring classical conditioning of HR in rabbits we found that: (a) the original response (OR) to the CS consisted of bradycardia that habituated within a few trials; (b) the CR also consisted of bradycardia that developed within 10 pairings of the CS and US and was not confounded by nonassociative responses; and (c) the CR was mediated entirely by an increase in vagal tone (Downs et al., 1972; Schneiderman, Smith, Smith, & Gormezano, 1966; Schneiderman et al., 1969; Yehle, Dauth, & Schneiderman, 1967).

We have used neuroanatomical and extracellular single-neuron recording techniques to define the CNS pathways that provide the anatomical substrate of classically conditioned bradycardia. A large part of this research has involved the tracing of a central descending pathway from the amygdalar central (ACE) nucleus through the lateral hypothalamus, lateral zona incerta of the subthalamus and parabrachial nucleus to the preganglionic vagal motoneurons in the medulla. We have also examined the specificity of this pathway in terms of conditioning. Another part of this research has involved examining the role of the auditory cortex and medial geniculate nucleus in conditioning, as well as the nature of the projections from structures in the central auditory CS pathway to the descending central efferent pathway that mediates the bradycardiac CR.

In order to trace the central bradycardia pathways, the approach of first defining the motor outflow and then working back into the CNS has been used. During an initial study using this tack, Schwaber and Schneiderman (1975) determined that the extracellular single-neuron recordings could be obtained from the cells of origin of vagal preganglionic cardioinhibitory motoneurons in the dorsal vagal nucleus (DVN) of rabbits. Jordan, Khalid, Schneiderman, and Spyer (1982) replicated these findings and also were able to record from preganglionic vagal cardioinhibitiory motor neurons in nucleus ambiguus (NA). Experiments in which the cervical vagus nerve has been dipped in HRP have indicated that the distribution of vagal preganglionic cell bodies in NA is far sparser than in the DVN for rabbits (Ellenberger, Haselton, Liskowsky & Schneiderman, 1982). In addition, bradycardiac responses can be elicited by low-intensity (<30 μA) stimulation in the DVN and in the NA.

Injection of HRP into the dorsal medulla, including DVN (Wallach et al., 1979), produced pronounced retrograde cell-body labeling in the ACE as well as in the lateral hypothalamus. Other investigations (Schwaber, Kapp, Higgins, & Rapp, 1982) have reported similar findings. Furthermore, Kapp and his colleagues (Kapp, Gallagher, Underwood, McNall, & Whitehorn, 1982) showed that electrical stimulation of ACE nucleus produced marked bradycardia that was either abolished or markedly attenuated by intravenous injections of atropine methylnitrate. The bradycardia was shown not to be an artifact of respiratory changes or gross motor activity, as it persisted after artificial ventilation and immobilization with Flaxedil.

Interestingly, we have also found that train stimulation of the ACE nucleus in lightly anesthetized rabbits elicits bradycardia and a depressor response. This suggested that the bradycardia elicited by stimulation of the hypothalamus might be attributable to fibers of passage originating in ACE nucleus. Consequently, we lesioned the ACE nucleus unilaterally and then stimulated the ipsilateral and contralateral hypothalamus either 30 minutes or 10-14 days after the lesion (Gellman, Schneiderman, Wallach, & LeBlanc, 1981). We found that stimulation of the lateral hypothalamus only failed to elicit bradycardiac responses when the stimulation was presented ipsilateral to the lesion site 10-14 days postlesion. Since fibers in the hypothalamus would be expected to be degenerated by 10 days after destruction of their cell bodies in the amygdala, the results of the Gellman et al. study suggest that the bradycardia elicited by stimulation of the hypothalamus is due to fibers originating in the ACE nucleus.

In exploring more caudal aspects of the diencephalon of rabbits for cardiovascular responsiveness, we found that train microstimulation of the lateral zona incerta of the subthalamus produced bradycardia that in turn slightly decreased blood pressure (Kaufman, Hamilton, Wallach, Petrik, & Schneiderman, 1979). These changes were abolished by bilateral vagotomy. Stimulation of the medial zona incerta produced a pronounced pressor response.

Stimulation of bradycardia-producing sites in the lateral zona incerta activated cardioinhibitory motoneurons in DVN. Although mean onset latency of these medullary neurons to lateral zona incerta stimulation was relatively short (6 msec), these stimuli did not follow repeated stimuli faithfully. Therefore, the connection between the lateral zona incerta and the dorsal medulla is probably not monosynaptic. However, a short train of pulses elicited greater firing rates than single pulses did. Therefore, it is possible that some connections between lateral zona incerta and the dorsal medulla may be monosynaptic but may require a high degree of temporal summation.

Another structure that showed retrograde cell-body labeling in the Wallach et al. (1979) experiment after injection of HRP into the dorsal medulla was the parabrachial nucleus of the pons. Train stimulation of either medial or lateral parabrachial nucleus produced primary bradycardia associated with a pressor response of longer latency (Hamilton, Ellenberger, Liskowsky, & Schneiderman, 1981). Injections of HRP into parabrachial nucleus revealed direct anatomical projections from regions of the forebrain previously implicated in the mediation of bradycardia. These included the ACE nucleus, lateral preoptic region, medial forebrain bundle, bed nucleus of stria terminalis, anterior and lateral hypothalamus, and lateral zona incerta. The correspondence between these HRP findings and the results of our previous functional studies implicating the ACE nucleus, lateral hypothalamus, and lateral zona incerta in the mediation of bradycardia is quite striking. Important correspondence also exists between the results of injecting HRP into the parabrachial nucleus in our study and into the dorsal medulla (Schwaber, Kapp, & Higgins, 1980; Schwaber et al., 1982; Wallach et al., 1979).

The previous studies suggest the presence of an oligosynaptic bradycardia pathway from ACE through LH, LZI, and PBN to cardiomotor cells in DVN and NA. Kapp and his colleagues (Kapp, Frysinger, Gallagher, & Haselton, 1979) have reported that ACE lesions attenuate the acquisition of conditioned bradycardia. Using a similar strategy, we examined the role of ACE in the retention of differentially conditioned bradycardia (Gentile, Jarrell, Teich, McCabe, & Schneiderman, 1986a). Electrodes were implanted bilaterally in ACE or in control sites just dorsal or rostral to ACE. Two days following surgery, animals were subjected to differential conditioning in which one tone (CS+) was paired with periorbital shock and a second tone (CS−) was presented alone. Each animal received one conditioning session per day until evidence of differential HR responses was obtained. Bilateral electrolytic lesions were then made. Thirty minutes after lesioning, animals received an additional conditioning session. Both control and ACE groups demonstrated differential HR responses prior to lesioning. In the control group, lesions had no effect on HR responses or bradycardiac response magnitude. However, the ACE lesion group failed to demonstrate differential HR responses after lesioning. Furthermore, the bradycardia-conditioned response was abolished. In both groups, lesions had no effect on the HR OR, magnitude of the UR, or baseline. These findings suggest that ACE also plays a role in the retention of differential Pavlovian conditioning of bradycardia in rabbits. In order to demonstrate that ACE lesions did not disrupt some general learning process, coreno-retinal potential responses (CRP) were conditioned in the same animals. The CRP is a potential change produced by extension of the nictitating membrane and retraction of the eyeball. In rabbits, the CRP is almost pefectly correlated with the nictitating membrane response. ACE lesions had no effect on the CRP CR, thereby suggesting that the lesions selectively abolished HR CRs but did not affect another simultaneously conditioned response.

Although the previous study implicates ACE in conditioned bradycardia, it was not clear whether the results were due to destruction of cell bodies in ACE or fibers of passage. Therefore, we undertook a study in which ibotenic acid, a substance that selectively destroys cell bodies but spares fibers of passage, was injected bilaterally into ACE or control sites (Gentile, Romanski, Jarrell, McCabe, & Schneiderman, 1986b). After approximately 17 days of recovery, animals were exposed to differential Pavlovian conditioning. ACE and control lesions had no effect on HR baseline, OR, UR, or CRP conditioning. Animals with control lesions showed differentially conditioned bradycardiac responses. However, animals in the ACE lesion group did not demonstrate differential bradycardiac responses to the acoustic stimuli. In addition, the bradycardiac response magnitude to both the CS+ and the CS− was attenuated in the ACE lesion group relative to controls. These findings indicate that intrinsic neurons in ACE and not fibers of passage play an important role in differentially conditioned bradycardiac responses but not CRP conditioned responses.

Recent work in our laboratory indicates that the lateral zona incerta lesions in rabbits selectively abolish an existing HR CR (Jarrell et al., 1986c). Electrodes were implanted bilaterally in lateral zona incerta or in control sites just dorsal or ventral to it. Two days following surgery, animals were subjected to Pavlovian conditioning or to pseudoconditioning. Subsequent bilateral electrolytic lesions did not influence either the baseline HR, HR OR, UR, or lack of response to pseudoconditioning. Bilateral lesions in lateral zona incerta alone but not nearby control lesions or unilateral zona incerta damage abolished the HR CR. In a follow-up experiment, the CRP and HR CRs were recorded. Bilateral lesions in lateral zona incerta abolished the HR CR without interfering with the CRP CR, indicating that the area is selectively involved in the conditioning of HR. This study also provides evidence that the amygdala-vagal bradycardiac pathway, which passes through lateral zona incerta, is the CR pathway.

Since the CS in our conditioning paradigm is a tone, the CS pathway involves the CNS sensory pathway for audition. This pathway originates in the hair cells of the inner ear and projects to the cochlear nuclei and superior olivary nucleus before ascending to the inferior colliculus, medial geniculate nucleus (MGN), and eventually the auditory cortex in the temporal lobe of the cerebral cortex. A recent study in our laboratory (Jarrell, Gentile, McCabe, & Schneiderman, 1986a) examined the role of MGN in differentially conditioned bradycardia. Injections of HRP into the ACE nucleus produced cell-body and fiber labeling at the ventral and medial borders of MGN. Kapp (Kapp, Schwaber, & Driscoll, 1984) has also reported HRP labeling in this area. The role of this region in the mediation of differential conditioning of bradycardia and CRP responses was then examined. Bilateral electrolytic lesions were made in the medial portion of MGN (mMGN) or in control sites dorsal or rostral to MGN. Ten days following surgery, lesioned animals and unoperated control animals were subjected to 7 days (1 session/day) of differential conditioning consisting of trials in which one tone (CS+) was paired with periorbital shock and a second tone (CS−) was presented alone. Each group demonstrated bradycardiac responses to both the CS+ and CS−. In the control-lesion and unoperated groups, the CS+ consistently elicited larger bradycardiac responses than did the CS−. However, animals with bilateral mMGN lesions did not demonstrate differential bradycardiac responses. The magnitude of the conditioned bradycardiac response was not significantly different among the three groups. Evidence of CRP differential conditioning was still present in each group, suggesting that the auditory projections for this CR are somewhat different than for bradycardiac CRs. These findings suggest that mMGN or fibers passing through this region selectively mediate HR differential conditioning in rabbits. The fact that bradycardiac responses are still present after lesions in mMGN suggests that other auditory regions may also be involved in the mediation of the bradycardiac CR.

A separate study was conducted to determine whether the results of our previous experiment were due to destruction of intrinsic neurons in mMGN or fibers of passage (Jarrell, Romanski, Gentile, McCabe, & Schneiderman, 1986d). Injections of ibotenic acid were made bilaterally in mMGN or in control sites. In addition, control injections of pontamine sky blue were made in mMGN. After 7 days of recovery, animals were subjected to differential Pavlovian conditioning. Each animal received one 60-trial conditioning session per day for 4 days. Ibotenic acid lesions had no effect on baseline HR, HR ORs, or HR URs. In the control-lesion and control-injection group, the CS+ elicited a larger bradycardiac response than did the CS−. However, animals with lesions in mMGN did not demonstrate differential bradycardiac responses to the CS+ and CS−. In this group, bradycardiac responses to the CS+ and CS− were similar in magnitude due to a reduction in the magnitude of the response to the CS+. These data suggest that cell bodies in mMGN were responsible for the observed effect, not fibers of passage. Since bradycardiac responses were still present after the lesion, other auditory regions may be involved in the mediation of the bradycardiac CR.

We have recently completed another study (Jarrell et al., 1986b) that examined further the role of mMGN in bradycardiac conditioning using a retention paradigm. This experiment also examined the possible contributions of the ventral division of the medial geniculate nucleus (vMGN) and auditory cortex to differential conditioning of bradycardia to tonal stimuli. Electrodes were chronically implanted bilaterally in mMGN, vMGN, or auditory cortex. After 7 days of recovery from surgery, each animal received one differential Pavlovian conditioning session. At the end of this session, electrolytic lesions were produced through the implanted electrodes. On the following day, the animals received another conditioning session. Lesions had no effect on baseline HR or the bradycardiac OR. Each group of animals demonstrated differential bradycardiac conditioning during the prelesion session. During the postlesion session, animals with lesions in vMGN continued to demonstrate differential CRs. However, animals with mMGN or auditory cortex lesions failed to demonstrate differential conditioning during the postlesion session due to the fact that the postlesion response to the CS− was significantly larger. The results of this study indicate that lesions in mMGN abolish the retention of previously established differential HR CRs to acoustic CS. The fact that either auditory cortex or mMGN lesions enhanced reponses to the CS− suggests that a corticothalamic pathway may be involved in the inhibition of responses to the CS−.

It has been argued that vMGN and mMGN are part of separate auditory pathways involved in parallel processing of acoustic stimulus information. Weinberger (1984) has suggested that the secondary leminiscal system that includes mMGN may play a role in processing of stimulus significance during conditioning. Although mMGN seems to be involved in both the retention and acquisition of differential bradycardiac CRs, it appears that the mechanism may be different in each case. In acquisition paradigms, mMGN lesions attenuated the magnitude of the response to the CS+; however, in retention paradigms, mMGN lesions enhanced the magnitude of the response to the CS−. Thus, it is possible that during the initial acquisition of the response, mMGN neurons serve to enhance the response to the CS+; whereas with repeated training, mMGN may play a role in the inhibition of the response to the CS−, perhaps via a corticothalamic pathway originating in the auditory cortex.

In summary, programmatic research examining the CNS integration of learned cardiovascular responses has begun to provide useful information concerning the integration of associative learning processes and the elaboration of cardiovascular responses. Aspects of the CNS efferent pathways mediating sympathetically driven cardiovascular CRs in the baboon and pigeon and parasympathetically mediated bradycardiac CRs in the rabbit have been identified. In addition, the integration of associative information in central sensory pathways with cardiac responses as well as the nature of the projections from central sensory structures to the central efferent pathways have begun to be explored.

The nature of the pathways mediating cardiovascular CRs appears to be quite specific. Specific lesions in the hypothalamus of the baboon abolished the cardiovascular components of the CER without influencing the conditioned suppression of lever-pressing (Smith et al., 1980). Similarly, specific lesions in ACE or in the lateral zona incerta of the rabbit abolished the bradycardiac CR without disrupting the CRP CR (Gentile et al., 1986a; Jarrell et al., 1986c). Perhaps most interestingly of all, lesions in the mMGN of the rabbit, which is primarily a sensory nucleus, abolished the bradycardiac CR without interfering with the CRP CR (Jarrell et al., 1986a). This, of course, suggests that specific sensorimotor integration of CRs is occurring within sensory CNS structures, as well as in the CNS efferent pathway.

LEARNED MODIFICATION OF ELICITED CARDIOVASCULAR RESPONSES

In addition to studies in which instrumental conditioning procedures have been used to modify tonic levels of cardiovascular activity, there has been a number of studies that have examined the extent to which operant procedures can be used to modify cardiovascular responses to imperative stimuli or to classically conditioned stimuli. Recently, in our laboratory we have begun to examine the extent to which classical conditioning leading to bradycardiac and/or depressor responses can be used to attenuate sympathetically mediated responses to imperative stimuli (e.g., exercise, peripheral electric shock). The potential clinical importance of such studies is considerable: If individuals can learn to control autonomic functions, it may be possible for them to reduce their cardiovascular reactivity to otherwise arousing stimuli.

In an initial study, Ainslie and Engel (1974) assessed the ability of monkeys to modify the cardiac response to impending electric shock. In this paradigm, animals were first classically conditioned by presenting a period of clicks at a fast rate (2/sec) that was always followed by shock, and periods of clicks at a slow rate (20/sec) that were never followed by shock. During the clicks followed by shock, the animal's HR was reliably faster than during the clicks not followed by shock. After this differential response had been established, the monkeys were trained operantly to slow or speed HR, and then the clicks were presented during the operant conditioning session. It was found that animals trained to increase their HR were able to further increase it during the aversive clicks, and animals trained to decrease their HR were able to lower it during aversive clicks even though tachycardia usually occurred during the clicks.

In separate studies, monkeys were trained to slow or speed HR in the face of challenges either via baroreflex stimulation (Engel & Joseph, 1982) or via intracranial electrical stimulation of CNS regions known to elicit tachycardia and a pressor response (Joseph & Engel, 1981). The operantly conditioned monkeys were able to attenuate the gain of the baroreflex elicited by phenylephrine injection (vasoconstriction) during periods when the animals were increasing HR to avoid shock. Conversely, monkeys were also able to attenuate the gain of the baroreflex elicited by nitroglycerin injections (vasodilation) during periods when they were slowing their HR to avoid tail shock. During intracranial stimulation, animals were able to maintain a conditioned bradycardia even though the stimulation-elicited response was usually tachycardia. Taken together, these studies suggest that operant procedures may be effective in modifying cardiac responses to a variety of imperative stimuli.

Several human studies have examined the effects of biofeedback on stress-related HR responses. In an early study (Sirota et al., 1974), female subjects were trained to raise or lower HR. At the end of the training session, two tones were presented—one paired with forearm shock and one followed by no shock. In the group receiving feedback to decrease HR, subjects were able to decelerate the heart during either tone. In the group trained to increase HR, subjects exhibited tachycardia during the tones. Therefore, the direction of HR response during anticipation of shock was modified by the direction of the feedback.

In a somewhat related study (Williams & Adkins, 1974), male college students were trained alternatively to increase and decrease HR. This operant training was followed by aversive classical conditioning in which shock was paired with a light. In the subsequent session, subjects could avoid the occurrence of shock by emitting an appropriate HR response determined by the investigators. In this situation, shock served as a stressful stimulus and a reinforcing stimulus. It was reported that the tachycardia seen in anticipation of shock was attenuated when subjects received feedback to decrease HR and augmented when given feedback to accelerate the heart.

Despite the success of these early studies in attenuating HR responses to aversive stiumuli, a number of recent studies have reported negative results (Bouchard & Labelle, 1982; Magnusson, Hedberg, & Tunved, 1981; Malcuit & Beaudry, 1980). Perhaps one problem with the earlier studies (e.g., Sirota et al., 1974) is that the investigators assumed that the classically conditioned HR response (i.e., anticipation of shock) was accelerative. However, it has been well established that the classically conditioned HR response in humans is decelerative (Obrist, 1968; Obrist, Wood, & Perez-Reyes, 1965). Thus, the deceleration obtained during the feedback and anticipation of shock was probably the classically conditioned response and not the operantly conditioned attenuation of tachycardia. In studies that have used stressors (e.g., mental arithmetic, ischemic arm pain) that elicit HR acceleration (Bouchard & Labelle, 1982; Malcuit & Beaudry, 1980), biofeedback has been effective in attenuating the stress-induced tachycardia. In a few studies that have achieved some degree of attenuation, it has been demonstrated that instructions to decrease HR were as effective as biofeedback (Reeves & Shapiro, 1982). Therefore, it appears that biofeedback does not produce direct reduction of cardiovascular reactivity elicited by aversive stressors. Instead, any degree of control over the cardiovascular response may be an indirect modification of the response to a stressor, as is seen in relaxation therapy (Jacob & Chesney, 1986).

An area of research that has proven more successful in terms of operant control over phasic responses is the modification of cardiovascular responses to exercise. In one study, subjects were trained to decrease the tachycardia induced by treadmill exercise (Goldstein et al., 1977). There was a significant within-session attenuation of the exercise-induced tachycardia, systolic BP, and the heart rate-pressure product in the feedback group compared to a control group. In a similar study, Perski and Engel (1980) reported that subjects in a feedback group were able to significantly attenuate HR responses elicited by submaximal bicycle ergometer exercise as compared to a control group. The control group, which did not receive feedback during initial sessions, later was successfully trained to attenuate HR reactivity during exercise. The original feedback group was withdrawn from feedback and subsequently exhibited only a small increase in reactivity compared to earlier feedback sessions. Although these studies have established the ability to mofidy dynamic exercise responses, attempts to attenuate cardiovascular reactivity elicited by static exercise have not been as convincing (Clemens & Shattock, 1979; Riley & Furedy, 1981).

One other use of biofeedback to modify reactivity that deserves mention is biofeedback-assisted relaxation. Patel (1977) compared biofeedback-assisted relaxation to an attention control in hypertensive patients. It was found that the biofeedback-assisted relaxation group showed significantly attenuated blood pressure responses to a cold pressor task and to exercise. These results were replicated in a similar study (Datey, 1980). Interestingly, however, the treatment had no effect on reactivity in normotensive controls.

In our laboratory we have recently begun a series of experiments in rabbits that is examining the extent to which responses mediated by the sympathetic nervous system, can be attenuated by classical conditioning. Previously, we had paired a tone CS with low frequency, 10-second train stimulation of the lateral hypothalamus as the US (Brickman & Schneiderman, 1977). This resulted in a depressor CR. In our present research we are using lateral hypothalmic stimulation as the US to condition a depressor CR. The depressor CR is then elicited during concomitant procedures that elicit sympathetic activation (e.g., peripheral tail shock). By pitting the conditioned activation of the CNS pathways mediating the depressor CR against activation of the CNS pathways mediating the sympathetic responses to imperative stimuli, we intend to study the manner by which the CNS permits relaxation training and similar procedures to counteract sympathetically mediated responses to stressful stimuli.

REFERENCES

Ainslie, G. W., & Engel. B. T. (1974). Alteration of classically conditioned heart rate by operant reinforcement in monkeys. *Journal of Comparative and Physiological Psychology, 87,* 373–382.
Anderson, D. E., & Brady, J. V. (1973). Prolonged pre-avoidance effects upon blood pressure and heart rate in the dog. *Psychosomatic Medicine, 35,* 4–12.
Anderson, D. E., Kearns, W. D., & Better, W. E. (1983). Progressive hypertension in dogs by avoidance conditioning and saline infusion. *Hypertension, 5,* 286–291.
Anderson, D. E., & Tosheff, J. (1973). Cardiac output and total peripheral resistance changes during preavoidance periods in the dog. *Journal of Applied Physiology, 34,* 650–654.
Anderson, D. E., & Yingling, J. E. (1979). Aversive conditioning of elevations in total peripheral resistance of dogs. *American Journal of Physiology, 236,* H880-H887.
Bali, L. R. (1979). Long-term effect of relaxation on blood pressure and anxiety levels of essential hypertensive males: A controlled study. *Psychosomatic Medicine, 41,* 637.
Bell, I. R., & Schwartz, G. E. (1975). Voluntary control and reactivity of human heart rate. *Psychophysiology, 12,* 339–348.
Benson, H., Herd, J. A., Morse, W. H., & Kelleher, R. T. (1969). Behavioral induction of arterial hypertension and its reversal. *American Journal of Physiology, 217,* 30–34.
Benson, H., Rosner, B. A., Marzetta, B. R., & Klemchuck, H. M. (1974). Decreased blood pressure in pharmacologically treated hypertensive patients who regularly elicited the hypertensive response. *Lancet, 1,* 289.
Bergman, J. S., & Johnson, H. J. (1971). The effects of instructional set and autonomic perception on cardiac control. *Psychopsysiology, 8,* 180–190.
Bergman, J. S., & Johnson, H. J. (1972). Sources of information which affect training and raising of heart rate. *Psychophysiology, 9,* 30–39.
Blanchard, E. B., Young, L. D., Scott, R. W., & Haynes, M. R. (1974). Differential effects of feedback and reinforcement in voluntary acceleration of human heart rate. *Perceptual and Motor Skills, 38,* 683–691.
Bouchard, M. A., & Labelle, J. (1982). Voluntary heart rate deceleration: A critical evaluation. *Biofeedback and Self-Regulation, 7,* 121–137.
Brickman, A., & Schneiderman, N. (1977). Classically conditioned blood pressure decreases induced by electrical stimulation of posterior hypothalamus in rabbits. *Psychophysiology, 14,* 287–292.
Clemens, W. J., & Shattock, R. J. (1979). Voluntary heart rate control during static muscular effort. *Psychophysiology, 16,* 327–332.
Cohen, D. H. (1982). Central processing time for a conditioned response in a vertebrate model system. In C. D. Woody (Ed.), *Conditioning.* New York: Plenum Press.
Cohen, D. H. & Obrist, P. A. (1975). Interaction between behavior and cardiovascular system. *Circulation Research, 37,* 693–706.
Cohen, D. H., & Randall, D. C. (1984). Classicial conditioning of cardiovascular reponses. *Annual Review of Physiology, 46,* 187–197.
Corley, K. C., Mauck, H. P., Shiel, F. O., Barber, J. H., & Clark, L. S. (1979). Myocardial dysfunction and pathology associated with environmental stress in squirrel monkey: Effect of vagotomy and propranolol. *Psychophysiology, 16,* 554–560.
Corley, K. C., Shiel, F. O., & Mauck, H. P. (1980). Stress-induced cardiomyopathy in squirrel monkey. In S. S. Kalter (Ed.), *The use of nonhuman primates in cardiovascular diseases.* Austin, TX: Austin University Press.
Datey, K. K. (1980). Role of biofeedback training in hypertension and stress. *Journal of Postgraduate Medicine, 26*(1), 68–73.
Davidson, R. J., & Schwartz, G. E. (1976). The psychobiology of relaxation and related states: A multiprocess theory. In D. I. Mostofsky (Ed.), *Behavior control and modification of physiological activity.* Englewood Cliffs, NJ: Prentice-Hall.

DiCara, L. B., & Miller, N. E. (1968). Instrumental learning of SBP responses by curarized rats: Dissociation of cardiac and vascular changes. *Psychosomatic Medicine, 40,* 276-293.
Downs, D., Cardozo, C., Schneiderman, N., Yehle, A. L., VanDercar, D. H., & Zwilling, G. (1972). Central effects of atropine upon aversive classical conditioning in rabbits. *Psychopharmacologia, 23,* 319-333.
Ellenberger, H. H., Haselton, J. R., Liskowsky, D. R., & Schneiderman, N. (1982). Localization of cardioinhibitory motor neurons in the medulla of the rabbit. *Federation Proceedings Abstracts, 41,* 1517.
Engel, B. T., & Joseph, J. A. (1982). Attenuation of baroreflexes during operant cardiac conditioning. *Psychophysiology, 19,* 609-614.
Ernst, F. A., Kordenat, R. R., Sandman, M. S., & Sandman, C. A. (1979). Learned control of coronary blood flow. *Psychosomatic Medicine, 41,* 79-85.
Forsyth, R. P. (1969). Blood pressure responses to long term avoidance schedules in the restrained rhesus monkey. *Psychosomatic Medicine, 31,* 300-309.
Forsyth, R. P. (1971). Regional blood flow changes during 72-hour avoidance schedules in the monkey. *Science, 173,* 546-548.
Francis, J., Hernandez, L. L., & Powell, D. A. (1981). Lateral hypothalamic lesions: Effects on Pavlovian cardiac and eyeblink conditioning in the rabbit. *Brain Research Bulletin, 6,* 155-163.
Friedman, R., & Iwai, J. (1976). Genetic predisposition and stress-induced hypertension. *Science, 193,* 161-162.
Friedman, R., & Iwai, J. (1977). Dietary sodium, psychic stress, and genetic predisposition to experimental hypertension. *Proceedings of the Society of Experimental Biology and Medicine, 155,* 449-452.
Gellman, M., Schneiderman, N., Wallach, J., & LeBlanc, W. (1981). Cardiovascular responses elicited by hypothalamic stimulation in rabbits reveal a medio-lateral organization. *Journal of the Autonomic Nervous System, 4,* 301-317.
Gentile, C. G., Jarrell, T. W., Teich, A., McCabe, P. M., & Schneiderman, N. (1986a). Amygdaloid central nucleus as mediator of differential Pavlovian conditioning of bradycardia in rabbits. *Behavioural Brain Research, 20,* 263-273.
Gentile, C. G., Romanski, L. M., Jarrell, T. W., McCabe, P. M., & Schneiderman, N. (1986b). Ibotenic acid lesions in amygdaloid central nuclesus prevent the acquisition of differentially conditioned bradycardia responses in rabbits. *Society for Neuroscience Abstracts, 12,* 755.
Goldstein, D. S., Ross. R. S., & Brady, J. V. (1977). Biofeedback heart rate training during exercise. *Biofeedback and Self-Regulation, 2,* 107-126.
Grignolo, A., Koepke, J. P., & Obrist, P. A. (1982). Renal function, heart rate, and blood pressure during exercise and avoidance in dogs. *American Journal of Physiology, 242,* R482-R490.
Hamilton, R. B., Ellenberger, H., Liskowsky, D., & Schneiderman, N. (1981). Parabrachial area as mediator of bradycardia in rabbits. *Journal of the Autonomic Nervous System, 4,* 261-281.
Harris, A. H. (1980). Conditioned blood pressure elevations in the baboon. In G. Adam, I. Meszaro, & E. I. Banyai (Eds.), *Advances in physiological sciences, Volume 17: Brain and behavior.* Budapest: Akademiai, Kaido.
Harris, A. H., Gilliam, W. J., Findley, J. D., & Brady, J. V. (1973). Instrumental conditioning in large-magnitude, daily 12-hour blood pressure elevations in the baboon. *Science, 182,* 175-177.
Harris, A. H., & Turkkan, J. S. (1981a). Generalization of conditioned blood pressure elevation: Schedule and stimulus control effects. *Physiology & Behavior, 26,* 935-940.
Harris, A. H., & Turkkan, J. S. (1981b). Performance characteristics of conditioned blood pressure elevations in the baboon. *Biofeedback and Self-Regulation, 6,* 11-24.
Harris, A. H., & Turkkan, J. S. (1982). Plasma lactate levels during baseline and blood pressure conditioning in the baboon. *Physiology & Behavior, 29,* 657-663.
Herd, J. A., Morse, W. H., Kelleher, R. T., & Jones, L. G. (1969). Arterial hypertension in the squirrel monkey during behavioral experiments. *American Journal of Physiology, 217,* 24-29.

Jacob, R. G., & Chesney, M. A. (1986). Psychological and behavioral methods to reduce cardiovascular reactivity. In K. A. Mathews (Ed.), *Handbook of stress reactivity, and cardiovascular disease*. New York: Wiley.

Jarrell, T. W., Gentile, C. G., McCabe, P. M., & Schneiderman, N. (1968a). The medial geniculate region as mediator of differential Pavlovian conditioning of bradycardia in rabbits. *Brain Research, 374*, 126–136.

Jarrell, T. W., Gentile, C. G., Romanski, L. M., Rose, B. J., McCabe, P. M., & Schneiderman, N. (1986b). The role of cortical and thalamic auditory regions in differential bradycardiac conditioning to acoustic stimuli in rabbits. *Society for Neuroscience Abstracts, 12*, 755.

Jarrell, T. W., McCabe, P. M., Teich, A., Gentile, C. G., VanDercar, D. H., & Schneiderman, N. (1986c). Lateral subthalamic area as mediator of classically conditioned bradycardia in rabbits. *Behavioral Neuroscience, 100(1)*, 3–10.

Jarrell, T. W., Romanski, L. M., Gentile, C. G., McCabe, P. M., & Schneiderman, N. (1986d). Ibotenic acid lesions in the medial geniculate region prevent the acquisition of differential Pavlovian conditioning of bradycardia to acoustic stimulus in rabbits. *Brain Research, 382*, 199–203.

Jordan, D., Khalid, M. E. M., Schneiderman, N., & Spyer, K. M. (1982). Localization and properties of ganglionic cardiomotor neurons in rabbits. *Pflugers Archiv-European Journal of Physiology, 395*, 244–250.

Joseph, J. A., & Engel, B. T. (1981). Instrumental control of cardioacceleration induced by central electrical stimulation. *Science, 214*, 341–343.

Julius, S., & Cottier, C. (1983). Behavior and hypertension. In T. M. Dembroski, T. H. Schmidt, & G. Blumchen (Eds.), *Biobehavioral bases of coronary heart disease* (pp. 271–289). Basel, Switzerland: Karger.

Kapp, B. S., Frysinger, R. C., Gallagher, M., & Haselton, J. R. (1979). Amygdala central nucleus lesions: Effect on heart rate conditioning in the rabbit. *Physiology and Behavior, 23*, 1109–1117.

Kapp, B. S., Gallagher, M., Underwood, M. D., McNall, C. D., & Whitehorn, D. (1982). Cardiovascular responses elicited by electrical stimulation of the amygdala central nucleus in the rabbit. *Brain Research, 234*, 251–262.

Kapp, B. S., Schwaber, J. S., & Driscoll, P. A. (1984). Subcortical projections to the amygdaloid central region in the rabbit. *Society of Neuroscience Abstracts, 10*, 831.

Katkin, E. S., & Murray, E. H. (1968). Instrumental conditioning of autonomically mediated behavior: Theoretical and methodological issues. *Psychological Bulletin, 70*, 52–68.

Kaufman, M. P., Hamilton, R. B., Wallach, J. H., Petrik, G. K., & Schneiderman, N. (1979). Lateral subthalamic area as mediator of bradycardia responses in rabbits. *American Journal of Physiology, 236*, H471–H479.

Kristt, D. A., & Engel, B. T. (1975). Learned control of blood pressure in patients with high blood pressure. *Circulation, 51*, 370–378.

Lang, P. J., & Twentyman, C. T. (1974). Learning to control heart rate: Binary versus analogue feedback. *Psychophysiology, 11*, 619–629.

Lang, P. J., & Twentyman, C. T. (1976). Learning to control heart rate: Effects of varying incentive and criterion of success on task performance. *Psychophysiology, 13*, 378–385.

Lawler, J. E., Barker, G. F., Hubbard, J. W., & Allen, M. T. (1980a). The effects of conflict on tonic levels of blood pressure in the genetically borderline hypertensive rat. *Psychophysiology, 17*, 363–370.

Lawler, J. E., Barker, G. F., Hubbard, J. W., & Schaub, R. G. (1980b). Pathophysiological changes associated with stress-induced hypertension in borderline hypertensive rat. *Clinical Science, 59* (Supplement) 307–310.

Lawler, J. E., Barker, G. F., Hubbard, J. W., & Schaub, R. G. (1981). Effects of stress on blood pressure and cardiac pathology in rats with borderline hypertension. *Hypertension, 3*, 496–505.

Lawler, J. E., Obrist, P. A., & Lawler, K. A. (1975). Cardiovascular functions during pre-avoidance, avoidance and post-avoidance in dogs. *Psychophysiology, 12*, 4–11.

Lisina, M. I. (1965). The role of orientation in the transformation of involuntary reactions into voluntary ones. In L. G. Voronin, A. N. Leontier, A. R. Luria, E. N. Sokolov, & O. S. Vinogradova (Eds.), *Orienting reflex and exploratory behavior*. Washington: American Institute of Biological Sciences.

Magnusson, E., Hedberg, B., & Tunved, J. (1981). Heart rate control and aversive stimulation. *Biological Psychiatry, 12*, 211–222.

Malcuit, G., & Beaudry, J. (1980). Voluntary heart rate following a cardiovascular arousing task. *Biological Psychiatry, 10*, 201–210.

Miller, N. E. (1969). Learning of visceral and glandular responses. *Science, 163*, 434–445.

Miller, N. E., & Dworkin, B. R. (1974). Visceral learning: Recent difficulties with curarized rats and significant problems for human research. In P. A. Obrist, A. H. Black, J. Brener, & L. V. DiCara (Eds.), *Cardiovascular physiology*. Chicago: Aldine.

Obrist, P. A. (1968). Heart rate and somatic-motor coupling during classical aversive conditioning in humans. *Journal of Experimental Psychology, 77*, 180–193.

Obrist, P. A. (1981). *Cardiovascular psychophysiology: A perspective*. New York: Plenum Press.

Orbist, P. A., Gaebelein, C. J., Shanks-Teller, E., Langer, A. W., Grignolo, A., Light, K. C., & McCubbin, J. A. (1978). The relationship between heart rate, carotid dp/dt, and blood pressure in humans as a function of the type of stress. *Psychophysiology, 15*, 102–115.

Obrist, P. A., Galosy, R. A., Lawler, J. E., Gaebelein, C. J., Howard, J. L., & Shanks, E. M. (1975). Operant conditioning of heart rate: Somatic correlates. *Psychophysiology, 12*, 445–455.

Obrist, P. A., Lawler, J. E., Hoard, J. L., Smithson, K. W., Martin, P. L., & Manning, J. (1974). Sympathetic influences on the heart in humans: Effects on contractility and heart rate of acute stress. *Psychophysiology, 11*, 405–427.

Obrist, P. A., Light, K. C., McCubbin, J. A., & Hoffer, J. L. (1979). Pulse transmit time: Relationship to blood pressure and myocardial performance. *Psychophysiology, 16*, 292–301.

Obrist, P. A., & Webb, R. A. (1967). Heart rate during conditioning in dogs: Relationship to somatic-motor activity. *Psychophysiology, 4*, 7–34.

Obrist, P. A., Wood, D. M., & Perez-Reyes, M. (1965). Heart rate during conditioning in humans: Effects of UCS intensity, vagal blockade, and adrenergic block of vasomotor activity. *Journal of Experimental Psychology, 70*, 32–42.

Patel, C. (1975). Twelve-month follow up of yoga and biofeedback in the management of hypertension. *Lancet, 7898*, 62–64.

Patel, C. (1977). Biofeedback-aided relaxation in the management of hypertension. *Biofeedback and Self-Regulation, 2*, 1–41.

Patel, C. H., & North, W. R. S. (1975). Randomized controlled trial of yoga and biofeedback in management of hypertension. *Lancet, 7925*, 93–95.

Perski, A., & Engel, B. T. (1980). The role of behavioral conditioning in the cardiovascular adjustment to exercise. *Biofeedback and Self-Regulation, 5*, 91–104.

Reeves, J. L., & Shapiro, D. (1982). Heart rate biofeedback and cold pressor pain. *Psychophysiology, 19*, 393–403.

Riley, D. M., & Furedy, J. J. (1981). Effects of instructions and contingency of reinforcement on the operant conditioning of human phasic heart rate change. *Psychophysiology, 18*, 75–81.

Schneiderman, N. (1970). Determinants of heart-rate conditioning. In J. H. Reynierse (Ed.), *Current issues in animal learning* (pp. 85–115). Lincoln: University of Nebraska Press.

Schneiderman, N., McCabe, P. M., Haselton, J. R., Ellenberger, H. E., Jarrell, T. W., & Gentile, C. G. (1986). Neurobiological bases of conditioned bradycardia. In R. F. Thompson, W. R. Prokasy, & I. Gormezano (Eds.), *Classical conditioning III: Neuropsychology and behavior of the rabbit*. Hillsdale, NJ: Lawrence Erlbaum Associates.

Schneiderman, N., Smith, M. C., Smith, A. C., & Gormezano, I. (1966). Heart-rate classical conditioning in rabbits. *Psychonomic Science, 6*, 241–242.

Schneiderman, N., VanDercar, D. H., Yehle, A. L., Manning, A. A., Golden, T., & Schneiderman, N. E. (1969). Vagal compensatory adjustment: Relationship to heart-rate classical conditioning in rabbits. *Journal of Comparative and Physiological Psycholoy, 68*, 176–183.

Schwaber, J. S., Kapp, B. S., & Higgins, G. (1980). The origin and extent of direct amygdala projections to the region of the dorsal motor nucleus of the vagus and thenucleus of the solitary tract. *Neuroscience Letters, 20*, 15–20.

Schwaber, J. S., Kapp, B. S., Higgins, G. A., & Rapp, P. R. (1982). Amygdaloid and basal forebrain direct connections with the nucleus of the solitary tract and the dorsal motor nucleus. *Journal of Neurociences, 2*, 1414–1438.

Schwaber, J., & Schneiderman, N. (1975). Aortic nerve activated cardioinhibitory neurons and interneurons. *American Journal of Physiology, 229*, 783–789.

Shapiro, D. (1977). A monologue or biofeedback and psychophysiology. *Psychophysiology, 14*, 213–227.

Shapiro, D., Tursky, B., Gershon, E., & Stern, M. (1969). Effects of feedback and reinforcement on the control of human systolic blood pressure. *Science, 163*, 588–590.

Shapiro, D., Tursky, B., & Schwartz, G. E. (1970). Differentiation of heart rate and systolic blood pressure in man by operant conditioning. *Psychosomatic Medicine, 32*, 417–423.

Shearn, D. W. (1962). Operant conditioning of heart rate. *Science, 137*, 30–31.

Sideroff, S., Elster, A. J., & Schneiderman, N. (1972). Cardiovascular conditioning in rabbits using appetitive or aversive hypothalamus stimulation as the US. *Journal of Comparative and Physiological Psychology, 81*, 501–508.

Sirota, A. D., Schwartz, G. E., & Shapiro, D. (1974). Voluntary control of human heart rate: Effect on reaction to aversive stimulation. *Journal of Abnormal Psychology, 83*, 261–267.

Sirota, A. D., Schwartz, G. E. & Shapiro, D. (1976). Voluntary control of human heart rate: Effect on reaction of aversive stimulation—a replication and extension. *Journal of Abnormal Psychology, 85*, 473–477.

Smith, O. A., Astley, C. A., Hohimer, A. R., & Stephenson, R. B. (1980). Behavioral and cerebral control of cardiovascular function. In M. J. Hughes & C. D. Barnes (Eds.), *Neural control of circulation*. New York: Academic Press.

Smith, O. A., Devito, J. L., & Astley, C. H. (1982). The hypothalamus in emotional behavior and associated cardiovascular correlates. In A. R. Morrison & P. L. Strick (Eds.), *Changing concepts of the nervous system* (pp. 569–584). New York: Academic press.

Snyder, C., & Noble, M. E. (1968). Operant conditioning of vasoconstriction. *Journal of Experimental Psychology, 77*, 263–268.

Surwit, R. S., Hager, J. L., & Feldman, J. (1977). The role of feedback in voluntary control of blood pressure in instructed subjects. *Psychophysiology, 14*, 97 (abstract).

Surwit, R. W., Williams, R. B., & Shapiro, D. (1982). *Behavioral approaches to cadiovascular disease*. New York: Academic Press.

Turkkan, J. S., & Harris, A. H. (1981). Shaping blood pressure elevations: An examination of acquisition. *Behavioral and Analytical letters, 1*, 97–106.

Turkkan, J. S., Lukas, S. E., & Harris, A. H. (1982). Hemodynamic effects of intravenous clonidine in the conscious, normotensive baboon. *Journal of Cardiovascular Pharmacology, 4*, 863–869.

VanDercar, D. H., Feldstein, M. A., & Solomon, H. (1977). Instrumental conditioning of human heart rate during free and controlled respiration. *Biological Psychology, 5*, 221.

Wallach, J. H., Ellenberger, H. H., Schneiderman, N., Liskowsky, D. R., Hamilton, R. B., & Gellman, M. D. (1979). Preoptic-anterior hypothalamic area as a mediator of bradycardia responses in rabbits. *Neuroscience Abstracts, 5*, 52.

Weinberger, N. M. (1984). The neurophysiology of learning: A view from the sensory side. In L. R. Squire & N. Butters (Eds.), *Neuropsychology of memory* (pp. 489–503). New York: Guilford Press.

Wells, D. T. (1973). Large magnitude voluntary heart rate changes. *Psychophysiology, 10*, 260–269.

Williams, J. L., & Adkins, J. R. (1974). Voluntary control of heart-rate during anxiety and oxygen deprivation. *Psychological Record, 24*, 3–16.

Wood, D. M., & Obrist, P. A. (1968). Minimal and maximal sensory intake and exercise as unconditioned stimuli in human heart rate conditioning. *Journal of Experimental Psychology, 76,* 254.

Yehle, A., Dauth, G., & Schneiderman, N. (1967). Correlates of heart rate conditioning in curarized rabbits. *Journal of Comparative and Physiological Psychology, 64,* 98–104.

Young, L. D., & Blanchard, E. B. (1974). Effects of auditory feedback of varying information content on the self control of heart rate. *Psychophysiology, 11,* 527–534.

2
PAVLOVIAN CONDITIONING OF ENDOCRINE RESPONSES

Mark E. Stanton
Seymour Levine
Stanford University School of Medicine

Neuroendocrinology has been described by Krieger and Hughes as "a discipline concerned with (a) the neural control of endocrine secretion, (b) the effects of target organ hormones on the brain, (c) the effects of hormones on behavior, and (d) the broader problems of interaction between the CNS and environment" (Krieger & Hughes, 1980, p. xv). This last aspect of neuroendocrinology which involves the interaction between CNS, environment, and endocrine function has revealed that one characteristic of almost all known endocrine systems is that they are sensitive and responsive to a variety of changes in environmental conditions. Mason (1975), while attempting to understand the common factors between the heterogeneity of environmental circumstances which activate the pituitary-adrenal system, proposed that psychological factors play the most definitive role. Thus, the emotional arousal occurring in conscious subjects exposed to different stressful situations appears to be responsible for the activation of the pituitary-adrenal system. Although the pituitary-adrenal system has been the major focus of most stress research, there has now been an increasing number of studies which have measured numerous other hormones now well known to be responsive to stressful stimuli. These include plasma growth hormone, prolactin, and testosterone. Although stress has produced the most extensive body of information on how psychological and environmental factors can influence the endocrine system, there are other important environmental and psychological influences on endocrine function. Thus, there are important psychological factors related to sociability which influence testosterone and estrogen-progesterone secretion. Furthermore, there are important zeitgebers, zeit time, and geber, given environmental factors which affect both the circadian and circannual rhythms of many known CNS, pituitary, and target-organ hormones. It is not the purpose of this brief introduction to catalogue all of the known environmental events which influence neuroendocrine function. This in itself takes up whole volumes.

When one considers the pervasiveness of environmental influences on endocrine function together with the extent to which environmental influences, as a general rule, are mediated through learning, one naturally comes to expect that learning can influence endocrine function. The issue of conditioned endocrine responses has recently been reviewed by Woods and Burchfield (1980). In this review, they note that most studies in this area have been poorly controlled and that it is often not possible to exclude nonassociative interpretations of endocrine responses which are observed in conditioning experiments. The major conclusion of this review was that as long as one accepts these limitations, the literature indicates that almost any endocrine system can probably be conditioned.

In this chapter we would like to approach the issue of conditioned endocrine responses in a different way. This approach will emphasize the *psychology* of endocrine conditioning with a view toward uncovering general principles, rather than providing an exhaustive empirical survey of different endocrine systems. We will focus only on those demonstrations of hormonal conditioning which are well controlled. We will then further examine, so far as is possible, the nature and properties of conditioning in these systems. Our aim is to show not only what is known in this area but, perhaps more importantly, what is not known about conditioned endocrine responses.

Psychologists have traditionally subdivided learning into two major categories: operant or instrumental learning, and classical or Pavlovian conditioning. As the title of this chapter implies, we will restrict discussion to the second category—Pavlovian conditioning. We have chosen to do this for two reasons. First, Pavlovian conditioning experiments permit a better assessment of the relative contribution of associative and nonassociative processes to endocrine secretion than do instrumental learning experiments. Second, instrumental learning contingencies have Pavlovian contingencies imbedded within them (Mowrer, 1947; Overmier & Lawry, 1979; Rescorla & Solomon, 1967). There is almost universal agreement among learning psychologists that instrumental learning is mediated, at least to some degree, by Pavlovian associations. This point is a very important one because the available evidence suggests that these Pavlovian associations are responsible for the learned endocrine effects that occur in instrumental learning situations.

This is illustrated in a study that we performed recently on operant conditioning and adrenal corticoids (Coe, Stanton, & Levine, 1983; see Figure 2.1). Rats given rewarded sessions in an operant chamber on a continuous reinforcement schedule show a dramatic decline in corticosterone relative to presession levels. This also occurs in yoked-control animals which receive similar apparatus exposure and reward presentation but are not required to (and do not) make the lever-press response. The effect of the association between placement in the operant chamber and presentation of reward can be seen when reward is withheld during extinction of operant conditioning. When reward is withheld, there is a dramatic increase in adrenal output. Figure 2.1 indicates this increase in corticosterone levels in both the lever-press animals and their yoked controls. Since this hormonal response does not depend on the operant response, it is probably the Pavlovian association between apparatus cues and reinforcement which accounts for corticoid changes in operant conditioning situations. Thus, it appears that of the two types of contingencies inherent in operant situations—instrumental and Pavlovian—the Pavlovian contingency is sufficient to account for the endocrine responses which are observed.

CONDITIONED ENDOCRINE RESPONSES

In this section we review those studies of Pavlovian conditioning of endocrine responses which include adequate control groups for the assertion that endocrine responses are associative in nature. The assertion that an endocrine conditioned response (CR), as with any kind of CR, is, in fact, a product of associative conditioning rests on evidence that the response reflects an association between conditioned stimulus (CS) and unconditioned stimulus (US), as opposed to other aspects of experience with these stimuli (e.g., Mackintosh, 1974, pp. 26–31). Nonassociative processes such as habituation, sensitization, and pseudoconditioning to either the CS, the US, or both must be excluded as possible causes of changed endocrine responsiveness. This is usually achieved by between-subjects designs which compare the response of conditioned animals with that of other animals which receive presentations of only the CS, only the US, and/or unpaired (or randomized) presentations of both. Alternatively, one can employ within-subjects "discrimination" designs which compare the response to one CS which is paired with the US with the response to another CS which is presented alone.

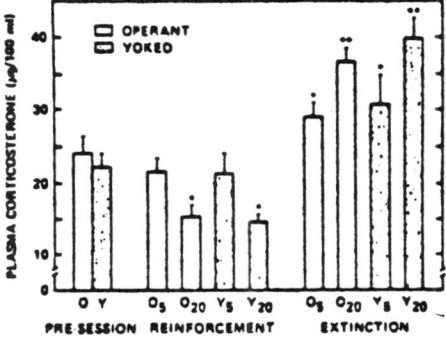

FIGURE 2.1. Mean corticosterone levels of operant (O) and yoked (Y) subjects obtained immediately prior to training sessions as well as after 5 or 20 minutes of reinforcement or extinction (Coe, Stanton, & Levine, 1983).

Only a few endocrine systems have been studied by means of conditioning experiments which were adequately designed to control for nonassociative factors. These systems are insulin, the pituitary-gonadal axis, and the pituitary-adrenal axis.

Conditioning of insulin secretion has been extensively investigated, and excellent reviews of this literature already exist (Eikelboom & Stewart, 1982; Woods & Burchfield, 1980; Woods & Kulkosky, 1976). In the majority of these studies, the CS is placement in a distinctive environment, usually with a novel odor present, the US is an injection of insulin, and the response measure is blood glucose level (from which changes in insulin secretion are inferred). Although there is no question that changes in blood glucose can be conditioned in this manner, the *direction* of these changes remains controversial. Some investigators have observed a conditioned decrease in blood glucose which resembles the response to the insulin US (e.g., Hutton, Woods, & Makous, 1970). Other investigators have observed a conditioned increase in blood glucose which opposes (or "compensates for") the response to the insulin US (e.g., Siegel, 1975). This discrepancy has been attributed to differences in the dose of insulin employed; high doses leading to conditioned hypoglycemia and low doses leading to conditioned hyperglycemia (Woods & Kulkosky, 1976). However, this has not been borne out by more recent investigations which have additionally shown that the CS environment which is paired with insulin can determine whether hyperglycemic or hypoglycemic conditioned responses (CRs) will be observed (Flaherty et al., 1980). Novel CS environments tend to produce conditioned hyperglycemia, whereas less novel conditioning environments tend to produce conditioned hypoglycemia (Flaherty & Becker, 1984). At present, there seems to be no simple explanation for the entire range of these findings. Recent attempts to reconcile this literature have emphasized either the multiple actions of insulin (Eikelboom & Stewart, 1982, pp. 518–519) or the multiple determinants of changes in blood glucose (Flaherty, Becker, Rowan, & Voelker, 1984). What is clear is that Pavlovian conditioning with exogenous insulin as the US is neither a simple phenomenon nor a particularly good model for studying conditioning of endocrine responses.

A more straightforward way to study conditioning of insulin responses is to employ more "natural" stimuli for insulin secretion as the US and assay for changes in insulin directly (rather than by inference from blood glucose). This has been done in a study by Woods et al. (1977). In this study, hungry rats were presented with a daily meal as the US. In three conditioning groups, this meal was paired with one of three conditioned stimuli: the time of day, the odor of mentholatum, or both in compound. In a fourth pseudoconditioning control group, daily meals were randomly presented with respect to both the odor and time of day. On the test day, animals received 5 minutes of exposure to their CS followed by blood sampling for subsequent assay of immunoreactive insulin. The insulin levels of these four groups are illustrated in the left part of Figure 2.2. It is apparent when daily meals associated with an explicit cue, presentation of that cue alone led to insulin levels which were elevated over those of the pseudoconditioning

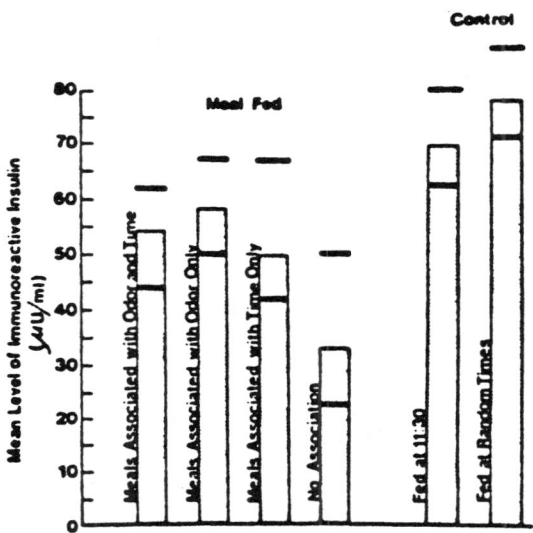

FIGURE 2.2. Mean levels of immunoreactive insulin in response to test presentations of a conditioned stimulus (CS) of four treatment groups (left part of figure). The horizontal bars represent the range of values for each group. See text for further explanation. (From Woods et al., 1977.)

control group (No Association). This was true irrespective of which cue was employed. (The two bars on the right of Figure 2.2 labeled "Control" represent the insulin levels of rats fed ad lib and are unimportant for the present purposes.) This experiment shows that conditioned cues for feeding promote insulin secretion. This conditioned effect is similar to the unconditioned effect of feeding on insulin secretion.

Another endocrine system for which there is convincing evidence of Pavlovian conditioning is the pituitary-gonadal axis. Graham and Desjardins (1980) measured luteinizing hormone (LH) and testosterone in male rats which were exposed to an olfactory CS and a sexually receptive female US. Briefly, males were placed in one cage containing vapors of methylsalicylate for 7 minutes and then placed in another cage with a sexually receptive female for 15 minutes. After 14 daily pairings of CS and US, males were blood sampled after exposure to the CS alone. In addition to this group which received pairings of the CS and US (CS-US), blood was also collected from four comparison groups. One of these groups (CS) received exposures to the odor only; another group (CS/US) received presentations of the CS followed 6 hours later by presentations of the US; another group (H) received handling only; and a fourth group (US) was sampled after 7 minutes of exposure to a receptive female in order to provide an assessment of the unconditioned response (UR) of the pituitary-gonadal axis to the US in this experiment. As shown in Figure 2.3, conditioned elevations of both LH and testosterone were found only in the group which received CS-US pairings. Moreover, the CR of the pituitary-gonadal axis was the same in direction and magnitude as the UR to simple exposure to a receptive female. The failure of the males in Group CS/US to show elevated LH and testosterone indicates that CRs in this system were not artifacts of pseudoconditioning or sensitization.

Yet another hormonal system for which there is convincing evidence of Pavlovian conditioning is the pituitary-adrenal system. In the case of the pituitary-adrenal system, two types of CRs have been observed, depending on whether appetitive or aversive conditioning procedures are used. With appetitive conditioning procedures, the conditioned response consists of a decrease in cor-

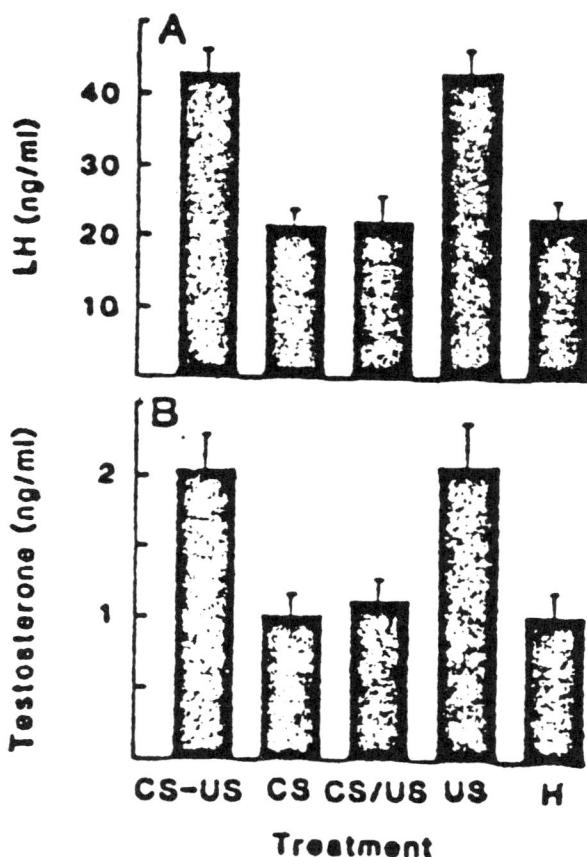

FIGURE 2.3. Mean concentrations of immunoreactive luteinizing hormone (LH) and testosterone in blood serum from independent groups of male rats. Error bars represent the standard error of the mean. See text for further explanation. (From Graham & Desjardins, 1980.)

ticosterone levels. This is illustrated in a study by Coover, Sutton, and Heybach (1977). In this study, the CS consisted of placement in a distinctive environment (a sound attenuating chamber) for 30 minutes. The US consisted of the animals' daily ration of food served as wet mash. Three groups of food-deprived rats received one conditioning trial a day for 1, 6, 14, or 24 days. Two groups (CD and F) received daily pairings of chamber placement and food. Another group (PC) received a pseudoconditioning regimen consisting of apparatus exposures and food presentations in an unpaired fashion. On the test day, all animals were placed in the CS chambers. Animals in Group F were fed, providing a measure of the UR to food presentation. Animals in Groups CD and PC were not fed, providing an assessment of the CR to cues associated with food. Figure 2.4 shows the change

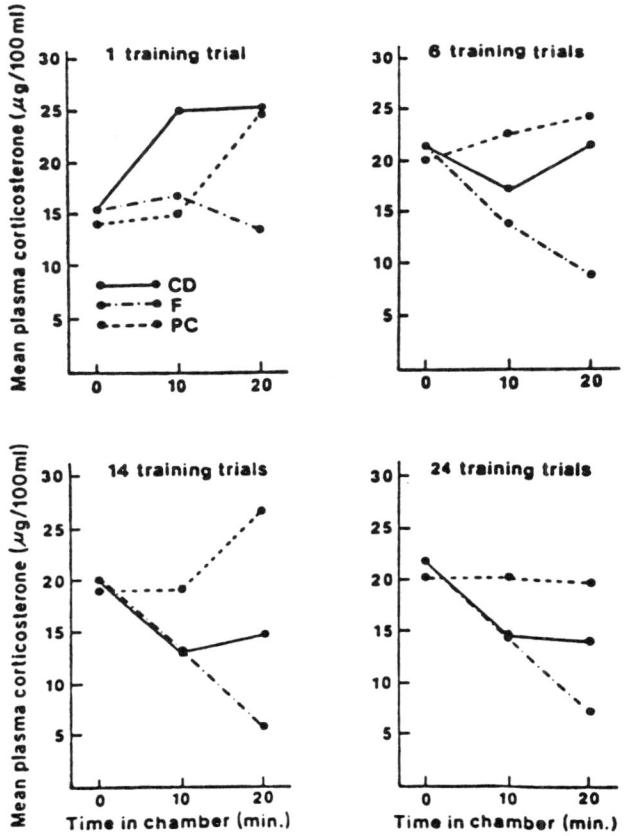

FIGURE 2.4. Mean plasma corticosterone levels as a function of time after presentation of the conditioned stimulus (placement in a sound-attenuating chamber), number of training trials, and treatment group (CD = conditioned but not fed on sample day; F = conditioned and fed on sample day; PC = never fed in chamber or pseudoconditioned). (From Coover, Sutton, & Heybach, 1977.)

in plasma corticosterone of these three groups as a function of number of training trials and time in the CS chamber. After one training trial, the response to apparatus exposure was an elevation in corticosterone in animals which were not fed, whereas hormone levels in animals which were fed remained unchanged. In the pseudoconditioned animals (Group PC) this response habituated with further training trials. With further training, animals which were fed (Group F) showed a marked decline in corticoids from 20 to 5 $\mu g\%$ during the first 20 minutes of exposure to the CS chamber. The conditioned animals (Groups CD), but not controls (Groups PC), showed a similar decline in corticoids in response to the CS chamber, but this response did not emerge until after 14 training trials. This study indicates decreases in adrenal glucocorticoids can be conditioned to cues that are associated with food. These conditioned decreases are similar in magnitude to unconditioned decreases in corticoids during the first 20 minutes after CS exposure.

The direction of the adrenal response in appetitive Pavlovian conditioning contrasts sharply with that observed in aversive Pavlovian conditioning. When neutral stimuli are paired with a noxious US, conditioned activation of the pituitary-adrenal system is observed. This is demonstrated in a study by Ader (1976) which employed a conditioned taste aversion paradigm (Figure 2.5). Rats were placed on a deprivation regimen in which access to water was restricted to a period of 15 minutes each day. The left panel of Figure 2.5 shows plasma corticosterone levels before conditioning in animals injected with lithium chloride [LiCl (i.p.)],

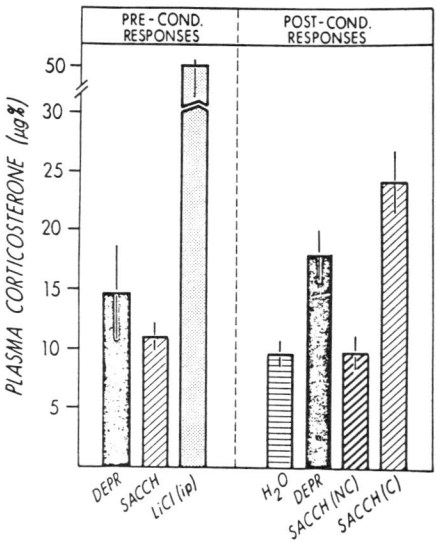

FIGURE 2.5. Mean plasma corticosterone levels as a function of treatment condition (see text for further explanation). Error bars represent standard errors of the mean. (From Ader, 1976.)

animals presented with a saccharin solution (SACCH), and a basal condition consisting of animals which were deprived but were otherwise not treated before blood sampling (DEPR). Clearly, lithium chloride injection results in a dramatic elevation in plasma corticoids, and saccharin consumption results in a small reduction relative to the deprived basal condition. The right-hand panel of Figure 2.5 shows corticosterone levels after conditioning. Three groups of animals had received a single pairing of saccharin with a lithium chloride injection 3 days prior to blood sampling. On the day that samples were taken, one of these groups was provided with tap water to drink (H_2O); one was similarly deprived but otherwise not treated (DEPR); and one was presented with a sodium saccharin solution to drink [SACCH(C)]. A fourth group did not receive a pairing of saccharin with lithium chloride and was presented with saccharin on the day of blood sampling [SACCH(NC)]. The data from these groups indicate consumption of a nonaversive fluid—water in the previously conditioned group; saccharin in the previously not-conditioned group—reduces corticosterone values over a deprived basal condition (DEPR). This is consistent with the effect of consummatory behavior on corticosterone levels discussed previously (Figure 2.4). Consumption of saccharin which was previously paired with lithium-chloride induced illness, on the other hand, led to an elevation of corticosterone over deprived-basal levels, and even more dramatically over levels shown by unconditioned animals which drank saccharin. This elevation in corticosterone cannot be attributed simply to a prior injection of lithium chloride (compare with H_2O condition) or to sensitization because animals which have received only an injection of lithium chloride on the conditioning day fail to show corticosterone elevations to CS consumption on the test day (Smotherman, Hennessy & Levine, 1976).

Taken as a whole, these studies indicate that endocrine systems are indeed subject to Pavlovian conditioning. Those endocrine systems which have been examined by means of well-controlled conditioning experiments are insulin, the pituitary-gonadal axis, and the pituitary-adrenal axis. In all of these endocrine systems (excepting the problematic case of conditioning with insulin injections), the CR resembles the UR.

DISSOCIATIONS OF CONDITIONED BEHAVIORAL AND ENDOCRINE RESPONSES

It is possible to learn something about the nature of endocrine conditioning from studies which have examined both behavioral CRs and endocrine CRs within the same experiment. These studies show behavioral and endocrine CRs can often be dissociated. That is, conditions which lead to clear behavioral learning often fail to produce conditioned hormonal responses. The appearance of endocrine CRs appears to depend on a number of additional factors. Examples of these factors can be seen at several levels of causal analysis. We will illustrate this diversity by examining four types of factors—psychological, endocrine, neural, and social—which modulate conditioned adrenal responses, independently of conditioned behavior.

In the case of conditioned adrenocortical responses associated with flavor aversion learning, a study performed by Smotherman et al. (1976) points to the importance of a psychological factor that is crucial for the conditioned endocrine response, namely approach–avoidance conflict. This study employed a special experimental protocol which made it possible to study flavor aversion learning in the absence of water deprivation. In a typical flavor aversion test situation, animals are faced with conflicting approach and avoidance tendencies. They are motivated by thirst to approach and drink the flavored solution on the one hand, and they are motivated to avoid the flavored solution because of its prior association with gastrointestinal malaise on the other. By using an experimental procedure which did not involve thirst, Smotherman et al. (1976) were able to study the conditioned adrenal response of animals experiencing the avoidance tendency in the absence of a counteracting approach tendency (i.e., to drink). Alternatively, animals could be deprived of water and tested with both the avoidance tendency and the counteracting approach tendency. The central finding of this study is shown in Figure 2.6.

Corticosterone values are indicated in the bar chart; dark bars correspond to the conditioned animals and white bars correspond to controls. Milk consump-

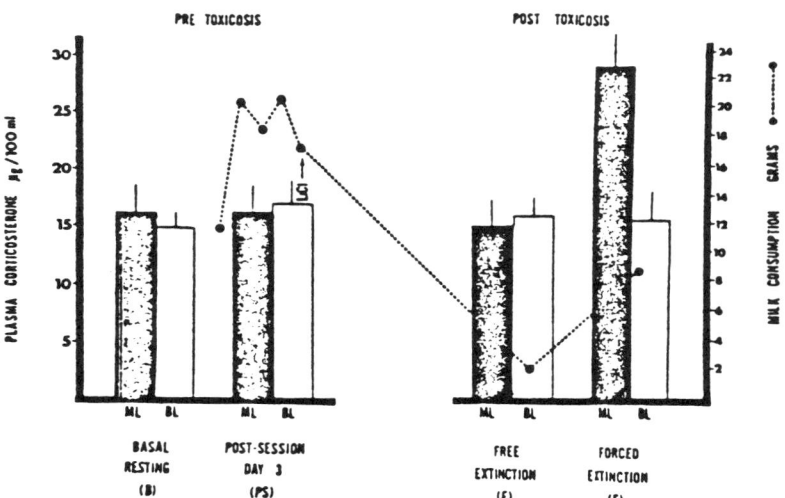

FIGURE 2.6. Mean milk consumption (in milliliters) of the conditioned animals (dark circles connected by dotted lines) and mean plasma corticosterone levels of conditioned (ML) and control (BL) groups as a function of treatment phase (see text for further explanation). Error bars represent standard error of the mean. (From Smotherman, Hennessy & Levine, 1976.)

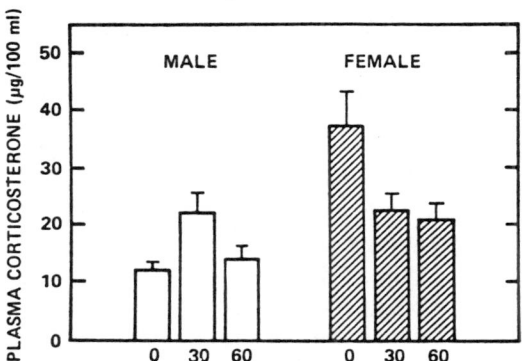

FIGURE 2.7. Plasma corticosterone levels (mean ± SEM) of male and female rats as a function of time after exposure to a saccharin solution which was previously paired with LiCl injection. (From Weinberg, Gunnar, Brett, Gonzalez, & Levine, 1982.)

tion in the conditioned animals (Group ML) is indicated by the dark circles connected by the dotted line. The left-hand panel shows that there were no differences between experimental groups in levels of plasma corticosterone either before (Basal Resting) or after (Post-Session Day 3) the initiation of daily drinking sessions in which animals were exposed to the to-be-conditioned flavor. Following the lithium chloride injection (note vertical arrow), drinking was suppressed, but there was no elevation in corticosterone levels when animals were not thirsty (Free Extinction). When animals were subsequently deprived of water (Forced Extinction), flavor consumption increased but was nonetheless below pretoxicosis levels. More importantly, conditioned elevations of plasma corticosterone appeared in the conditioning animals (ML) but not in controls (BL).

These data indicate an additional psychological factor, namely conflict, which determines whether or not conditioned adrenocortical activity will be seen. We now turn to a study indicating that the endocrine status of an animal also modulates conditioning of the pituitary-adrenal axis. Weinberg, Gunnar, Brett, Gonzalez and Levine (1982) have shown there are sex differences in the pattern of adrenocortical secretion elicited by saccharin exposure following flavor aversion conditioning, even though there are ⁻ɔx differences in the conditioned behavior. The basic finding is illustrated in Figure 2.7. Male rats, which have learned a flavor aversion and are deprived of water during testing, show an elevation in plasma corticosterone 30 minutes following flavor presentation which returns to baseline at 60 minutes. This is the same conflict-induced elevation in corticosterone which was demonstrated by Smotherman et al. (1976; Figure 2.6). Female rats, on the other hand, show a very different pattern of pituitary-adrenal activity. First, at the onset of flavor exposure, their levels of plasma corticosterone are very much higher than the corresponding values for males. Second, the response to flavor presentation, which is seen both 30 and 60 minutes later, is a marked decrease in hormone rather than the increase which is shown by males. In a subsequent experiment, Weinberg et al. (1982) showed that this sex difference in the pattern of hormone secretion to an aversive flavor can be attributed to sexually dimorphic steroid hormones, specifically the male hormone, testosterone. Ovariectomy did not change the pattern of response shown by females. However, castrated males showed the female pattern rather than the typical pattern illustrated in Figure 2.7 for noncastrated males. It should be emphasized that this modulation of the conditioned adrenal response by testosterone was not accompanied by a corresponding modulation of conditioned suppression of drinking behavior.

In addition to the psychological and endocrine factors outlined above, there are also forebrain neural systems which mediate conditioned adrenal activity independently of conditioned behavior. Smotherman, Kolp, Coyle, and Levine (1981) examined conditioned taste aversion and pituitary-adrenal activity in rats which received either bilateral hippocampectomy, control lesions involving overlying cortex, or no surgical operation whatsoever. They used the procedure involving forced drinking after food and water deprivation, which produces conflict-induced elevations in corticosterone. There were no differences associated with brain lesions in the behavioral suppression of flavor consumption following pairing of the flavor with lithium chloride injection. There were also no differences in the magnitude of the unconditioned adrenocortical response to lithium chloride injection across the different lesion conditions. There was, on the other hand, a very clear effect of lesion on conditioned elevations of plasma corticosterone, as indicated in Figure 2.8.

Conditioned rats from the unoperated and cortically lesioned groups showed

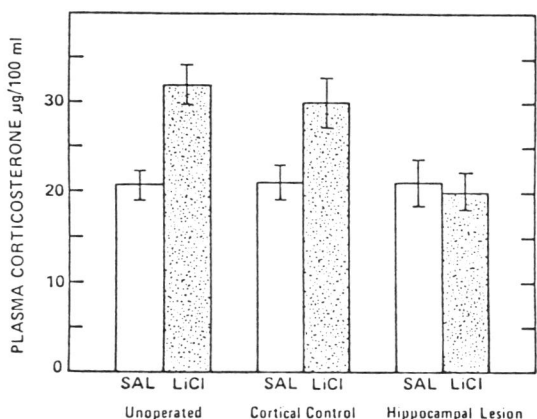

FIGURE 2.8. Mean plasma corticosterone levels (± SEM) in response to saccharin exposure as a function of lesion condition in animals which previously received saccharin paired with an injection of LiCl (LiCl) or saline (SAL). (From Smotherman, Kolp, Coyle, & Levine, 1981.)

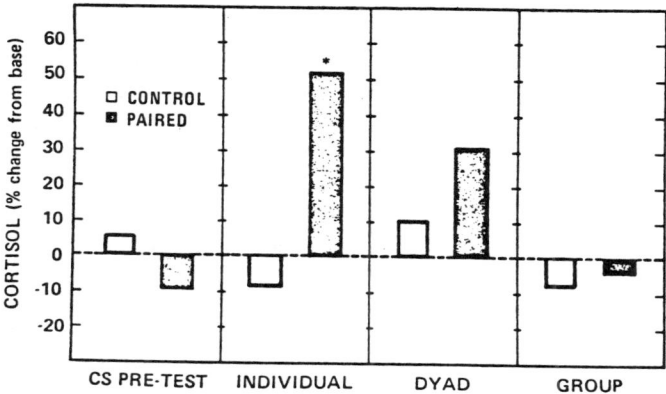

FIGURE 2.9. Cortisol responses of adult male squirrel monkeys to 10 nonreinforced conditioned stimulus (CS) presentations before training (CS Pre-Test) and after training as a function of social housing condition. The CS Pre-Test occurred under individual housing. Separate groups of monkeys were trained with the CS followed by shock (Paired) or the CS without shock (Control). *Differs from control and from zero-percent baseline, $p < .05$. (From Stanton, Patterson, & Levine, 1985.)

elevations in corticosterone over their respective (conditioning) controls. Conditioned rats with hippocampal lesions, in contrast, showed no such elevations of plasma corticosterone. Apparently, the hippocampal formation is part of the neural pathway for the conditioned pituitary-adrenal response, but not the unconditioned hormonal response to lithium chloride or the conditioned or unconditioned behavioral response.

We have seen that, in contrast to behavioral CRs, endocrine CRs can depend on factors at the psychological, endocrine, and neural levels. In this final example, we turn to evidence indicating that social factors can modulate conditioned endocrine secretion in the squirrel monkey. As is true generally of primate species, squirrel monkeys are a group-living species with a highly evolved communication system and repertoire of social behaviors. This characteristic of squirrel monkeys makes them ideal animals in which to study social modulation of stress responses, particularly the way in which social affiliation reduces an individual's response to stress. Stanton, Patterson, and Levine (1985) performed a study to determine whether social affiliation could modulate the squirrel monkey's cortisol response to a conditioned fear stimulus. The conditioned fear stimulus was a flashing light which was paired with footshock for one group of animals (Paired), but was presented without shock for another group of animals (Control). Tests of fear conditioning were conducted with animals housed either individually (Individual), with one partner (Dyad), or with several social partners (Group). The basic finding of this study is shown in Figure 2.9.

Tests of the cortisol response always occurred in the home cage. Animals in both the Paired and Control groups received 10 nonreinforced presentations of the CS. Prior to fear conditioning, CS presentations failed to elicit a change in cortisol secretion from basal levels in either group of animals, as indicated in the left panel of Figure 2.9 (CS Pre-Test). Following fear conditioning, the appearance of conditioned elevations of cortisol depended on whether subjects were housed individually or with social partners. When housed individually, animals that had received the CS paired with shock showed significant elevations of cortisol relative to Control animals and to zero-percent baseline. When animals were housed as dyads, that is, with one other conspecific in the home cage, cortisol elevations to the conditioned fear stimulus were attenuated somewhat and did not differ from those of Control animals. When housed as a group of 6 animals, the response to the conditioned fear stimulus was virtually absent. It is noteworthy that these differences in cortisol secretion across social conditions cannot be attributed to differences in the level of fear conditioning, which was clearly evident behaviorally in all social contexts. These findings indicate that there are social factors which can modulate endocrine CRs independently of behavior.

The fact that a variety of social, psychological, endocrine, and neural factors can influence endocrine CRs independently of behavioral CRs is instructive about the mechanisms of endocrine conditioning. For example, these findings rule out a simple stimulus substitution mechanism in which both behavioral and endocrine responses are a necessary consequence of activation of a conditioned aversive emotional state (Figure 2.10-A). In the case of flavor-aversion learning, for instance, this hypothesis would state the lithium chloride US unconditionally elicits an aversive emotional state that and the arousal of this state then leads unconditionally to activation of the pituitary-adrenal axis. Once saccharin and lithium-chloride-induced illness become associated, exposure to saccharin alone leads to activation of this aversive state, which in turn unconditionally activates the pituitary-adrenal axis and the behavioral aversion to saccharin. The fact that conditioned pituitary-adrenal activity often fails to accompany conditioned aversive behavior suggests that additional processes are necessary to translate the *conditioned* aversive emotional state into endocrine activity (Figure 2.10-B).

The dissociation between behavioral and pituitary-adrenal CRs is also instructive with regard to the neural substrates of Pavlovian conditioning. Recent progress in this area indicates that aversive Pavlovian conditioning "involves two memory trace systems that have distinct neuronal substrates" (Thompson et al., 1987). One system serves as the substrate for a nonspecific "conditioned fear" response (Konorski, 1967; Mowrer, 1947). This system is mediated by neural circuitry involving the brain stem, hypothalamus, and limbic areas such as the amygdala. In the terminology of Konorski (1967), this is the "preparatory response" system. The other memory trace system subserves conditioning of discrete, specific, adaptive, striated-muscle CRs. This system is mediated by a well-delineated circuit involving the cerebellum (Thompson, McCormick, & La-

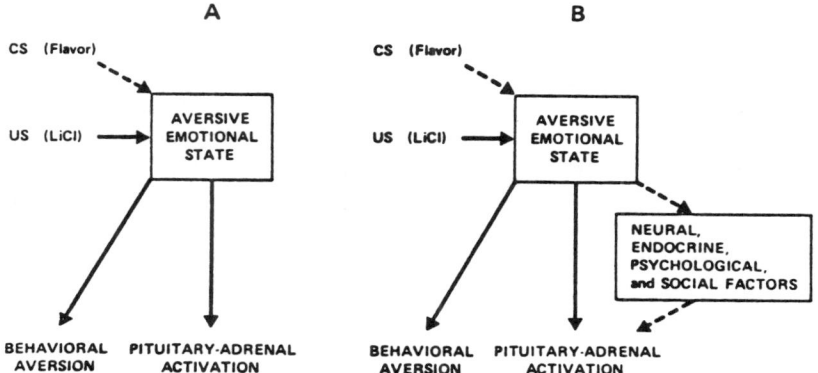

FIGURE 2.10. Schematic diagram indicating how Pavlovian conditioning of behavioral and endocrine responses is mediated by a hypothetical aversive emotional state. Arrows indicate causal pathways which occur either unconditionally (solid lines) or as a result of conditioning (dashed lines). (A) Conditioned behavioral and endocrine responses are both mediated by a conditioned pathway between CS and the aversive emotional state in conjunction with a "hard-wired" pathway between this state and behavioral and endocrine systems. (B) Conditioned endocrine responses are mediated as in (A) except that an independent conditioned pathway links the emotional state with the endocrine system. It is in this pathway that neural, endocrine, psychological, and social factors reviewed here exert their effects. This pathway is distinct from the pathway mediating unconditioned effects on endocrine function because these latter effects are not modulated by the same factors which modulate the conditioned pathway.

vond, 1986). In the terminology of Konorski (1967), this is the "consummatory response" system. Both traditional analysis at the behavioral level (Konorski, 1967; Mowrer, 1947; Rescorla & Solomon, 1967) and more recent analysis at the neural level (Thompson et al., 1987) suggest these two memory systems are clearly distinct, although they may interact under certain circumstances.

The evidence that we have reviewed in this chapter indicating endocrine CRs can easily be dissociated from behavioral ones lends additional support to the distinction between these memory systems. We believe that pituitary-adrenal activity is a valuable index of the "conditioned fear" system (Hennessy & Levine, 1979). As we have already stated, however, pituitary-adrenal activity cannot be viewed as a "hard-wired" index of conditioned fear. Rather, a multiplicity of additional factors determine whether conditioned fear states result in hormone secretion (Figure 2.10-B).

The dissociation between behavioral and endocrine CRs is also instructive with respect to another issue, namely that of endocrine modulation of behavior. The idea that endocrines feed back on the brain and subsequently influence behavior is one which has been actively investigated (Krieger & Hughes, 1980; Martinez, Jensen, Messing, Rigter, & McGaugh, 1981). It has been amply demonstrated that pharmacological doses of various exogenously administered hormones can produce certain behavioral effects. In the case of changes in the animal's endogenous endocrine levels, however—changes which are most often phasic and in the physiological range—the modulation of behavior by endocrines is more problematic. Certainly, if pituitary-adrenal CRs can be prevented without any detectable effect on behavioral CRs, then it seems any role pituitary-adrenal hormones might have in generating behavioral CRs may be minimal at best. This is not to say that pituitary-adrenal hormones do not play a role in other conditioning processes. In fact, exogenous administration of pituitary-adrenal hormones appears to affect the extinction of conditioned responding rather than conditioned responding, per se (Levine, Smotherman, & Hennessy, 1977).

PROPERTIES OF ENDOCRINE CONDITIONING

Pavlovian CRs obey a definite set of laws. These laws, or properties, relate various stimulus manipulations to the strength of conditioned responding. A list (not necessarily exhaustive) of these properties would include CS-US contiguity, partial reinforcement, extinction, latent inhibition, conditioned inhibition, inhibition of delay, overshadowing, blocking, US preexposure effects, sensory preconditioning, second-order conditioning, cue-to-consequence specificity, and so forth (see Pavlov, 1927).

In this section, we would like to examine the properties of conditioned endocrine responses. Understanding the properties of endocrine conditioning is important for at least three reasons. First, since many properties are unique to Pavlovian conditioning (as opposed to other forms, such as instrumental conditioning), they help serve to define this type of conditioning. In order to designate a particular learned response as a Pavlovian CR, it is helpful to demonstrate that this response possesses the properties of Pavlovian conditioning. The more of these properties the response can be shown to have, the more convincing is the conclusion that this response is Pavlovian in nature. Second, knowledge of the properties of conditioning can reveal much about underlying mechanisms. This is true at both the psychological and neural levels. For example, the question of whether endocrine CRs are the product of stimulus-response (S-R) or stimulus-stimulus (S-S) associations can be revealed by studies of sensory preconditioning and second-order conditioning. As another example, since different properties of conditioning are mediated at different levels of the neuraxis, a survey of the properties of endocrine conditioning may provide hints as to the neural circuitry involved. Finally, it is important to understand the properties of endocrine conditioning simply as a point of comparison with what is currently known about Pavlovian conditioning. One need only consider the analysis of ingestional aversion learning as a unique versus general form of conditioning to see the rich potential of this approach (Domjan, 1980; Revusky, 1977).

As will soon become apparent, much too little work has been done in this area.

2. PAVLOVIAN CONDITIONING OF ENDOCRINE RESPONSES   41

Indeed, what we do not know is much more impressive than what we do know. We can only present three examples, all from studies of the pituitary-adrenal system.

Habituation

The first example concerns habituation to novelty. Although habituation is not, strictly speaking, a property of Pavlovian conditioning, it is a form of stimulus processing which has been of theoretical interest to Pavlovian investigators. Stern, Erskine, and Levine (1973) habituated rats to exposure to an open field. Both behavioral (locomotor activity) and corticoid measures were taken. As indicated in Figure 2.11, the first exposure to the open field elicited high levels of locomotor activity and a substantial pituitary-adrenal response. With repeated exposures to the open field, locomotor activity declined substantially. This habituation of locomotor activity in the open field is well documented (Hinde, 1970). On the other hand, there was little evidence of habituation of the pituitary-adrenal response. Corticosterone levels were as high on the last day of open field exposure as they were on the first day. This finding is consistent with many others which indicate that the pituitary-adrenal response to novelty is very difficult to habituate. It is probably premature to conclude that pituitary-adrenal responses show no habituation whatsoever. It does, however, seem warranted to conclude that adrenocortical responses habituate much more slowly than do behavioral ones.

Latent Inhibition

The other property of Pavlovian conditioning which has been examined in an endocrine conditioning paradigm is latent inhibition. Pavlov (1927) was the first

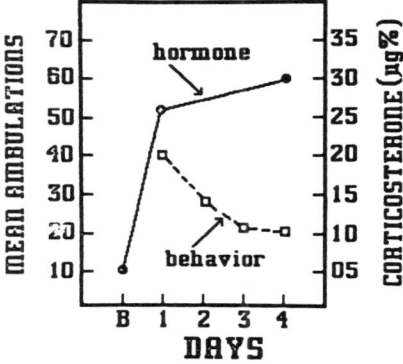

FIGURE 2.11. Mean ambulations in the open field (open squares) and levels of plasma corticosterone (closed circles) as a function of days of exposure ("B" indicates basal condition). (Adapted from Stern, Erskine, & Levine, 1973.)

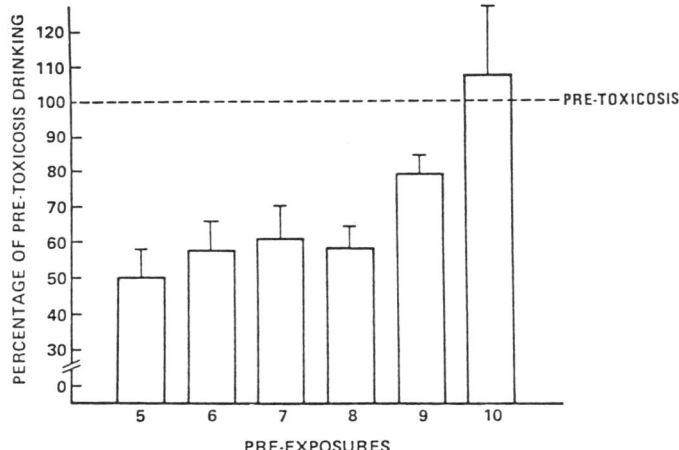

FIGURE 2.12. Mean (± SEM) milk consumption during test sessions as function of number of milk preexposures. Consumption is expressed as a percentage of individual subjects' consumption prior to LiCl injection. (From Smotherman, Margolis, & Levine, 1980.)

to demonstrate that repeated preexposure to a CS prior to pairings of that CS with a US impairs the rate of conditioning which subsequently occurs. The phenomenon of latent inhibition was studied by means of a flavor toxicosis paradigm by Smotherman, Margolis, and Levine (1980). The general procedures were similar to those used in the flavor aversion studies previously reviewed in this chapter (Figures 2.6 and 2.8), except that the number of flavor preexposures prior to pairings with lithium chloride injection was the major independent variable. As illustrated in Figure 2.12, latent inhibition was obtained in the drinking measure. As the number of preexposures increased, the behavioral aversion to the flavored solution decreased. In the case of the conditioned endocrine response (Figure 2.13), CS preexposure produced an impairment which was evident after even fewer exposures than was the case in the behavioral measure.

Opponent Process Theory

A theory which has arisen in the past decade in connection with the study of Pavlovian conditioning states that presentation of a US may, in some instances, activate a response system which opposes the UR. This opponent process may be the result of conditioning, or it may be an innate or "slave" process which is directly activated by the US (Schull, 1979; Solomon & Corbit, 1974; Wagner, 1981). We have already briefly alluded to conditioning studies, in which the US is an injection of exogenous insulin, as one instance where conditioned compensatory responses may be seen (Siegel, 1975). There is also some evidence that

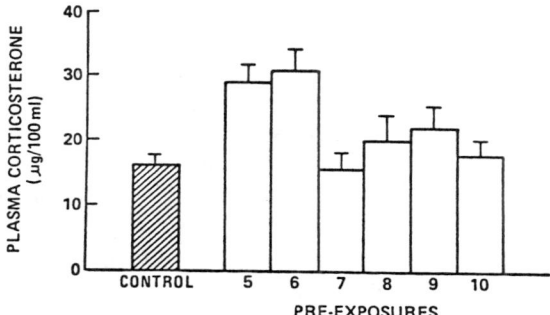

FIGURE 2.13. Mean (± SEM) plasma corticosterone levels in response to milk presentation during testing of a control (not conditioned) group and of 6 conditioned groups, given differing numbers of milk preexposures prior to conditioning. (From Smotherman, Margolis, & Levine, 1980.)

opponent processes may govern the activity of the pituitary-adrenal system. Levine and Coover (1976) measured the pituitary-adrenal response of fasted rats to a daily meal. They found that the adrenocortical response had two components. The first component was a decline in hormone which occurred over the first 10–20 minutes after the meal or the presentation of cues associated with the meal (see also Figure 2.4). The second component was a marked increase or rebound in hormone which overshot basal levels. This second component was evident in animals presented only with feeding-related cues approximately 50-60 minutes following presentation of these cues. This second component seems to reflect the omission of the food US on the test day and is similar to the frustration-elicited corticosterone increases seen in operant situations (Coe et al., 1983; Levine, Goldman & Coover, 1972; Figure 2.1). This compensatory rebound in hormone level suggests that the pituitary-adrenal system may be sensitive to conditioned-opponent processes elicited by appetitive stimuli.

These three examples indicate that hormonal responses may show the same properties as do behavioral ones, although they may follow a different time course across trials. These examples also further demonstrate the point which was made earlier that behavioral and endocrine measures of conditioning are easily dissociated. But by far the most noteworthy feature of these studies is their limited number. This illustrates the severe paucity of information on the properties of endocrine CRs. The main point that we would like to make is that currently the data are too limited to permit any real characterization of the properties of endocrine CRs.

SUMMARY AND CONCLUSIONS

This review of endocrine conditioning is based on a limited amount of data. Nevertheless, some conclusions are possible.

First, Pavlovian conditioning has been demonstrated according to rigorous criteria in a limited number of endocrine systems. These systems include insulin, the pituitary-gonadal system, and the pituitary-adrenal system. We would like to emphasize, however, that the absence of evidence for conditioning in other endocrine systems does not mean that these systems are not capable of being conditioned. We agree with Woods and Burchfield (1980) that practically any endocrine system is probably capable of being conditioned. We only mean to point out the current lack of rigorous evidence.

Second, endocrine responses which are observed in operant conditioning experiments are probably attributable to the Pavlovian contingencies which are imbedded in operant procedures. Again, this is a relatively unexplored issue. We know of no experiments on control of endocrine levels by operant or biofeedback techniques, perhaps because of the methodological limitation that such experiments would require nearly instantaneous assessment of endocrine levels, something which goes beyond the current state of technology. The fact that Pavlovian associations appear to account for endocrine responses which occur in operant conditioning situations recalls classic two-process learning theory (Mowrer, 1947) which relates Pavlovian versus instrumental learning mechanisms to autonomic versus skeletal response classes. Skeletal responses are subject to instrumental conditioning, whereas autonomic responses are subject to Pavlovian conditioning. Viewed from this perspective, control of endocrine responses by the Pavlovian component of instrumental learning situations is in some sense consistent with this aspect of two-process theory. This is not a trivial point for practitioners of behavioral medicine seeking to modulate endocrine levels by means of conditioning techniques.

Third, endocrine CRs are very easily dissociated from behavioral ones. In many cases, clear behavioral conditioning is not accompanied by conditioning in endocrine pathways. Consequently, stimulus substitution, as a rule for response generation, is not sufficient to account for endocrine CRs. Stimulus substitution probably sets the stage for endocrine CRs, but a broad range of additional factors apparently determines whether such CRs will ultimately be generated. A full understanding of endocrine conditioning must take these factors and their mechanisms of action into account.

Finally, much too little is known about how the laws of Pavlovian conditioning apply to endocrine responses. This is a very important question which remains to be pursued. Without this knowledge, it will not only be impossible to understand the mechanisms of endocrine conditioning, but it will also not be possible to use endocrine conditioning appropriately in the practice of behavioral medicine.

ACKNOWLEDGMENTS

This research was supported by HD-02881 from NICH&HD, MH-23645 from NIMH, and USPHS Research Scientist Award MH-19936 from NIMH to S.

Levine; and by Postdoctoral Training Grant MH-15147 from NIMH to M. E. Stanton.

REFERENCES

Ader, R. (1976). Conditioned adrenocortical steroid elevations in the rat. *Journal of Comparative and Physiological Psychology, 90*, 1156–1165.

Coe, C. L., Stanton, M. E., & Levine, S. (1983). Adrenal responses to reinforcement and extinction: Role of expectancy vs. instrumental responding. *Behavioral Neuroscience, 97*, 654–657.

Coover, G. D., Sutton, B. R., & Heybach, J. P. (1977). Conditioning decreases in plasma corticosterone level in rats by pairing stimuli with daily feedings. *Journal of Comparative and Physiological Psychology, 91*, 716–726.

Domjan, M. (1980). Ingestional aversion learning: Unique and general processes. In J. S. Rosenblatt, R. A. Hinde, C. Beer, & M. Busnel (Eds.), *Advances in the study of behavior* (pp. 275–336). New York: Academic Press.

Eikelboom, R., & Stewart, J. (1982). Conditioning of drug-induced physiological responses. *Psychological Review, 89*, 507–528.

Flaherty, C. F., & Becker, H. C. (1984). Influence of conditioned stimulus context on hyperglycemic conditioned responses. *Physiology and Behavior, 33*, 587–593.

Flaherty, C. F., Becker, H. C., Rowan, G. A., & Voelker, S. (1984). Effects of chlordiazepoxide on novelty-induced hyperglycemia and conditioned hyperglycemia. *Physiology and Behavior, 33*, 595–599.

Flaherty, C. F., Uzwiak, A. J., Levine, J., Smith, M., Hall, P., & Schuler, R. (1980). Apparent hyperglycemic and hypoglycemic conditioned responses with exogenous insulin as the unconditioned stimulus. *Animal Learning and Behavior, 8*, 382–386.

Graham, J. M., & Desjardins, C. (1980). Classical conditioning: Induction of luteinizing hormone and testosterone secretion in anticipation of sexual activity. *Science, 210*, 1039–1041.

Hennessy, J. W., & Levine, S. (1979). Stress, arousal, and the pituitary-adrenal system: A psychoendocrine hypothesis. In J. M. Sprague & A. N. Epstein (Eds.), *Progress in psychobiology and physiological psychology* (Vol. 8, pp. 133–178). New York: Academic Press.

Hinde, R. A. (1970). Behavioral habituation. In G. Horn & R. A. Hinde (Eds.), *Short-term changes in neural activity and behavior* (pp. 3–30). London: Cambridge University Press.

Hutton, R. A., Woods, S. C., & Makous, W. (1970). Conditioned hypoglycemia: Pseudoconditioning controls. *Journal of Comparative and Physiological Psychology, 71*, 198–202.

Konorski, J. (1967). *Integrative activity of the brain.* Chicago: University of Chicago Press.

Krieger, D. T., & Hughes, J. C. (1980). *Neuroendocrinology.* Sunderland, MA: Sinauer.

Levine, S., & Coover, G. D. (1976). Environmental control of suppression of the pituitary-adrenal system. *Physiology and Behavior, 17*, 35–37.

Levine, S., Goldman, L., & Coover, G. D. (1972). Expectancy and the pituitary-adrenal system. In R. Porter & J. Knight (Eds.), *Physiology, Emotion and psychosomatic illness* (pp. 281–296). Amsterdam: Elsevier.

Levine, S., Smotherman, W. P., & Hennessy, J. W. (1977). Pituitary-adrenal hormones and learned taste aversion. In L. H. Miller, C. A. Sandman, & A. J. Kastin (Eds.), *Neuropeptide influences on the brain and behavior* (pp. 163–177). New York: Raven Press.

Mackintosh, N. J. (1974). *The psychology of animal learning.* New York: Academic Press.

Martinez, J. L., Jr., Jensen, R. A., Messing, R. B., Rigter, H., & McGaugh, J. L. (Eds.). (1981). *Endogenous Peptides and learning and memory processes.* New York: Academic Press.

Mason, J. W. (1975). Emotion as reflected in patterns of endocrine integration. In L. Levi (Ed.), *Emotions: Their parameters and measurement* (pp. 143–181). New York: Raven Press.

Mowrer, O. H. (1947). On the dual nature of learning—a reinterpretation of "conditioning" and "problem solving". *Harvard Education Review, 17*, 102–148.

Overmier, J. B., & Lawry, J. A. (1979). Pavlovian conditioning and the mediation of behavior. In G. H. Bower (Ed.), *The psychology of learning and motivation* (Vol. 13, pp. 1-55). New York: Academic Press.

Pavlov, I. P. (1927). *Conditioned reflexes*. London: Oxford University Press.

Rescorla, R. A., & Solomon, R. L. (1967). Two-process learning theory: Relationships between Pavlovian conditioning and instrumental learning. *Psychological Review, 74*, 151-182.

Revusky, S. (1977). Learning as a general process with an emphasis on data from feeding experiments. In N. W. Milgram, L. Krames, & T. M. Alloway (Eds.), *Food aversion learning* (pp. 1-51). New York: Plenum Press.

Schull, J. (1979). A conditioned opponent theory of Pavlovian conditioning and habituation. In G. H. Bower (Ed.), *The psychology of learning and motivation* (Vol. 13, pp. 57-90). New York: Academic Press.

Siegel, S. (1975). Conditioning insulin effects. *Journal of Comparative and Physiological Psychology, 89*, 189-199.

Smotherman, W. P., Hennessy, J. W., & Levine, S. (1976). Plasma corticosterone levels during recovery from LiCl produced taste aversions. *Behavioral Biology, 16*, 401-412.

Smotherman, W. P., Kolp, L. A., Coyle, S., & Levine, S. (1981). Hippocampal lesion effects on conditioned taste aversion and pituitary-adrenal activity in rats. *Behavioral & Brain Research, 2*, 33-48.

Smotherman, W. P., Margolis, A., & Levine, S. (1980). Flavor preexposures in a conditioned taste aversion situation: A dissociation of behavioral and endocrine effects in rats. *Journal of Comparative and Physiological Psychology, 94*, 25-35.

Solomon, R. L., & Corbit, J. D. (1974). An opponent-process theory of motivation: I. Temporal dynamics of affect. *Psychological Review, 81*, 119-145.

Stanton, M. E., Patterson, J. M., & Levine, S. (1985). Social influences on conditioned cortisol secretion in the squirrel monkey. *Psychoneuroendocrinology, 10*, 125-134.

Stern, J. M., Erskine, M. S., & Levine, S. (1973). Dissociation of open-field behavior and pituitary-adrenal function. *Hormones and Behavior, 4*, 149-162.

Thompson, R. F., Donegan, N. H., Clark, G. A., Lavond, D. G., Lincoln, J. S., Madden, J., IV, Mamounas, L. A., Mauk, M. D., & McCormick, D. A. (1987). Neuronal substrates of discrete, defensive conditioned reflexes, conditioned fear states, and their interactions in the rabbit. In I. Gormezano, W. F. Prokasy, & R. F. Thompson (Eds.), *Classical conditioning III: Behavioral, neurophysiological, and neurochemical studies in the rabbit* (pp. 371-399). Hillsdale, NJ: Lawrence Erlbaum Associates.

Thompson, R. F., McCormick, D. A., & Lavond, D. G. (1986). Localization of the essential memory trace system for a basic form of associative learning in the mammalian brain. In S. H. Hulse & B. F. Green Jr. (Ed.), *100 years of psychological research in America* (pp. 125-171). Baltimore: Johns Hopkins University Press.

Wagner, A. R. (1981). SOP: A model of automatic memory processing in animal behavior. In N. E. Spear & R. R. Miller (Eds.), *Information processing in animals: Memory mechanisms* (pp. 5-47). Hillsdale, NJ: Lawrence Erlbaum Associates.

Weinberg, J., Gunnar, M. R., Brett, L. P., Gonzalez, C. A., & Levine, S. (1982). Sex differences in biobehavioral responses to conflict in a taste aversion paradigm. *Physiology and Behavior, 29*, 201-210.

Woods, S. C., & Burchfield, S. R. (1980). Conditioned endocrine responses. In J. M. Ferguson & C. Barr Taylor (Eds.), *The comprehensive handbook of behavioral medicine* (Vol. I, pp. 239-254). Jamaica, NY: Spectrum Publications.

Woods, S. C., & Kulkosky, P. J. (1976). Classically conditioned changes of blood glucose level. *Psychosomatic Medicine, 38*, 201-219.

Woods, S. C., Vasselli, J. R., Kaestner, E., Szakmary, G. A., Milburn, P., & Vitiello, M. V. (1977). Conditioned insulin secretion and meal-feeding in rats. *Journal of Comparative and Physiological Psychology, 91*, 128-133.

3
THE PLACEBO EFFECT AS A CONDITIONED RESPONSE

Robert Ader
University of Rochester School of Medicine and Dentistry

There have been many descriptions of a placebo and the "placebo effect" (Beecher, 1965; Gadow & Poling, 1986; Shapiro, 1971; Turner, Gallimore, & Fox-Henning, 1980; White, Tursky, & Schwartz, 1985). The placebo, itself, is usually an inert substance or an active drug that is (as far as is known) inneffective in modifying the response or treating the particular ailment under study. If a physician gives you a pill that contains no ingredients known to influence your rash, your cold symptoms, or your pain, for example, but you experience relief from whatever it is that ails you, that's the "placebo effect." The phenomenon has been variously described as yesterday's cure; a treatment for the patient rather than the disease; or a nuisance, that is, a psychological factor that, in influencing the response to active medications, needs to be controlled in evaluating drug effects. There is a voluminous literature documenting responses to placebo treatment and the variables that influence that response. These include, with various degrees of reliability, the size, shape, and color of the pill; whether the effect is being assessed in a clinical or in an experimental situation; the intensity of a patient's symptoms; the sex and personality characteristics of the subject or patient; the qualities of the physician; and the nature of the patient-physician relationship. Although demonstrably effective in a number of clinical situations and in a number of people (Beecher, 1965), the phenomenon is frequently attributed to trickery; magic; the healing power of faith; the "art" of medical practice; an immeasurable aspect of therapy; the suggestibility of the subject or patient; or, most frequently, to, the rapport and personal interaction between physician and patient (Casey, 1968; Liberman, 1962; Shapiro, 1971).

For Spiro (1984), "the placebo stands at the center of the conflict between science and intuition, reminding physicians that science alone may not be sufficient for medical practice" (p. 2). The point of Spiro's essay is that physicians should be aware of what they do not know. His discussion of the placebo effect is merely a vehicle for illustrating his point. Most certainly, clinicians should come to recognize what they do not know, and a consideration of the placebo effect emphasizes what we do not know. Not knowing, however, does not define a conflict between science and intuition because not knowing does not make a phenomenon unmeasurable or unknowable. The fact that we are unable to specify the mechanisms underlying the psychobiological interactions that influence pathophysiological processes, for example, reflects more on our ignorance and ingenuity than on the validity of such phenomena. The placebo effect may be a case in point. Unwittingly, perhaps, arguing that the placebo effect is unmeasurable but nonetheless real reinforces a dichotomy that is premature and almost certainly misdirecting. No progress will be achieved in our understanding of placebo effects by ignoring or rejecting such phenomena as unmeasurable and therefore unscientific or, at the other extreme, by the uncritical acceptance and definition of such phenomena as beyond the ken of science.

The lack of scientific attention being paid to placebo effects may reflect the lack of any theoretical position(s) within which to organize the existing data and upon which to base the design of new research. I am not, however, going to offer a new conceptualization or definition of the placebo effect. I hope, merely, to prompt reexamination of the notion that the complex of stimuli that accompany the administration of a drug and the placebo constitute conditioned stimuli and that the placebo effect is a conditioned response. This analysis has remained a descriptive one. If one were to accept this description, though, what would one do about it? How would it dictate new research strategies designed to elaborate the placebo effect? I was led to consider these questions because data were obtained suggesting that there would be considerable heuristic value in adopting a conditioning model for manipulating, controlling, and predicting placebo effects in pharmacotherapeutic situations.

Several authors have likened the placebo effect to a conditioned response or, at least, alluded to learning in influencing the response to placebos (Beecher, 1965; Evans, 1974; Gadow et al., 1985; Gleidman, Gantt, & Teitelbaum, 1957; Herrnstein, 1962; Knowles, 1962; Kurland, 1957; Lasagna, Mosteller, von Pelsinger & Beecher, 1954; Petrie, 1960; Pihl & Altman, 1971; Ross & Schnitzer, 1963; Skinner, 1953; Stanley & Schlosberg, 1953; Wikler, 1973; Wolf, 1950). One recent and denotative description of the placebo effect as a conditioned response is given by Wickramasekera (1980) who, like others in the past, proposes that the entire ritual surrounding drug administration can become a conditioned stimulus by virtue of the repeated association of such neutral events with drug administration in the developmental history of the individual.

There have been a few experimental studies specifically directed to the placebo effect as a conditioned response (Deutsch, 1974; Herrnstein, 1962; Hayashi, Ohashi, & Takadoro, 1980; Lang, Ross, & Glover, 1967; Numan, Smith, & Lal,

1975; Pihl & Altman, 1971; Roffman, Reddy, & Lal, 1973; Ross & Schnitzer, 1963). Herrnstein (1962), for example, reported that, under some temporal circumstances, a rat would show suppression of behavioral responding to an injection of saline that had previously characterized its response to scopolamine hydrobromide. Others (Pihl & Altman, 1971; Ross & Schnitzer, 1963) have demonstrated that after one or more injections of d-amphetamine, the (unconditional) increase in activity could be observed after an injection of saline, a placebo (i.e., a conditioned stimulus), the magnitude of the "placebo" response being a function of the number of repeated injections of the drug. In still other studies (Numan et al., 1975; Roffman et al., 1973), the repeated pairing of a tone with injections of morphine subsequently enabled presentation of the tone alone to alleviate the hypothermia and body shakes associated with morphine withdrawal in the rat.

In addition to such experimental analyses of the placebo effect, numerous studies and reviews have dealt with the conditioning of pharmacologic and physiologic responses (Eikelboom & Stewart, 1982; Harris & Brady, 1974; Lynch, Fertiziger, Teitelbaum, Cullen, & Gantt, 1973; Miller, 1969; Siegel, 1977). The work of Siegel and his colleagues (reviewed elsewhere in this volume) is one example of the systematic study of the role of conditioning in determining the behavioral and physiological responses to drugs and to the withdrawal of drugs—and the clinical implications of such phenomena. All of this literature should be considered part of the same body of data that bears on an analysis of placebo effects.

To argue that a placebo response is a conditioned response is not new, and the author is not the first to note the paucity of data on how the placebo effect might be exploited for therapeutic purposes. It is surprising, therefore, that so few studies have attempted a systematic analysis of placebo effects as conditioned responses or have taken advantage of conditioning in designing pharmacotherapeutic protocols. This essay describes briefly the use of conditioning to alter immunologic reactivity and how these conditioning operations were applied in a pharmocotherapeutic regimen designed to retard the development of autoimmune disease in animals and then discuss the implications of these data for experimental and clinical research.

BEHAVIORALLY CONDITIONED IMMUNOSUPPRESSION AND THE PHARMACOTHERAPY OF AUTOIMMUNE DISEASE IN ANIMALS

In an effort to explore the conditioning of alterations in immunologic reactivity, a taste aversion learning paradigm was used in which rats were first subjected to a single pairing of a novel, distinctively flavored drinking solution (saccharin), the conditioned stimulus (CS), with the effects of an immunosuppressive drug, cyclophosphamide (CY), the unconditioned stimulus (UCS). Subsequently, animals were immunized with sheep red blood cells (SRBC). Conditioned animals that were reexposed to saccharin had lower hemagglutinating antibody titers six days after the injection of SRBC than conditioned animals that were not reexposed to the CS, nonconditioned animals that were exposed to saccharin, and a saline-treated group. These original data (Ader & Cohen, 1975) were taken as evidence of a conditioned immunosuppressive response and have since been verified by other investigators (Rogers, Reich, Strom, & Carpenter, 1976; Wayner, Flannery, & Singer, 1978) (Figure 3.1).

Although the effects of conditioning in modifying immunologic reactivity have been relatively small, they have been quite consistent. Changing the CS or changing the magnitude of the UCS (which alters the kinetics of the antibody response) still results in conditioned immunosuppression (Ader & Cohen, 1981). Since conditioned animals reexposed to the saccharin solution previously paired with CY do not drink very much of the CS solution, it was necessary to control for the differential fluid intake of experimental and control groups. This was accomplished by permitting animals to choose between bottles containing plain or saccharin-flavored water. Under these preference testing conditions, the total fluid intake of experimental and control groups does not differ, but conditioned animals reexposed to the CS previously paired with CY still show an aversion to saccharin and still show a conditioned immunosuppressive response (Ader, Cohen, & Bovb-

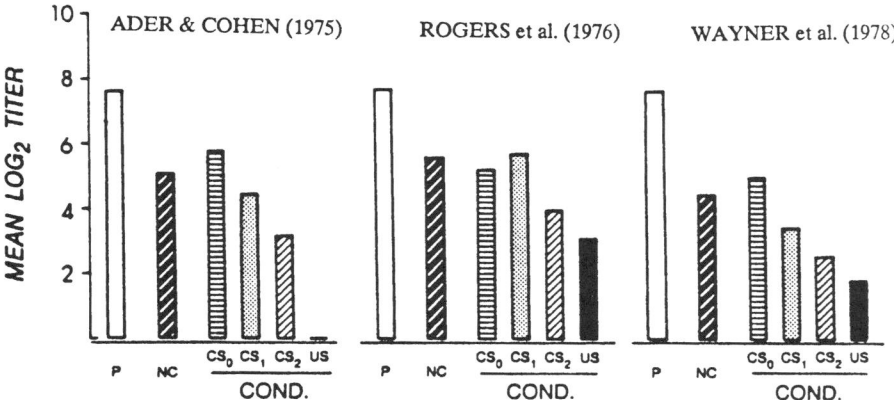

FIGURE 3.1. Hemagglutinating antibody titers (mean ± SE) measured six days after immunization with SRBC. P = placebo-treated animals; NC = nonconditioned rats provided with saccharin on Day 0 (day of antigen) and/or Day 3; CS_0 = conditioned animals that were not reexposed to saccharin after antigen treatment; CS_1 = conditioned animals that were reexposed to saccharin on Day 0 or 3; CS_2 = conditioned animals reexposed to saccharin on Days 0 and 3; US = conditioned animals injected with CY on the day of immunization. (Reprinted with permission of Pergamon Press, Inc. from Ader, *Advances in immunopharmacology*, 1981, Vol. 1, p. 430.)

jerg, 1982). In other experiments, lithium chloride was used instead of CY as the UCS (Ader & Cohen, 1975) or and elevation in corticosterone was superimposed on the residual immunosuppressive effects of CY (Ader, Cohen, & Grota, 1979). These studies provided no support for the hypothesis that the conditioned suppression of an antibody response was mediated by an increase in adrenocortical steroids.

The response to SRBC is a humoral response involving an interaction between T and B lymphocytes. However, a conditioned attenuation of the antibody response to a T-cell (thymus) independent antigen in mice can be observed (Cohen, Ader, Green, & Bovbjerg, 1979). Behaviorally conditioned immunosuppression can also be observed in the case of a cell-mediated response, another class of immune reactions (Bovbjerg, Ader, & Cohen, 1982). In addition, experimental extinction of the conditioned response has been demonstrated (Bovbjerg, Ader, & Cohen, 1984). There have now been several additional reports confirming conditioned alterations in humoral and cell-mediated immunity (Gorczynski, Macrae, & Kennedy, 1982, 1984; Klosterhalfen & Klosterhalfen, 1983; Kusnecov, Sivyer, King, Husband, Cripps, & Clancy, 1983; Sato, Flood, & Makinodan, 1984; Smith & McDaniels, 1983).

Because the magnitude of the effects of conditioning in altering immunologic reactivity have been relatively small, we sought to examine the biologic significance of a conditioned immunosuppressive response using an experimental model of autoimmune disease (Ader & Cohen, 1982). The female New Zealand hybrid $(NZB \times NZW)F_1$ mouse has become a standard experimental model for systemic lupus erythematosus (SLE) in man (Steinberg, Huston, Taurog, Cowdrey, & Raveche, 1981; Talal, 1976; Theolopolous & Dixon, 1981). These animals spontaneously develop a lethal glomerulonephritis between approximately 8 and 14 months of age. Treatment with cyclophosphamide, however, retards the progression of disease (Casey, 1968; Hahn, Knotts, Ng, & Hamilton, 1975; Lehman, Wilson, & Dixon, 1976; Morris, Esterly, Chase, & Sharp, 1976; Russell & Hicks, 1968; Steinberg, Gelfand, Hardin, & Lowenthal, 1975) by suppressing immunologic reactivity, thereby prolonging survival of the organism. Since several studies have indicated that immunologic reactivity could be suppressed by conditioning, we considered the possibility that by pairing a neutral (conditioned) stimulus with injections of CY and inducing a conditioned immunosuppressive response it might be possible to substitute CSs for some proportion of the active drug usually received by lupus-prone mice in the course of pharmacotherapy. Specifically, it was hypothesized that conditioned mice reexposed to the neutral stimuli associated with immunosuppressive medication (CY) would be more resistant to the development of autoimmune disease than nonconditioned mice treated with the same amount of drug.

New Zealand hybrid mice born in the laboratory were individually caged under a 12-hour light-dark cycle and provided with food and water ad libitum. An 8-week pharmacotherapeutic regimen was begun when the animals were four months old.

All mice were given a .15% solution of sodium saccharin in plain water by pipette. Cyclophosphamide was injected intraperitoneally (ip) according to the following schedule:

1. Group C100% received an ip injection of 30 mg/kg CY immediately after being given saccharin. Saccharin-CY pairings occurred at the same time of day and on the same day of each week. This sequence of events, equivalent to a standard pharmacotherapeutic protocol, was administered for a period of eight weeks.[1]
2. Group C50%, another conditioned group, also received saccharin weekly, but an ip injection of CY (30 mg/kg) followed saccharin on only 2 of each 4 weeks (in a random sequence). On the remaining trials, these mice received an ip injection of physiological saline.
3. Group NC50%, a nonconditioned group, was also exposed to saccharin weekly and ip injections of saline or CY on 2 of each 4 weeks, but the CY or saline injections were not paired with saccharin; they were administered on different days of the same week.
4. Control animals received no immunosuppressive therapy. They were, however, exposed to unpaired saccharin and ip injections of saline each week.

Pharmacologically, there is no difference between Groups C50% and NC50%; both groups receive the same amount and number of exposures to saccharin and CY. Nonconditioned mice treated with only half the amount of CY administered to Group C100% were expected to manifest symptoms of SLE (proteinuria) and die sooner than animals in Group C100%. Group C50% also received only half the amount of CY administered to Group C100%. However, to the extent that reexposure to the conditioned stimuli paired with CY is capable of eliciting a conditioned immunosuppressive response, it was predicted that conditioned mice would show a greater resistance to the development of autoimmune disease than nonconditioned mice, even though both groups received the same amount of drug.

Weekly treatment with CY delayed the onset of proteinuria and prolonged the survival of $(NZB \times NZW)F_1$ mice, as expected. As can be seen in Figure 3.2, the different chemotherapueutic regimens significantly influenced the development of proteinuria and mortality. Inclusion of the total population of each group may underestimate the impact of conditioning because all of these hybrid mice could be expected to develop autoimmune disease and die. Thus, the longer one monitors the progression of disease, the more difficult it is to discern treatment effects.

Statistically significant differences were also obtained using as a reference point the rate of development of proteinuria in the initial 50% of the mice that developed

---

[1] This dose of drug and duration of treatment proved to be effective in prolonging survival, but were not sufficient to obviate the development of autoimmune disease.

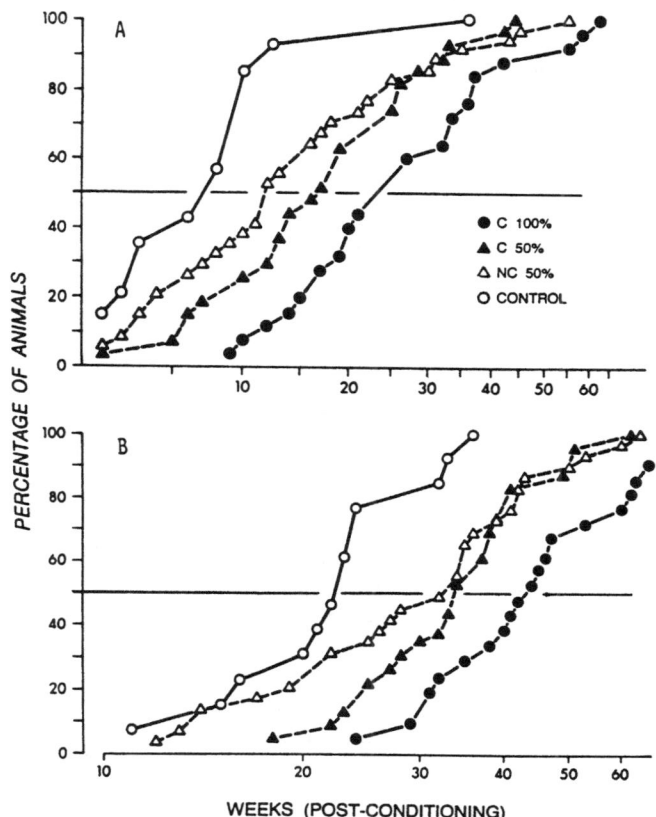

FIGURE 3.2. (A) Rate of development of an unremitting proteinuria in (NZB × NZW)F_1 female mice under different chemotherapeutic protocols. Group C100% ($n = 25$) received saccharin followed by CY each week; Group C50% ($n = 27$) received CY following half the weekly saccharin trials; Group NC50% ($n = 34$) received the same saccharin and CY as Group C50%, but saccharin and CY were not paired; Control mice ($n = 14$) received saccharin and unpaired injections of saline. (B) Cumulative mortality rate in these same (NZB × NZW)F_1 female mice. (Reprinted with permission of the American Association for the Advancement of Science from Ader and Cohen, *Science*, 1982, *215*, p. 1535.)

lupus or the rate at which a 50% mortality was reached. Animals treated with CY every week developed proteinuria more slowly than mice in any of the other groups. Nonconditioned mice treated with half the amount of CY received by animals maintained under a standard pharmacotherapeutic regimen did not differ from controls that received no CY. However, conditioned mice treated with the same total amount of drug developed proteinuria more slowly than did nonconditioned animals. The effects of the different treatment schedules on mortality yielded the same pattern of results. Nonconditioned animals did not differ from animals that received no immunosuppressive therapy, whereas conditioned mice survived significantly longer than untreated controls and did not differ from animals in Group C100%. Again, the critical comparision is between conditioned and nonconditioned animals that were treated with the *same* amount of drug and, like the difference in the rate of development of proteinuria, Group C50% survived significantly longer than Group NC50%. These results are consistent with previous studies of conditioned immunosuppression and with predictions that might be derived from such data regarding the application of conditioning in a pharmacotherapeutic situation. In conditioned mice, reexposure to a CS previously paired with an immunosuppressive UCS delayed the onset of autoimmune disease under a regimen of immunosuppressive therapy that was not, in itself, sufficient to influence the development of disease.

Based on these results, we suggested that there might be some heuristic value in viewing some pharmacotherapeutic regimens as conditioning paradigms (Ader & Cohen, 1982). If a pharmacotherapeutic regimen can be construed as a series of conditioning trials (i.e., CS-UCS pairings), the conditioned pharmacotherapeutic response should be sensitive to the manipulation of any number of experimental variables. It should, for example, be subject to experimental extinction, and resistance to extinction might be a function of the schedule of reinforcement. In the present pharmacotherapeutic paradigm, experimental extinction procedures, operationally defined as unreinforced presentations of the CS, would consist of reexposing conditioned animals to saccharin that was not followed by CY. Preliminary data on extinction were obtained in a second experiment.

During the initial period of therapy, the procedures were the same as those in the above study, except that the critical experimental group (Group C33%) received CY following saccharin on only one third of the weekly trials on which saccharin was presented. Nonconditioned animals (Group NC33%) received the same exposures to saccharin and CY, but in an unpaired fashion. At the end of the 12-week treatment period, Groups C100%, C33%, and NC33% were divided into three subgroups. One third of each group continued to receive saccharin and ip injections of saline and/or CY on the same schedule that existed during the initial chemotherapy period; one third continued to receive saccharin and ip injections of saline (CS), but CY treatment was discontinued; and one third received neither saccharin nor CY. Based on studies of conditioned immunosuppression, it was predicted that unreinforced CS presentations would influence the development of SLE in conditioned mice but not in nonconditioned animals.

Although the number of animals in this preliminary study was relatively small, the results yielded statistically significant differences that conformed to these predictions. Mortality was delayed in animals that continued to receive chemotherapy relative to mice that were taken off CY. Mice that continued to receive CS exposures after the termination of CY treatment, however, died more slowly than did mice deprived of all "medication" (Figure 3.3). In fact, the mortality rate of mice that continued to receive CS presentations without the UCS did not differ from that in mice that continued to receive saccharin *and* CY.

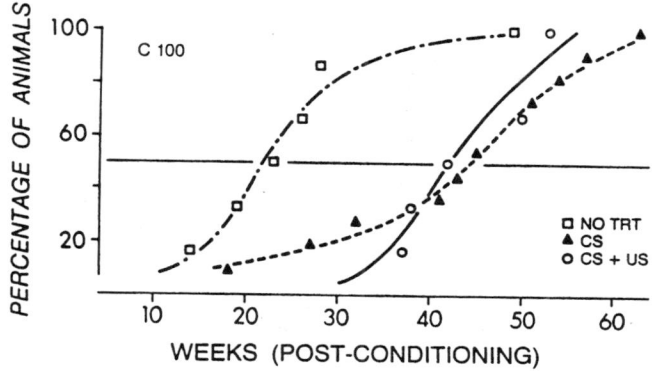

FIGURE 3.3. Mortality rate in (NZB × NZW)F_1 female mice treated with saccharin and CY weekly and then continued on a regimen of saccharin and CY (Group CS + US; $n = 6$), continued on placebo medication, alone (Group CS; $n = 11$), or deprived of both saccharin and CY (No treatment; $n = 6$). (Reprinted with permission of Guilford Press from Ader, in *Placebo: Theory, Research and Mechanisms*, 1985, p. 315.)

As in our initial study, the informative comparison is between the results obtained from conditioned and nonconditioned animals that receive the same amount of chemotherapy. These data are shown in Figure 3.4. For both Groups C33% and NC33%, mice deprived of both saccharin and CY died relatively rapidly compared to animals that continued to receive chemotherapy. Conditioned mice (Group C33%) that were taken off CY but continued to receive weekly exposures to the CS died more slowly than did animals deprived of both saccharin and CY, and, at least for the initial 50% of these populations, the mortality rate among mice that were reexposed to the CS did not differ from mice that continued to receive active drug treatment. In constrast, continued exposure to saccharin in nonconditioned animals had no effect on survival. The mortality rate in these mice did not differ from that in animals that received neither saccharin nor CY.

These results do not provide evidence of conditioned immunosuppression, per se, since we did not directly measure immune function. Nonetheless, these preliminary data involving the effects of chemotherapy and drug withdrawal provide presumptive evidence for the operation of conditioning processes and are consistent with the acquisition and extinction effects reported by Bovbjerg et al. (1984), and Gorczynski et al. (1982).

The direct implication of these data is that behavioral factors are capable of altering immune function; that is, that the immune system is subject to some regulation or modulation by the brain. This issue has been elaborated elsewhere (Ader, 1981; Ader & Cohen, 1985; Guillemin, Melnechuk, & Cohn, 1984). These data can also be considered an extension of the conditioning of drug-induced physiological responses (Eikelboom & Stewart, 1982). It is within the latter context that these data have implications for our understanding of placebo effects and for the conduct of psychopharmacologic and pharmacotherapeutic research.

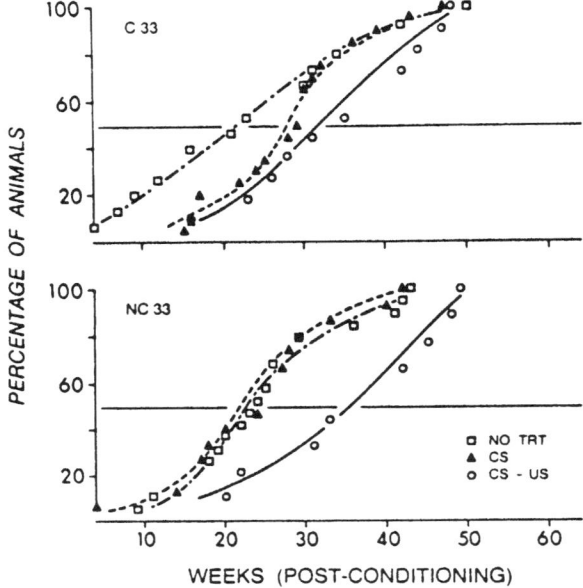

FIGURE 3.4. Mortality rate in conditioned (C33) and nonconditioned (NC33) (NZB × NZW)F_1 female mice that continued to receive saccharin and CY (Group CS + US), continued to receive only saccharin (Group CS), or received neither saccharin nor CY (No treatment); $ns = 11$ to 20 per subgroup. (Reprinted with permission of Guilford Press from Ader, in *Placebo: Theory, Research and Mechanisms*, 1985, p. 315.)

A CONDITIONING MODEL OF PHARMACOTHERAPY

Applying a behavioral terminology to a pharmacologic treatment regimen, those physiologic effects unconditionally elicited by the introduction of a drug are referred to as "unconditioned responses." The drug may be referred to as the "unconditioned stimulus" (UCS). Those environmental or behavioral events or stimuli that are either coincidentally or purposely associated with and reliably precede the voluntary or involuntary receipt of a drug (but which are neutral with respect to the unconditioned effects of the drug) are referred to as "conditioned stimuli" (CS). Repeated pairing of a CS and a UCS can eventually enable the CS to elicit a conditioned response (CR)—an approximation of the response previously evoked by the UCS.[2]

An experiment designed to evaluate drug effects usually involves two basic

---

[2] Drug-induced conditioned responses can be opposite in direction to the unconditioned effects of the drug. This issue, discussed elsewhere in this chapter and volume, represents one of the limiting factors in defining the pharmacotherapeutic situations in which conditioning might be of therapeutic value.

groups: an experimental group that receives an active drug and a control group that does not. The experimental group may be divided on the basis of dose, route, time, and/or frequency of administration, but it always receives a drug. In contrast, the control group does not receive the active pharmacologic agent but receives an inert or chemically irrelevant substance (placebo) instead. In all other respects, the experimental and control groups are not supposed to differ; that is, the stimuli that attend the administration of either active drug or placebo are the same. In conditioning terms, traditional pharmacotherapeutic protocols (in contrast to the evaluation of acute drug effects) involve continuous reinforcement. That is, experimental subjects experience the stimuli associated with the administration of medication that are invariably followed (reinforced) by the unconditioned psychophysiologic effects of the drug. At the other extreme, the voluntary or medically directed administration of an inert substance is never reinforced. Among experimental subjects, then, the probability of reinforcement is 100% whereas control subjects are under a 0% reinforcement schedule.

There is, however, an alternative to the administration of either drug *or* placebo—the administration of drug *and* placebo. Despite descriptions of the placebo effect as a conditioning phenomenon and data suggesting the utility of interspersing drug and placebo trials (e.g., Herrnstein, 1962), I know of no clinical studies of the therapeutic process that have varied schedules of pharmacologic reinforcement. Pharmacotherapeutic research has not systematically manipulated the stimuli associated with the administration of drugs and evaluated the effects of noncontinuous or partial schedules of pharmacologic reinforcement, that is, schedules of reinforcement in which the receipt of "medication" and the attendant environmental stimuli are pharmacologically reinforced on some occasions but not on others.

Varying reinforcement schedule (the "active drug:placebo ratio") represents an alternative means of manipulating drug dose. Under a long-term regimen of pharmaco-therapy, cumulative drug dose might be lowered by changing reinforcement schedule rather than by lowering the concentration of drug administered on the component drug trials. This strategy, which capitalizes on conditioned pharmacologic effects, could have several clinical advantages. If it can be shown that a partial reinforcement schedule can approximate the therapeutic effects of a continuous reinforcement schedule, total drug dose could be reduced, some side effects might be reduced (resulting in increased adherence to drug regimens), problems of dependence might be lessened or alleviated more easily, and the duration of the effects of pharmacotherapy might be extended. The cost of medication would also be reduced.

Returning to the animal studies described above, we found first that the immunosuppressive effects of cyclophosphamide could be conditioned. Then, conditioned stimuli were successfully substituted for some proportion of the active drug used in a pharmacotherapeutic regimen designed to protect animals against the development of autoimmune disease. One comparison group (Group C100%)

was treated under a standard therapeutic protocol in which the environmental stimuli associated with the receipt of a drug were invariably followed by the unconditioned immunosuppressive effects of the chemotherapeutic agent. Animals in Group C100% experienced continuous pharmacologic reinforcement. Animals in Group C50% were conditioned under a partial reinforcement schedule; the unconditioned effects of CY occurred on only 50% of the occasions on which these mice were exposed to the complex of stimuli that defined the CS. Since these mice received only half the total amount of drug received by animals in Group C100%, a nonconditioned group (NC50%) was also treated with half the amount of drug received by Group C100%. For the nonconditioned animals, however, there was no close temporal relationship between those stimuli that were purposely associated with and reliably preceded drug administration in Group C50%. Pharmacologically, the treatment of the conditioned and nonconditioned groups was identical. Manipulation of the environmental contingencies, however, resulted in a delay in the onset of lupus in conditioned animals using an amount of drug that was not, by itself, sufficient to alter the development of disease.

These studies on lupus-prone mice provided no evidence that a partial reinforcement schedule is as effective as continuous reinforcement. It should be recognized, though, that the selection of a 50% reinforcement schedule was an arbitrary one. Also, assuming that like skeletal responses, drug-induced physiological responses, conditioned under partial reinforcement are more resistant to extinction than those acquired under continuous reinforcement, it might have been expected that autoimmune disease would have developed more slowly in Group C50% than in Group C100% when active drug was discontinued and only the CS was presented. That is, it might have been hypothesized that pharmacologically unreinforced CS presentations would extend the pharmacotherapeutic effects of a partial reinforcement schedule to a greater extent than a continuous reinforcement schedule. This prediction would require comparing groups treated with the same amount of drug. Unfortunately, the extinction data reported here do not meet this criterion and do not, therefore, adequately address this hypothesis; mice treated under the continuous schedule of reinforcement (Group C100%) received three times as much drug as animals treated under the partial schedule of reinforcement (Group C33%). This prediction, then, remains to be tested. It is of interest, nonetheless, that a comparison of conditioned and nonconditioned animals that received the same cumulative amount of drug revealed different therapeutic outcomes. Continued exposure to the CS following the termination of active drug therapy delayed the onset of autoimmune disease only among conditioned animals.

These data on the pharmacotherapy of autoimmune disease in mice suggest that by titrating reinforcement schedule (along with other parameters of a treatment regimen), one might approximate the therapeutic effects of a continuous schedule of pharmacologic reinforcement using a lower cumulative amount of drug. It is also conceivable that pharmacotherapeutic effects could be extended or the gradual withdrawal of drugs facilitated (i.e., that resistance to extinction would be greater) in patients treated under partial schedules of reinforcement than in patients treated under a traditional, continuous regimen of pharmacotherapy.

It is generally believed, however, that resistance to extinction of classically conditioned responses is not greatly affected by variations in reinforcement schedule. Indeed, it has been suggested that the effect of partial reinforcement on resistance to extinction is one of the variables that differentiates between classical and instrumental conditioning (Kimble, 1961). Spence (1966) argued that a partial reinforcement effect in classical conditioning would only be seen in human subjects since such an effect was purportedly based on cognitive processes not present in lower animals. Historically, the effects of partial reinforcement in retarding extinction are less regularly observed in classical than in instrumental conditioning, but there are several examples of a partial reinforcement effect on extinction of classically conditioned responses in lower animals, and Macintosh (1974), for one, has argued that the available data do not provide sufficient grounds for distinguishing between classical and instrumental conditioning on this basis. The literature is mixed, but from the table provided by Farrell, Locurto, Duncan, and Terrace (1980), for example, it is evident that a greater resistance to extinction following partial as compared to continuous reinforcement is not an infrequent observation in classical conditioning studies involving different species performing different responses to different conditioned and unconditioned stimuli.

Since the rate of acquisition of a conditioned response is typically retarded under partial reinforcement, the imposition of different schedules of pharmacologic reinforcement in clinical situations might most profitably be introduced following a period of standard pharmacotherapy, a situation in which patients are reinforced consistently for taking prescribed medication. One example of the greater resistance to extinction that can follow partial as compared to continuous reinforcement occurred under comparable circumstances. Questioning the contention that partial reinforcement has little effect on the extinction of classically conditioned responses, Gibbs, Latham, and Gormenzano (1976) conducted a study of classical conditioning of the rabbit nictitating membrane in which partial schedules of reinforcement ranging from 50% down to 5% were introduced following acquisition of the conditioned response under continuous reinforcement. Performance remained high even under a 15% reinforcement schedule. During extinction, the highest response rates were displayed by animals that had been maintained under partial reinforcement schedules of 50% and 25%. In contrast, extinction was rapid among animals maintained under a continuous schedule of reinforcement and in animals on the lowest (15% and 5%) reinforcement schedules.

Thus, while there may be no strong argument for predicting that partial reinforcement would have longer lasting effects than continuous reinforcement in a pharmacotherapeutic situation, the available literature provides no grounds for rejecting such a possibility. Moreover, the distinction between classical and instrumental conditioning is blurred (Davis & Hurwitz, 1977; Mackintosh, 1974) and it might be difficult to define pharmacotherapeutic responses as pure illustrations of either classical or instrumental conditioning. Indeed, it would not be unreasonable to infer that there are elements of both classical and instrumental conditioning in the pharmacotherapeutic situation.

Would not the conditioning of pharmacotherapeutic effects also result in the conditioning of deleterious side effects? Indeed, they may. The presence of side effects illustrates the multiple effects of drugs and, excluding clinical situations, the labeling of what are to be considered primary and secondary or "side" effects is frequently determined by the interests of the investigator. Of course, side effects need not be injurious, in which case they may actually promote conditioning by increasing the detectability of UCS effects. The issue is, nonetheless, a meaningful one because even a "single" effect of a pharmacologic agent may show changes over time that reflect different effects of the drug on different organ systems or responses to the initial effects of the drug. Gantt (1953) described the phenomenon of schizokinesis, a dissociation in the rate of acquisition and/or extinction of different conditioned responses. We have observed such a dissociation in the extinction of conditioned taste aversion and immuno-suppressive responses (Bovbjerg et al., 1984). If one entertains the possibility that these multiple effects result from different conditioning processes (Eikelboom & Stewart, 1982), that is, that they are controlled by different conditioned and unconditioned stimuli, acquisition and/or extinction could proceed at different rates and be differentially reinforced.

Some side effects result from the direct action of drugs on a target organ, and some of these may not be relevant to the restoration of homeostasis for which the drug was prescribed. If such drug actions are not mediated by the CNS, they do not constitute unconditioned stimuli and will not induce conditioned responses directly. In turn, however, they may elicit changes in target organs that do constitute UCSs for CNS-mediated responses that are subject to conditioning. Eikelboom and Stewart (1982) and Miller and Dworkin (1980) have argued that the appropriate designation of conditioned and unconditioned stimuli would clarify observations of paradoxical (compensatory) conditioned responses, that is, conditioned responses that are opposite in direction to unconditioned responses (e.g., Siegel, this volume). Predicting the direction of drug-induced physiologic (and, presumably, pharmacotherapeutic) responses, then, would depend on knowledge of the site(s) of action of the pharmacologic agent.

Thus, with respect to a conditioning model of pharmacotherapy, conditioned side effects could not be more prevalent than the side effects unconditionally elicited by continuous administration of the therapeutic agent. Deleterious side effects elicited by the direct action of a drug on some organ system would, in a conditioning model, be less prevalent simply because fewer administrations of active drug might be necessary if patients were treated under a partial schedule of pharmacologic reinforcement. As a matter of conjecture, the elicitation of anticipatory (compensatory) responses to an external stimulus previously associated with the deleterious side effects that result from the direct action of a drug on some target organ might have a salutary effect. This may be beside the point because situations in which therapeutic effects are based on direct drug actions (e.g., replacement therapies) are not appropriate models for examining conditioned pharmacotherapeutic effects.

CONCLUSIONS

Having accepted previous *descriptions* of the "placebo effect" as a conditioning phenomenon, I have tried to address the issue of how one might proceed from the description to an experimental analysis of the placebo effect and how this analysis might apply to clinical situations. In this respect, our own data are quite preliminary, but they do suggest that there is an alternative to an analysis of pharmacologic and pharmacotherapeutic effects in terms of differences between groups that are treated with drug or placebo. Subjects or patients can be treated with drug and placebo by introducing partial schedules of pharmacologic reinforcement. This alternative represents a shift from a concern for defining "pure" pharmacologic effects to a concern for the potentially beneficial effects of placebo administration.

In contrast to the present analysis based on the conceptualization of the placebo effect as a learned response, placebo studies have, for the most part, concentrated on the individual's initial responses to inert medication. These acute studies which implicitly capitalize on the experiential (reinforcement) history of the individual have yielded interesting and important data, including information about individual differences. These may, however, represent only a small proportion of the variance involved in understanding and exploiting placebo effects. The factors that contribute to the initial or essentially pre-experimental responses to a placebo may be no more than variables on which subjects or patients should be matched in studies designed to describe the acquisition and extinction of conditioned pharmacologic and pharmacotherapeutic responses under circumstances in which one can exercise explicit control over the reinforcement history of the individual. In addition to dose, route, frequency, and duration of medication, etc., an "active drug:placebo ratio" is, in this context, a relevant dimension of pharmacotherapeutic regimens. Partial reinforcement schedules provide an alternative means of adjusting dose of drug. It is an alternative which, based on a conditioning model, leads to testable hypotheses regarding the acquisition and/or extinction of the response to placebo medication, and, as such, should suggest innovative strategies for psychopharmacologic research and psychopharmacotherapeutic interventions.

I do not wish to quibble about labels; it is not my intent to redefine the "placebo effect" but to broaden the concept and suggest new strategies for the experimental analysis of the phenomenon. One could, for example, reserve the designation "placebo effect" for those initial responses to inert or irrelevant substances that are substituted for active drug under a variety of experimental and clinical situations in humans. One could then describe the long-term pharmacotherapeutic effects that derive from conditioned pharmacologic responses without referring to these as placebo effects. It is difficult to redefine phenomena, especially those that have a long history and are inextricably bound to specific kinds of experimental paradigms. However, it would be a mistake not to broaden the concept of the placebo effect to include its role in long-term pharmacotherapeutic regimens and to take advantage of the experimental strategies of a learning perspective.

There are several potential advantages in adopting a conditioning perspective in the evaluation and construction of pharmacotherapeutic regimens. One of these would be the availability of animal models of disease which would facilitate basic research and testing of schedules of pharmacologic reinforcement. Clinically, prescription of partial schedules of reinforcement could reduce the total amount of drug required for the treatment of some pathophysiologic conditions, it might reduce side effects (and thereby increase adherence to a treatment protocol), it might attenuate drug dependence, and it might be used to extend the effects of pharmacotherapy or gradually reduce and eliminate the need for drug. To speculate even further, the imposition of partial schedules of pharmacologic reinforcement might influence the interaction between pharmacotherapeutic and psychotherapeutic interventions (Rounsaville, Klerman, & Weissman, 1981). It might, for example, enable psychotherapy to be accomplished during symptom-free periods that were not completely regulated by the continuous effects of pharmacologic agents. Psychotherapy conducted under these conditions might be more readily generalized to a subsequent drug-free period than psychotherapy conducted under the influence of drugs. Most generally, it would seem worthwhile to pursue the possibility of achieving short- and long-term therapeutic goals using lower maintenance levels of drugs, maximizing the benefits and reducing the risks (and the costs) of drugs prescribed for a variety of clinical disorders.

The placebo effect is not something mystical, nor does the administration of a placebo have to be a lie—and it is not my intent to deny the therapeutic impact of the faith and trust that can derive from the relationship between physician and patient. On the contrary, I would expect that an appropriate patient-physician relationship would facilitate the acquisition of conditioned pharmacotherapeutic responses in humans. However, as a bona fide learning phenomenon, it is being suggested that the placebo effect is amenable to experimental analysis and that its therapeutic potential has probably been underestimated.

The present analysis is, admittedly, highly speculative. I have constructed an elaborate scheme based on a modicum of data. Nevertheless, no special violence has been done to what we know about conditioning—or think we know about placebos. The available literature suggests that new and interesting data might be obtained by adopting a learning perspective in the experimental analysis of drug effects and of pharmacotherapeutic regimens. The clinical utility of this perspective in different pathophysiologic conditions and with different pharmacologic agents, however, remains to be determined.

ACKNOWLEDGMENTS

This chapter is based on the Presidential Address given at the Annual Meeting of the Academy of Behavioral Medicine Research. Preparation of this chapter and related research of the author were supported by a Research Scientist Award (K5-MH06318) from the National Institute of Mental Health and by research grants from the National Institute of Neurological and Communicative Disorders and Stroke and the Kroc Foundation.

The author wishes to acknowledge and thank Drs. Nicholas Cohen, Larry Guttmacher, Leonard Salzman, and Anthony Suchman, who provided critical comments on an initial draft of this chapter.

REFERENCES

Ader, R. (Ed.). (1981). *Psychoneuroimmunology*. New York: Academic Press.
Ader, R., & Cohen, N. (1975). Behaviorally conditioned immunosuppression. *Psychosomatic Medicine, 37*, 333–340.
Ader, R., & Cohen, N. (1981). Conditioned immunopharmacologic effects. In R. Ader (Ed.), *Psychoneuroimmunology* (pp. 281–319). New York: Academic Press.
Ader, R., & Cohen, N. (1982). Behaviorally conditioned immunosuppression and murine systemic lupus erythematosus. *Science, 215*, 1534–1536.
Ader, R., & Cohen, N. (1985). CNS-immune system interactions: Conditioning phenomena. *Behavioral and Brain Sciences, 8*, 379–426.
Ader, R., Cohen, N., & Bovbjerg, D. (1982). Conditioned suppression of humoral immunity in the rat. *Journal of Comparative and Physiological Psychology, 96*, 517–521.
Ader, R., Cohen, N., & Grota, L. J. (1979). Adrenal involvement in conditioned immunosuppression. *International Journal of Immunopharmacology, 1*, 141–145.
Beecher, H. K. (1959). *Measurement of subjective responses: Quantitative effects of drugs*. New York: Oxford.
Beecher, H. K. (1965). The powerful placebo. *Journal of the American Medical Association, 159*, 1602–1606.
Bovbjerg, D., Ader, R., & Cohen, N. (1982). Behaviorally conditioned suppression of a graft-vs.-host response. *Proceedings of the National Academy of Sciences, 79*, 583–585.
Bovbjerg, D., Ader, R., & Cohen, N. (1984). Acquisition and extinction of conditioned suppression of a graft-vs.-host response in the rat. *Journal of Immunology, 132*, 111–113.
Brody, H. (1982). The lie that heals: The ethics of giving placebos. *Annals of Internal Medicine, 97*, 112–118.
Casey, T. P. (1968). Immunosuppression by cyclophosphamide in NZB/NZW mice with lupus nephritis. *Blood, 32*, 436–444.
Cohen, N., Ader, R., Green, N., & Bovbjerg, D. (1979). Conditioned suppression of a thymus independent antibody response. *Psychosomatic Medicine, 41*, 487–491.
Davis, H., & Hurwitz, H. M. B. (1977). *Operant-Pavlovian interactions*. Hillsdale, NJ: Lawrence Erlbaum Associates.

Deutsch, R. (1974). Conditioned hypoglycemia: A mechanism for saccharin-induced sensitivity to insulin in the rat. *Journal of Comparative and Physiological Psychology, 86*, 350-358.

Eikelboom, R., & Stewart, J. (1982). Conditioning of drug-induced physiological responses. *Psychological Review, 89*, 507-528.

Evans, F. J. (1974). The placebo response in pain reduction. *Advances in Neurology, 4*, 289-296.

Farrell, L., Locurto, C. M., Duncan, H. J., & Terrace, H. S. (1980). Partial reinforcement in autoshaping with pigeons. *Animal Learning and Behavior, 8*, 45-59.

Gadow, K. D., & Poling, A. D. (1986). Placebo theory and experimental design. In K. D. Gadow & A. D. Poling (Eds.), *Advances in learning and behavioral disabilities* (Supl. 1, pp. 41-84). Greenwich CT: JAI Press.

Gantt, W. H. (1953). Principles of nervous breakdown in schizokinesis and autokinesis. *Annals of the New York Academy of Sciences, 56*, 143-163.

Gibbs, C. M., Latham, S. B., & Gormenzano, I. (1976). Classical conditioning of the rabbit nictitating membrane response: Effects of reinforcement schedule on response maintenance and resistance to extinction. *Animal Learning and Behavior, 6*, 209-215.

Gleidman, L. H., Gantt, W. H., & Teitelbaum, H. A. (1957). Some implications of conditional reflex studies for placebo research. *American Journal of Psychiatry, 113*, 1103-1107.

Gorczynski, R. M., Macrae, S., & Kennedy, M. (1982). Conditioned immune response associated with allogeneic skin grafts in mice. *Journal of Immunology, 129*, 704-709.

Gorczynski, R. M., Macrae, S., & Kennedy, M. (1984). Factors involved in the classical conditioning of antibody responses in mice. In R. Ballieux, J. Fielding, & A. L'Abbatte (Eds.) *Breakdown in human adaptation to stress: Towards a multidisciplinary approach* (pp. 704-712).

Guillemin, R., Melnechuk, T., & Cohn, M. (Eds.) (1984). *Neural regulation of immunity*. New York: Raven.

Hahn, B. H., Knotts, L., Ng, M., & Hamilton, T. R. (1975). Influence of cyclophosphamide and other immunosuppressive drugs on immune disorders and neoplasia in NZB/NZW mice. *Arthritis and Rheumatism, 18*, 145-152.

Harris, A. H., & Brady, J. V. (1974). Animal learning—visceral and autonomic conditioning. *Annual Review of Psychology, 25*, 107-133.

Hayashi, T., Ohashi, K., & Takadoro, S. (1980). Conditioned drug effects to d-amphetamine and morphine-induced motor acceleration in mice: Experimental approach for placebo effect. *Japanese Journal of Pharmacology, 30*, 93-100.

Herrnstein, R. J. (1962). Placebo effect in the rat. *Science, 138*, 677-678.

Kimble, G. A. (1961). *Hilgard and Marquis' conditioning and learning*. New York: Appleton-Century-Crofts.

Klosterhalfen, W., & Klosterhalfen, S. (1983). Pavlovian conditioning of immunosuppression modifies adjuvant arthritis in rats. *Behavioral Neuroscience, 97*, 663-666.

Knowles, J. B. (1962). Conditioning and the placebo effect. *Science, 138*, 677-678.

Kurland, A. A. (1957). The drug placebo: Its psychodynamic and conditioned reflex action. *Behavioral Science, 2*, 101-110,

Kusnecov, A. W., Sivyer, M., King, M., Husband, M. G., Cripps, A. W., & Clancy, R. L. (1983). Behaviorally conditioned suppression of the immune response by antilymphocyte serum. *Journal of Immunology, 130*, 2117-2120.

Lang, W. J., Ross, P., & Glover, A. (1967). Conditional response induced by hypotensive drugs. *European Journal of Pharmacology 2*, 169-174.

Lasagna, L., Mosteller, F., von Pelsinger, J. M., & Beecher, H. K. (1954). A study of the placebo response. *American Journal of Medicine, 16*, 770-779.

Lehman, D. H., Wilson, C. B., & Dixon, F. J. (1976). Increased survival times of New Zealand hybrid mice immunosuppressed by graft-vs.-host reactions. *Clinical and Experimental Immunology, 25*, 297-302.

Liberman, R. (1962). An analysis of the placebo phenomenon. *Journal of Chronic Diseases, 15*, 761-783.

Lynch, J. J., Fertiziger, A. P., Teitelbaum, H. A., Cullen, J. W., & Gantt, W. H. (1973). Pavlovian conditioning of drug reactions: Some implications for problems of drug addiction. *Conditional Reflex, 8,* 221–223.
Mackintosh, N. J. (1974). *The psychology of animal learning.* New York: Academic.
Miller, N. E. (1969). Learning of visceral and glandular responses. *Science, 163,* 434–445.
Miller, N. E., & Dworkin, B. (1980). Different ways in which learning is involved in homeostasis. In R. F. Thompson, L. H. Hicks, & V. B. Shvyrkov (Eds.), *Neural mechanisms of goal-directed behavior and learning* (pp. 57–73). New York: Academic Press.
Morris, A. D., Esterly, J., Chase, G., & Sharp, G. C. (1976). Cyclophosphamide protection in NZB/NZW disease. *Arthritis and Rheumatism, 19,* 49–55.
Numan, R., Smith, N., & Lal, H. (1975). Reduction of morphine-withdrawal body shakes by a conditioned stimulus in the rat. *Psychopharmacological Communications, 1,* 295–303.
Petrie, A. (1960). Some psychological aspects of pain and the relief of suffering. *Annals of the New York Academy of Sciences, 86,* 13–27.
Pihl, R. O., & Altman, J. (1971). An experimental analysis of the placebo effect. *Journal of Clinical Pharmacology, 11,* 91–95.
Roffman, M., Reddy, C., & Lal, H. (1973). Control of morphine-withdrawal hypothermia by conditioned stimuli. *Psychopharmacologia, 29,* 197–201.
Rogers, M. P., Reich, P., Strom, T. B., & Carpenter, C. B. (1976). Behaviorally conditioned immunosuppression: Replication of a recent study. *Psychosomatic Medicine, 38,* 447–452.
Ross, S., & Schnitzer, S. B. (1963). Further support for the placebo effect in the rat. *Psychological Reports, 13,* 461–462.
Rounsaville, B. J., Klerman, G. L., & Weissman, M. (1981). Do psychotherapy and pharmacotherapy for depression conflict? Empirical evidence from a clinical trial. *Archives of General Psychiatry 38,* 24–29.
Russell, P. J., & Hicks, J. D. (1968). Cyclophosphamide treatment of renal disease in (NZB × NZW)F_1, hybrid mice. *Lancet, 1,* 440–446.
Sato, K., Flood, J. F., & Makinodan, T. (1984). Influence of conditioned psychological stress on immunological recovery in mice exposed to low dose X-irradiation. *Radiation Research, 98,* 381–388.
Shapiro, A. K. (1971). Placebo effects in medicine, psychotherapy, and psychoanalysis. In A. E. Bergin & S. L. Garfield, (Eds.), *Handbook of psychotherapy and behavior change* (pp. 439–473). New York: Wiley.
Siegel, S. (1977). Learning and psychopharmacology. In M. E. Jarvik (Ed.), *Psychopharmacology in the practice of medicine* (pp. 61–70). New York: Appleton-Century-Crofts.
Skinner, B. F. (1953). *Science and human behavior.* London: MacMillan.
Smith, G. R., & McDaniels, S. M. (1983). Psychologically mediated effect on the delayed hypersensitivity reaction to tuberculin in humans. *Psychosomatic Medicine, 45,* 65–70.
Spence, K. W. (1966). Cognitive and drive factors in the extinction of the conditioned eyeblink in human subjects. *Psychological Review, 73,* 445–458.
Spiro, H. M. (1984). Placebos, patients, and physicians. *Pharos, 47*(2), 2–6.
Stanley, W. C., & Schlosberg, H. (1953). The psychophysiological effects of tea. *Journal of Psychology, 36,* 435–448.
Steinberg, A. D., Gelfand, M. C., Hardin, J. A., & Lowenthal, D. T. (1975). Therapeutic studies in NZB/W mice: III. Relationship between renal status and efficacy of immunosuppressive drug therapy. *Arthritis and Rheumatism, 18,* 9–14.
Steinberg, A. D., Huston, D. P., Taurog, J. D., Cowdery, J. S., & Raveche, E. S. (1981). The cellular and genetic basis of murine lupus. *Immunology Reviews, 55,* 121–154.
Talal, N. (1976). Disordered immunologic regulation and autoimmunity. *Transplantation Reviews, 31,* 240–263.
Theofilopoulos, A. N., & Dixon, F. J. (1981). Etiopathogenesis of murine SLE. *Immunology Reviews, 55,* 179–216.

Turner, J. L., Gallimore, R., & Fox-Henning, C. (1980). An annotated bibliography of placebo research. *JSAS Catalog of Selected Documents in Psychology, 10*, Ms. No. 2063.

Wayner, E. A., Flannery, G. R., & Singer, G. (1978). The effects of taste aversion conditioning on the primary antibody response to sheep red blood cells and *Brucella abortus* in the albino rat. *Physiology and Behavior, 21*, 995-1000.

White, L., Tursky, B., & Schwartz, G. (Eds). (1985). *Placebo: Theory, research and mechanisms.* New York: Guilford.

Wickramasekera, I. (1980). A conditioned response model of the placebo effect: Predictions from the model. *Biofeedback and Self Regulation, 5*, 5-18.

Wikler, A. (1973). Dynamics of drug dependence: Implications of a conditioning theory for research and treatment. *Archives of General Psychiatry 28*, 611-616.

Wolf, S. (1950). Effects of suggestion and conditioning on the action of chemical agents in human subjects—the pharmacology of placebos. *Journal of Clinical Investigation, 29*, 100-109.

4
THE TREATMENT OF SCOLIOSIS BY CONTINUOUS AUTOMATED POSTURAL FEEDBACK

Barry Dworkin
Susan Dworkin
The Pennsylvania State University College of Medicine

INTRODUCTION

Scoliosis is a pathological lateral curvature of the spine; in the idiopathic or familial variety, 80% of the patients are female. Figure 4.1 shows examples of the clinical manifestations of a severe and a mild curvature, and Figure 4.2 shows how a 35-degree scoliotic curve looks on x-ray measurement. In all its degrees of severity, scoliosis affects approximately 2%-4% of the adolescent population (Kane, 1977). In approximately 7% of those affected (2% of the general population), idiopathic scoliosis will produce a truncal deformity which progresses throughout the rapid growth period of adolescence (Rogala, Drummond, & Gurr, 1978).

In a child with a progressive deformity, if the curvature is detected early, while still mild, progression may be halted nonsurgically by the use of a scoliosis orthosis such as the Milwaukee Brace shown in Figure 4.3. These braces have been demonstrated to be effective for the majority of patients, provided that treatment is begun early enough and the orthosis is worn faithfully (Blount & Moe, 1980; Edmonson & Morris, 1977).

Conventional brace therapy has several significant drawbacks; because the brace stabilizes the spine by exerting pressure on the thorax at critical points, it must envelop the trunk, and to do so, it must be bulky and uncomfortable. In stabilizing the spine, the orthosis restricts truncal motion, causing atrophy of truncal musculature. As an end result, the spine becomes limited in its flexibility. Finally, the constant pressure of the brace, in some cases, may cause permanent deformation of the rib cage or the soft tissues directly under the pressure points. Such secondary deformities are less serious than the spinal deformity of scoliosis, but they are, nonetheless, of concern. For a scoliosis orthosis to be effective, it is generally believed that it must be worn 23 hours per day, 7 days a week, until

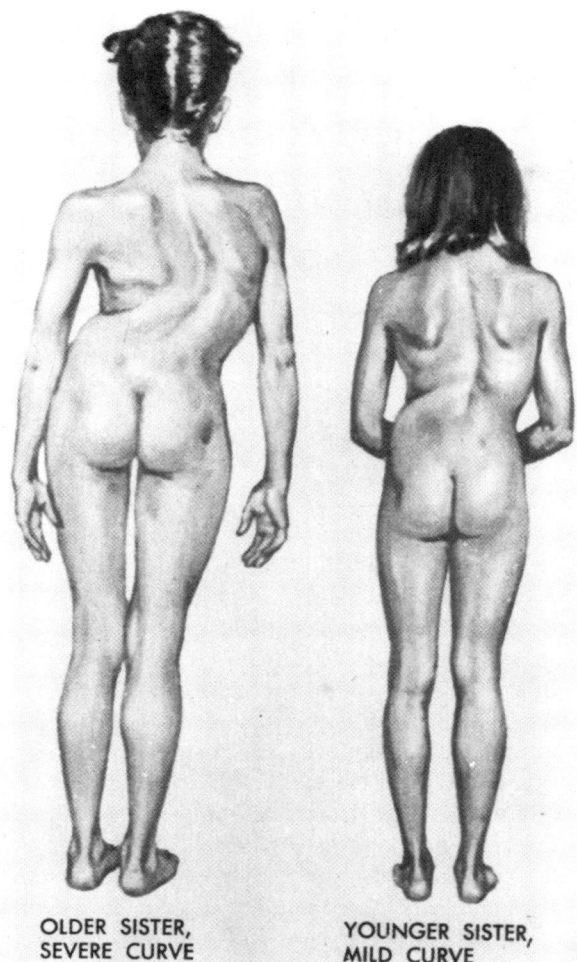

FIGURE 4.1 Two examples of a scoliotic curve. Left figure has a severe curve and right figure has a mild curve.

full skeletal maturity is reached, usually a period of 3–4 years. Unfortunately, this treatment must be undertaken during the most psychologically sensitive period of life. The bulkiness of the brace distorts the youngster's appearance at a time when outward appearance is of extreme importance. The brace identifies the child as different at a time of life when it is most painful to be different. It is, therefore, understandable that the chief cause of failure of brace treatment is failure of patient compliance.

One study, for instance, reported that only 59% (73 of 123) of patients demonstrated satisfactory compliance (Keiser & Shufflebarger, 1978). That cosmetic acceptability is an important aspect of compliance is shown by reports

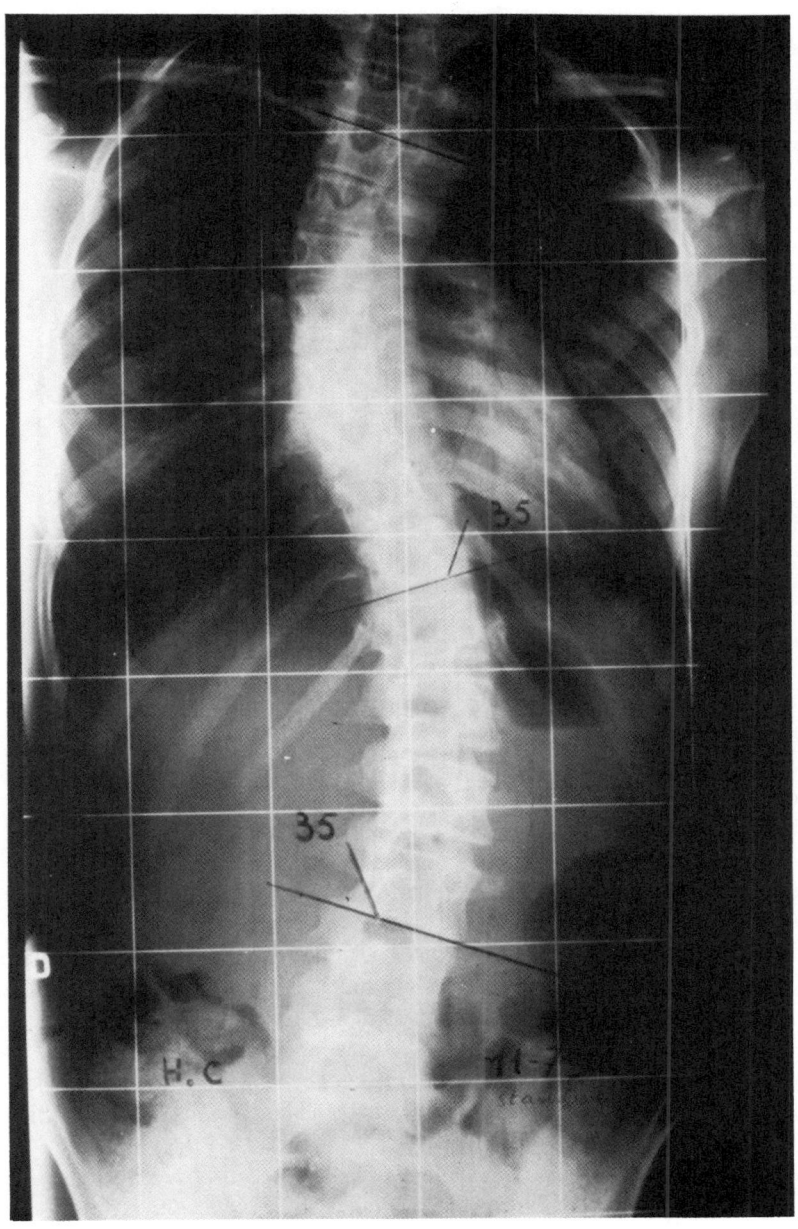

FIGURE 4.2 Typical radiograph of an S-shaped (double) 35° curve.

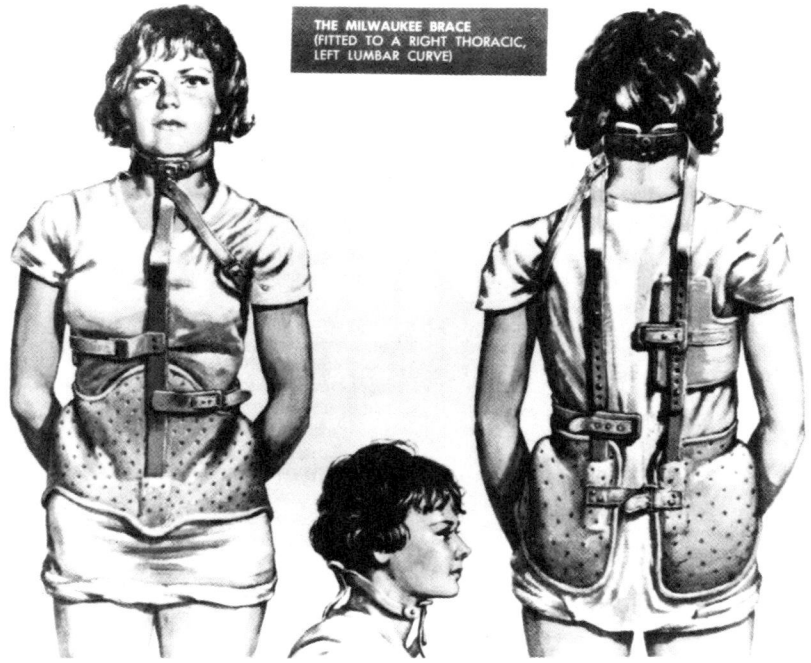

FIGURE 4.3 The Milwaukee brace.

that less objectionable bracing methods, such as the "Boston Bucket," are associated with higher levels of compliance (Sevastikoglou & Karlman, 1973; Wickers, Bunch, & Barnett, 1977).

The pathophysiology of scoliosis is unknown. However, certain features of the natural history and treatment suggested to us that an instrumental learning therapy could be developed as an alternative to bracing. Scoliosis usually begins with a single curve, as in Figure 4.4, which almost invariably becomes converted into a double curve shown in Figure 4.2. The existence of the second curve is possibly a consequence of the patient's attempt to correct her visual-vestibular error or to proprioceptively stabilize her center of mass. Since, this second curve is often thought to be compensatory, we reasoned that if a patient could learn to make a compensatory curve, it was at least conceivable that, given more salient information about the shape of her spine, she could learn to straighten the primary curve instead.

In addition to these physiological considerations, we discovered that there was controversy about how the brace actually functions to reduce the scoliotic curve. Those patients who passively slouch into it, developing thick enough calluses so that its pressure points cease to be uncomfortable, usually do not benefit from the brace. In fact, there is a growing conviction among orthopedists specializing in scoliosis that the brace's action is not primarily passive via direct mechanical

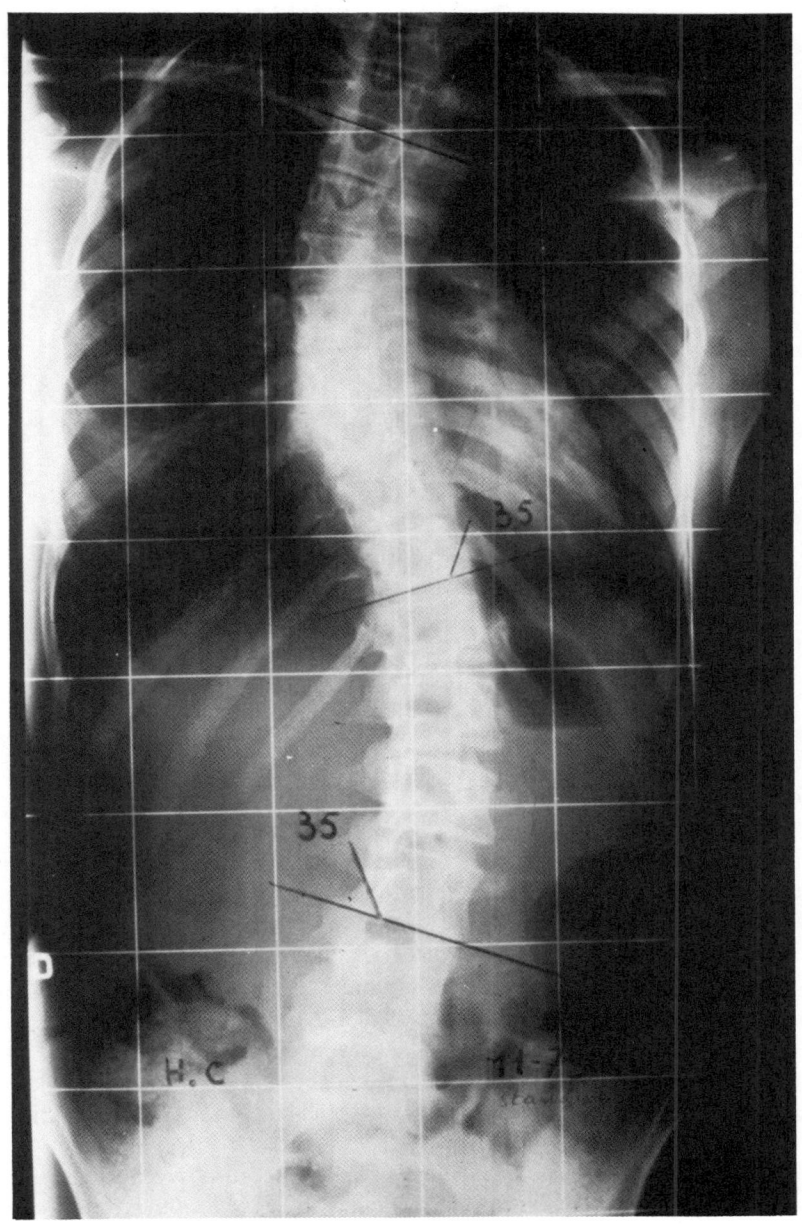

FIGURE 4.2 Typical radiograph of an S-shaped (double) 35° curve.

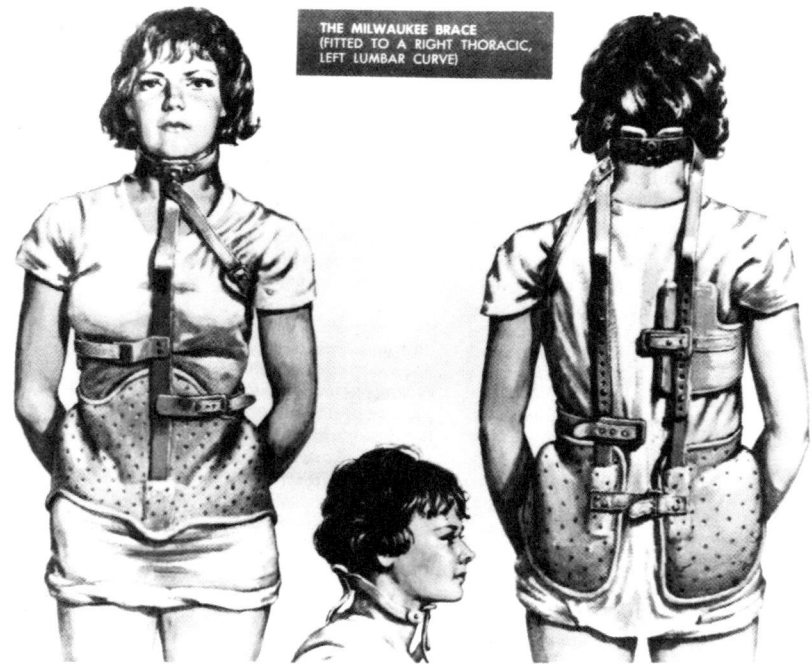

FIGURE 4.3 The Milwaukee brace.

that less objectionable bracing methods, such as the "Boston Bucket," are associated with higher levels of compliance (Sevastikoglou & Karlman, 1973; Wickers, Bunch, & Barnett, 1977).

The pathophysiology of scoliosis is unknown. However, certain features of the natural history and treatment suggested to us that an instrumental learning therapy could be developed as an alternative to bracing. Scoliosis usually begins with a single curve, as in Figure 4.4, which almost invariably becomes converted into a double curve shown in Figure 4.2. The existence of the second curve is possibly a consequence of the patient's attempt to correct her visual-vestibular error or to proprioceptively stabilize her center of mass. Since, this second curve is often thought to be compensatory, we reasoned that if a patient could learn to make a compensatory curve, it was at least conceivable that, given more salient information about the shape of her spine, she could learn to straighten the primary curve instead.

In addition to these physiological considerations, we discovered that there was controversy about how the brace actually functions to reduce the scoliotic curve. Those patients who passively slouch into it, developing thick enough calluses so that its pressure points cease to be uncomfortable, usually do not benefit from the brace. In fact, there is a growing conviction among orthopedists specializing in scoliosis that the brace's action is not primarily passive via direct mechanical

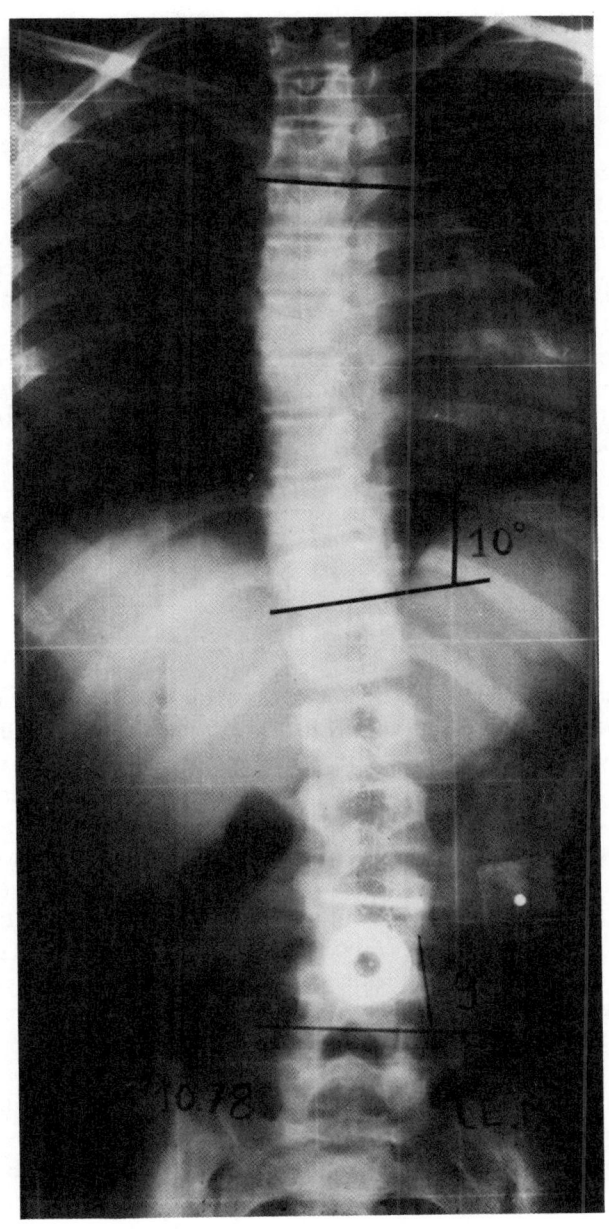

FIGURE 4.4 Radiograph of a single scoliotic curve.

forces on the spine, but that its effectiveness requires the active cooperation of the patient using it (Blount & Moe, 1980)—that is, that the patient use her own muscles to reduce the spinal curvature as she holds her body away from the pressure points.

In light of the foregoing, it seemed plausible to us that the effectiveness of the brace could depend on its ability to signal spinal curvature through increased discomfort at the pressure points. This would serve to inform a cooperative child of her poor posture as well as motivate her to straighten up. If this were the case, we thought that the postural training of a child might be performed as well or conceivably even better by a much less cumbersome, less cosmetically disfiguring, but more accurate device. That postural training can be easily accomplished with an automated electronic instrument was shown by Azrin and his associates (Azrin, Rubin, O'Brien, Ayllon, & Roll, 1968). These investigators successfully corrected common slouching in 25 subjects by an average of 86% through use of a warning tone that was activated by slouching.

We reasoned that provided with continuous information about the appropriateness of her posture, a scoliotic child could learn to use her trunk and paraspinal muscles to straighten her spine.

METHOD

Accurate and instantaneous assessment of the appropriate behavior is the initial and often most difficult requirement for any instrumental learning therapy. For a brace to be effective, most orthopedists believe that it must be worn 23 hours a day. Thus, a substitute for the brace required a portable and reliable method of measuring the spinal curvature on a moment-to-moment basis so that the patient could be rewarded when there was an improvement. The length of the spine is a good measure of the degree of curvature. The length of a loop wrapped from the shoulders and through the crotch (Figure 4.5A) is proportional to the length of the spine. A loop such as "A" measures only the circumference of the trunk and is unaffected by head and leg position; however, when we tried to train a scoliosis patient to straighten her spine using a simple technique based on this measure, her behavior immediately revealed that the measure was contaminated by respiration. We visually observed her to be expanding her chest by holding her breath, increasing the circumference of her body until she finally activated the transducer. These observations were confirmed by measurements taken from a second transducer placed around her chest represented by loop "B" in Figure 4.5.

We found that it was possible to combine algebraically these two transducer signals electronically, subtracting an appropriate fraction of the contaminating respiratory effect, and leaving a relatively pure measure of the length of the spine represented in Figure 4.6, trace C. A good approximation was achieved by a

4. THE TREATMENT OF SCOLIOSIS   73

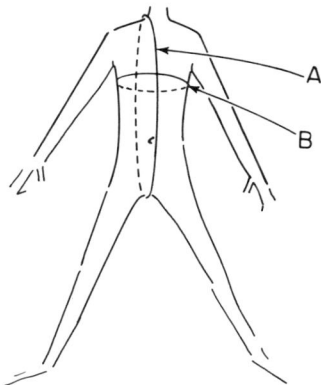

FIGURE 4.5 Torso showing the measuring loops. "A" is the circumferential harness from the seventh cervical vertebra to the pubis, which is lengthened as the patient extends the major axis of her body by straightening her spine. "B" measures the chest circumference.

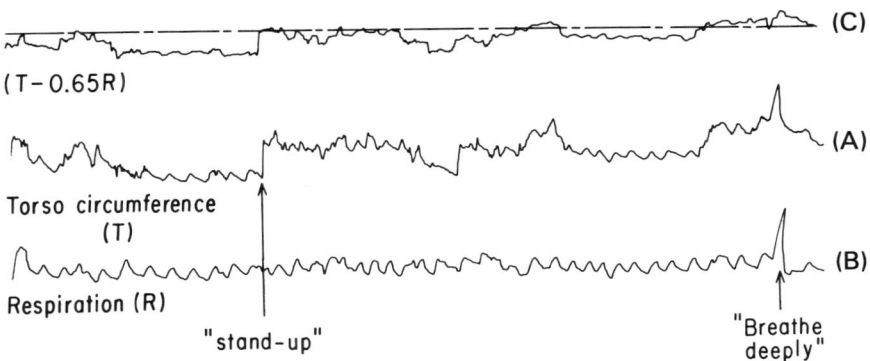

FIGURE 4.6 The relationship between torso circumference (A), respiration (B), and the derived measure of spinal length (C). At "stand-up," the patient was instructed to straighten spine, producing increase in vertical torso circumference and derived spinal length (C). Signal to "breathe deeply" affects torso circumference but not derived spinal length. Throughout, small flucuations in spinal length occur independently of respiration.

simple linear function, which we were able to analog compute by interconnecting conventional polygraph amplifiers. This trace shows the combined signal which reflects only spinal length.

Today we would employ a microprocessor, but in 1973 to accomplish the measurement and computation function in a relatively rugged and portable device, we developed a special mechanical switch: a two-dimensional isotonic displacement transducer in which the relationship between the criterion and the length of the chest and body loops could be arbitrarily set. This transducer draws no quiescent current and was durable enough to survive the normal activities of a teenage girl.

Because we initially focused our attention on the response measurement aspect of the training procedure, the first posture-training device (PTD) employed a very simple escape learning paradigm. When the special mechanical-analog-computer-switch was closed by poor posture, a signal in the form of a tone was turned on to warn the patient that the curvature of her spine was excessive. As soon as she corrected it, the tone was stopped.

Our pilot subject shown in Figure 4.7 was a 12-year-old girl who had already worn a Milwaukee Brace for several years. She was very eager to try something else. However, her first encounter with our prototype device was both disappointing for us and stressful for her. Her behavior indicated that she perceived

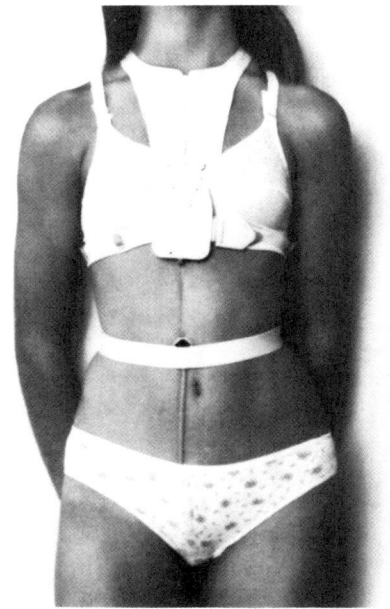

FIGURE 4.7 Pilot subject wearing an early version of the posture-training device (PTD).

the tone signal, which warned her that her posture was incorrect, to be increasingly annoying and unpleasant. Eventually, we realized that she was interpreting the tone as a punishment signal. When she performed the correct response, straightening her spine, the tone terminated and that rewarded her behavior, but the tone onset was an aversive stimulus contingent on incorrect behavior—a punishment, and consequently unpleasant. When we realized what was happening, we inserted a variable-interval 20-second delay between when her posture fell below criterion and when the tone was activated. This obscured the contingency between the onset of poor posture and the onset of the tone, and emphasized the contingency between the correct response and the offset of the tone. The result of inserting this delay was dramatic: At the next session, the young woman, at first apprehensive, soon relaxed. The punishment contingency had been effectively obscured, and she focused on the tone offset as the signal for successful behavior. Although both reward and punishment may be effective in changing behavior, the concomitant emotional consequences of the two procedures are very different: Reward is always preferable when the response is complex or difficult, and almost mandatory if the desired behavior has a low initial probability.

As we proceeded, several additional problems related to response shaping became evident. First, our patient discovered that by raising her shoulders, she could turn off the signal with less effort than was required when using her back muscles. Second, because the time-out began with a criterion response no matter how brief, she also learned that she could make a phasic response that would temporarily end the tone and could be repeated whenever necessary. Responses that achieve reinforcement most readily are learned—even if they are therapeutically undesirable. Both of these maneuvers terminated the tone and produced reinforcement, but neither would help her scoliosis.

By simply replacing the original wide bib-type neck piece with the narrow nylon cord shown in Figure 4.8, we greatly reduced the sensitivity of the instrument to shoulder movements. The problem of the preferred phasic response was more difficult. The easiest and most obvious solution would be to require a response of minimum duration, but postponing reinforcement of the initial phase of a desired behavior is detrimental to learning because delayed reinforcements are less effective than immediate ones. We found that by modifying the timing circuit so that the allotted initial delay, or time-out, was proportional to the time the patient remained in the correct posture, we could achieve an effective contingency. The first time the patient assumed an erroneous posture, the timer would start and, after 20 seconds, the signal would begin. When the posture was corrected, the tone signal would terminate immediately, but, if she quickly assumed an incorrect posture again, the tone would almost instantly return. On the other hand, if she maintained the correct posture, the signal would remain off while her posture was correct and would continue to do so for an equal amount of time up to a limit of 20 seconds after she returned to an incorrect posture. Consequently, the duration of the time-out which she could earn was contingent on the

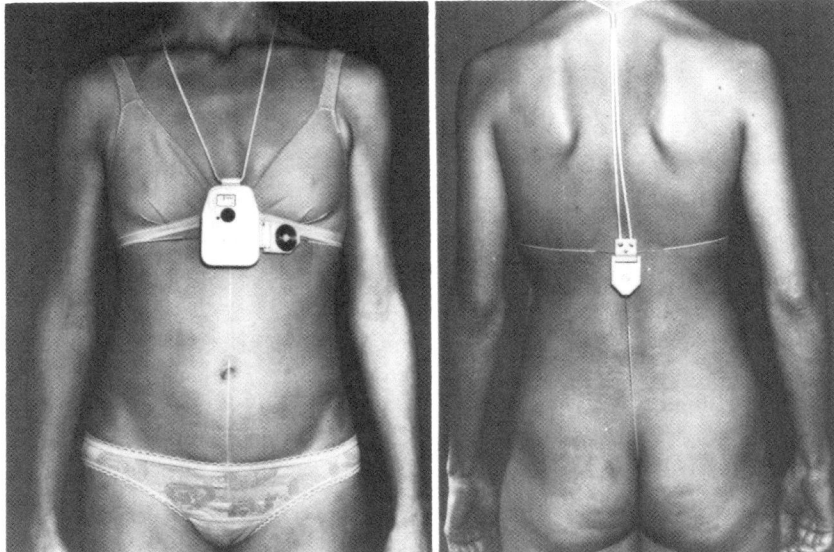

FIGURE 4.8 Front and back views of the current version of the PTD.

duration of her correct posture. She was differentially rewarded with longer time-outs for tonic responses and punished by an almost immediate tone onset for very brief phasic responses. Because the phasic response has low initial probability, punishment causes it to disappear rapidly, and the few necessary punishments occur early in training without disruptive emotional consequences.

A further problem was related to the perspicuousness and reinforcement value of the tone. We were concerned that if we made the tone audible only to the patient, many adolescents would simply ignore it. A louder tone might be a more effective reinforcer because of its potential social consequences; however, under an optimal reinforcement schedule, it was inevitable that the tone would be activated many times a day, and it seemed senseless to embarrass a conscientious patient unnecessarily. The solution was to use two tones, a quiet, "private" one and a considerably louder, "public" one. Activation of the loud tone was contingent on a lack of response to the quiet one. Most patients soon reached the point where the louder tone was never activated, and they were able to terminate even the first tone very quickly.

Since the correct postural behavior is a refined skill and there is a tendency for beginning patients to become flustered and to have difficulty, creating potentially embarrassing situations, we provided an easily reached "panic button" on the top of the instrument which, after a brief delay, terminates the tone and initiates a 20-second time-out. A random delay of 1–3 seconds between pressing the "panic button" and termination of the tone was very effective in preventing reinforcement and strengthening of this necessarily available but undesirable response. In the PTD, the response measurement and reinforcement delivery mechanisms are separate and extrinsically linked; thus, the relationship between response and reinforcement is accessible and easily manipulated.

Greater design flexibility is another dividend of this arrangement. For example, the actual measuring loops are thin nylon filaments. They do not touch the skin, but move within Teflon guides similar to bicycle cables. The length transducers are isotonic, producing little variation in the force applied to the body with changing position. This leads to rapid sensory adaptation, and within a month, the patients are easily able to wear the device comfortably all day and night. Thus, while accurate and persuasive, the PTD is also comfortable and inconspicuous. Except under the lowest-cut tops, the device is not noticed easily by other people while it is worn. As a consequence, it is possible to begin treatment sooner and to keep most patients cooperative and well motivated throughout a necessarily extended course of therapy.

For scoliosis, early treatment is particularly desirable because a smaller curve requires less countervailing force for correction. The learning therapy can be applied before the brace is mandatory, when reduced muscular effort is sufficient for correction, and, as the curve decreases with treatment, the correct postural response becomes progressively easier. Nevertheless, maintaining motivation derived from distant goals is never easy. The therapist must establish and support the link between the occurrence of the tone signal and future medical and cosmetic consequences. In this sense, the scoliosis treatment presents many of the problems of a conventional behavior therapy. However, it differs from most other behavior therapy in that the bulk of the actual learning is a result of direct interaction between the patient and the PTD.

To monitor the patient's behavior in her normal life situation, we built a miniature digital recording system into the instrument. Objective measurement using this system indicated that most scoliosis patients could learn to perform the required postural response competently. A typical record is shown in Figure 4.9. In the first panel, the recording system was active, but the reinforcing tones were not connected. The record shows that the postural measure is relatively stable and constant from day to day. At the end of the eighth day, the reinforcement signal was activated. Within the first 24 hours of reinforcement, there was a rapid initial improvement of posture, followed by more gradual, but consistent progress during the subsequent week. By the eighth day of training, the patient's performance was essentially asymptotic with respect to the criterion spinal length which we had established. At this point, the data recorder showed that the low-level "private" tone signal was activated less than once per hour, and then only for a few seconds—the louder "public" tone was almost never activated. By incrementing the criterion, the tone became again more frequent and the negative slope of the learning curve was reestablished.

Figure 4.10 (left) shows a silhouette photograph of a scoliosis patient, early in

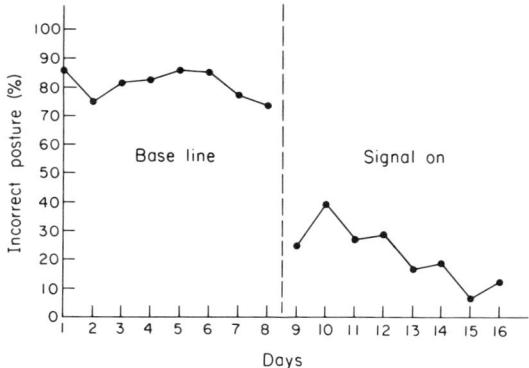

FIGURE 4.9 During baseline, the patient wears the PTD with the signal inactivated. At the vertical dashed line, the signal was activated. The data are taken from the digital timing system built into the instrument.

training after the tone signal had been disconnected for several hours. In Figure 4.10 (right), the tone was activated, and this silhouette photograph was automatically triggered by the criterion response which terminated the tone. The same pair of silhouettes is shown in Figures 4.11 (left) and 4.11 (right), but here the use of a mirror image superimposition technique makes it easier to see the effect of the PTD on postural symmetry. Data like these convinced us that the PTD could shape the desired response; however, the important question was whether this type of postural training would arrest or correct scoliosis.

We recently completed a seven-year pilot study. The 12 patients reported on here were selected from five private and institutional practices on the basis of being judged by the referring scoliosis specialist orthopedist to require bracing; that is, they were progressively deteriorating as judged from several examinations. All had flexible curves that could be easily reduced, and all patients and their parents gave informed consent.

The orthopedists agreed to follow these patients in the conventional manner—that is, as if they had been braced—and to supply us with duplicate records of periodic visits, including necessary radiographic data. One important measurement in the data set was the standard Cobb angle (James, 1967) determined from the anteroposterior radiograph, always taken in the same way on standard 14 × 17-inch (1 inch=2.54 cm) or 14 × 36-inch film with the patient instructed to stand straight and tall, facing the tube 40 inches from the plate. The interval between x-ray evaluations was, as usual, at the discretion of the referring orthopedist because the rate of progression varied significantly from patient to patient, and more frequent x-ray exposure might have been ethically questionable.

During the first two weeks of treatment, each child was adapted to the physical presence of the device and the routine associated with its use. The digital data-

4. THE TREATMENT OF SCOLIOSIS   79

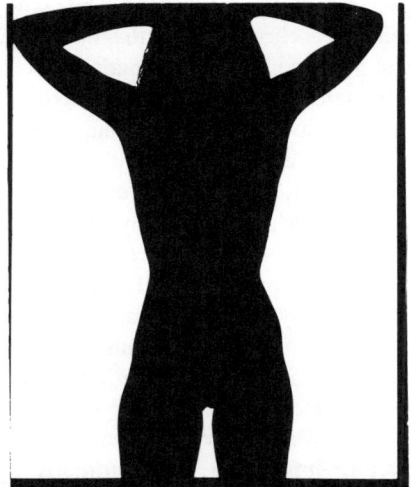 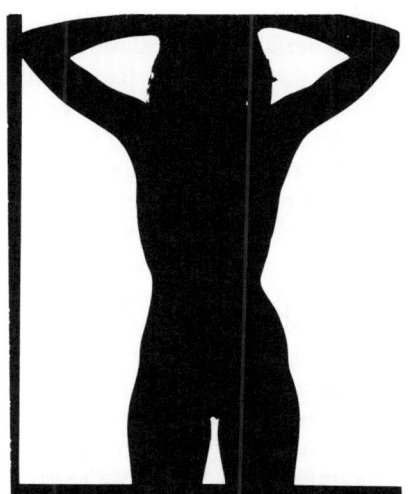

FIGURE 4.10 Two silhouette photographs of a scoliosis patient. The photograph on the left shows her posture after the tone signal has been inactivated for several hours. In the right photograph the tone is activated, and when she made the correct postural response, the picture was taken.

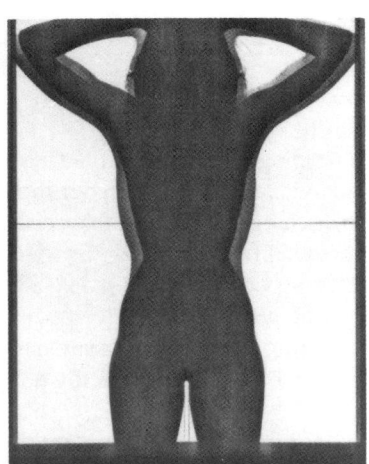 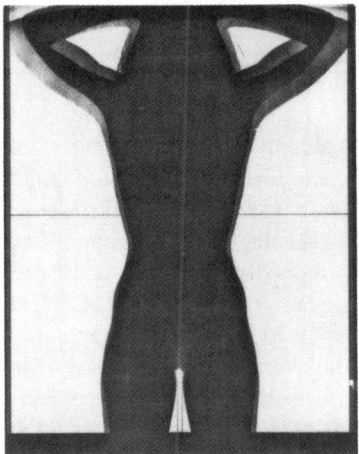

FIGURE 4.11 The same silhouette photographs as in Figure 4.10, with the addition of a mirror-image superimposition technique showing the effect of the PTD on postural symmetry.

recording system was operational, but the tone signal was inactivated. Data collected during this period were used to determine a baseline for the initial criterion setting (i.e., the trunk length that the patient was required to maintain).

Although the training device is specifically sensitive to the desired postural behavior (straightening of the spine), an initial period of guidance (shaping) is helpful in reducing frustration and increasing the rate at which the child acquires efficient use of her muscles. During this initial period, the patients were also instructed to observe themselves in a mirror in order to help eliminate any obviously bad posture. With an appropriate starting point established, the treatment consisted of gradually adjusting the criterion setting as the patient's skill and muscle strength developed. These adjustments were guided by the data from the digital recording apparatus and were only indirectly influenced by the patients' subjective estimates of difficulty. The accumulated time in an erroneous posture reflects the patient's performance, relative to the criterion, and coupled with the independent judgment of the referring orthopedists was sufficient to determine the periodic adjustment. If a patient's disease was arrested or improving, we required less effort of her and advanced the criterion quite slowly; greater effort was demanded only of patients with intractable curves. The device was worn for 2 hours per day for the first week, 4 hours the second, and so on, up to 23 hours per day for most patients. All patients learned rapidly to reach criterion while sleeping.

When and how each patient ended participation in the clinical program was determined by the consulting orthopedist. Although a few patients merely stopped wearing the device when they reached skeletal maturity, most were weaned slowly, just as is conventionally practiced in bracing.

RESULTS

Table 4.1 summarizes the results of the posture-training treatment on the Cobb angle for the 12 patients of this pilot study. Ten individuals remained in our program until they reached skeletal maturity and were discharged by their orthopedists as satisfactorily corrected. Two patients were removed from the study by their orthopedists and fitted with braces. The range of starting Cobb angles was $11°–28°$ (mean = $20.3°$; SD = $4.6°$); the range of final Cobb angles was $8°–30°$ (mean = $19.3°$; SD = $6.9°$). Overall, for the 12 patients during the period of treatment, the average change was a $1°$ improvement (SD = $7.5°$) in the measured Cobb angle; that is, the progression was stopped.

All patients initially found the use of the device for their treatment preferable to the thought of having to wear a brace. They learned very quickly to make necessary postural adjustments under the initial, easy-criterion settings. The most common complaint during the first few weeks of the training period was one of fatigue which, however, quickly lessened as they became more experienced with use of the device. After the initial few weeks, all found the device comfortable,

TABLE 4.1
Pilot Study of Posture-Training Device for Scoliosis

Patient (Months in Treatment)	Cobb angle, Degrees				
	Initial	Final*	Net Change*	Smallest†	Largest†
Patients remaining in study					
S.E. (35)	20	12	− 8	12	—
E.S. (21)	22	10	−12	10	—
A.S. (15)	16	15	− 1	15	—
H.H. (32)	26	22	− 4	22	28
A.V. (23)	21	8	−13	8	—
K.C. (14)	20	26	6	26	32
E.L. (23)‡	11	19	8	—	19
D.C. (10)‡	15	18	3	—	20
S.F. (26)	28	24	− 4	20	—
E.Z. (11)	23	22	−1	22	—
Patients removed from study					
B.G. (33)‡	20	30	10	13	30
M.U. (11)	21	25	4	—	25

Note. From the pilot study at Rockefeller University, 1977–1982. Patients within each group are listed in order of admission to clinical program.
* At termination of posture-training-device therapy.
† During posture-training-device therapy.
‡ These patients displayed motivational problems (see text).

except for a few sporadic problems with pressure soreness from part of the harness in the superior gluteal cleft. Although some individuals adopted inappropriate postures early in treatment, such as prolonged shrugging of their shoulders, these postures generally extinguished as the patients learned how to perform efficiently the specific and easier postural adjustments that terminated the tone. All children developed an upright, very straight posture.

In addition to the specific skeletomuscular behavior of posture, the children also learned very quickly that various body positions and/or use of some furniture made it practically impossible to control the device. For example, they found that sitting in very soft chairs made it difficult to lengthen their spine adequately, whereas sitting on a hard surface eased their task considerably. A number of individuals reported regularly sitting on the floor to do their homework, using their beds as desks. Because it is non-constraining and inconspicuous, patients were able to wear the device during almost every physical activity—exercise/dancing classes, cycling, and basketball—except swimming. Thus, using the signal from the instrument as a guide, they learned to reorganize their environment and their general behavior patterns to facilitate satisfactory spinal orientation. It is useful to think of this component of the learned behavior as somewhat distinct from the more specific spinal skeletomuscular behavior which we originally envisioned that the PTD would produce. This more general kind of learning underlines the potential usefulness of portable behavioral monitors in managing a wide range of behavioral problems.

Soon after we began our pilot study, a group of physiological and clinical psychologists headed by Niels Birbaumer at Tübingen University in West Germany joined in the evaluation of the PTD. They eventually treated 19 additional scoliosis and 8 kyphosis patients in collaboration with groups of orthopedists in Munich, Stuttgart, and at the German Scoliosis Center in Bad Wildungen. Kyphosis is another form of spinal curvature which results in an exaggerated, round-shoulder-type posture. The conventional treatment of surgery or bracing is similar to that for scoliosis. The protocol which the Tübingen group used differed from ours in several ways. Most importantly, there was more therapist intervention in the shaping process, and they required the patients to wear the device for much less time per day. In a report of their study, which has been submitted for publication, they divided their results by patient compliance and type of curvature. For 14 scoliosis patients who wore the device for at least 10 hours per day, 9 had excellent outcomes and 6 showed continued progression of the scoliotic curve, eventually requiring either bracing or surgery. Their results for kyphosis were quite dramatic—7 of the 8 patients wore the PTD for at least 10 hours per day, and none of these had any progression in their kyphotic curves. For all 8 patients treated for kyphosis, there was a mean decrease in curvature of $12.5°$; for the 7 patients who wore the device for at least 10 hours, the decrease was $15.7°$.

Because of the attitude of the committees overseeing human investigations, neither our pilot study nor the German one included active control groups. It was believed that a realistic "placebo" condition would be difficult to achieve and that there was adequate evidence in the orthopedic literature that intensive programs of exhortation, verbal instruction, and exercises are without any effect on the condition of the spine (Collins & Ponseti, 1969; Ponseti & Friedman, 1950). However, the difference between the protocols and compliance rates of American and German studies provides something of an opportunity to estimate the dose-response relationship of the PTD treatment of scoliosis. The German patients wore the device for 10–15 hours per day, and a number wore it less than 10 hours. In the American study, almost all of the patients wore the device for 23 hours per day. Figure 4.12 shows the combined results of the patients from both sides of the Atlantic by the number of hours the device was worn. Greater use is associated with a better therapeutic effect. While it is possible that this relationship is at least partially spurious because the data represent a correlation among observations rather than a true randomized experiment, the histories of individual patients also tended to confirm a connection between longer daily wearing time and the therapeutic efficacy in the posture training treatment. The following two cases are examples of this relationship.

Patient K.C. had a starting curve of $20°$ and initially took a somewhat non-

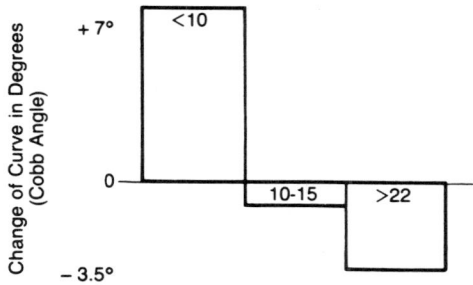

FIGURE 4.12 Combined results from American and German pilot studies on the relationship between hours per day that the PTD was used and final change in curvature.

chalant attitude toward working with the device. She wore it only while at home for 8–12 hours per day. Her curve progressively worsened to 32° as she approached the end of her growth. At this point, she was told by her orthopedist that if the trend continued, she would be braced. This exhortation stimulated her to work actively with the device and to wear it 23 hours a day. The record of her performance from the digital recorder showed dramatic improvement. Her next x-ray, 2 months later, showed a corresponding 6° improvement to 26° and she was discharged as satisfactorily treated a few months later.

The other patient, B.G., was treated for 33 months. She was extremely conscientious—almost to a fault. She figured out a clever method of anticipating the "private" tone by watching the digital display on the front of the device with a small mirror which she carried with her. Although we discouraged this rather compulsive behavior, for the first 21 months of treatment, her total time below the criterion posture as indicated by the digital recorder was close to zero. During this time, the radiographic measurements of her curve declined from an initial 20° to 13°. At that point, the referring orthopedist told her that her growth was almost completed and she was in little danger of deterioration. He set her next examination for a full year later—the normal follow-up time for post-treatment scoliosis. She remained in the study and retained the device, but wore it infrequently, and the digital recorder showed increasingly poorer performance. At the annual examination, her curve was found to have increased to 30°; the orthopedist removed her from the study and prescribed a brace.

DISCUSSION

The ultimate criterion of success for a new scoliosis treatment is whether a patient can pass through the critical period during adolescent growth without requiring bracing and/or spinal-fusion surgery. As described above, each of our patients was selected on the basis of exhibiting documented progressive changes that would soon mandate use of a brace. Untreated curves of this type are expected to worsen at a rate of one to two degrees per month; thus, if the experimental treatment was ineffective, we would have expected that all or most of the 12 children would have been removed from our program. The observed result of 10 individuals successfully avoiding wearing a brace strongly suggests that the PTD is effective ($p < 0.01$, χ^2 test).

Furthermore, the extensive experience of Blount and Moe (1980) would indicate that, in fact, we selected the most difficult curves to treat. This selection was determined by the fact that the Rockefeller Committee on Human Experimentation did not want pilot patients who had larger curves to use our experimental treatment instead of the brace. When small flexible curves such as those which were treated are braced, they often show little or no final correction, yet still may be prevented from progressing. In addition, flexible curves treated by bracing were found to stabilize later and lost more of the correction later. Thus, successful end results for the patients we report here are all the more impressive and suggest that treatment with a PTD offers a therapeutic result comparable to using a brace, at least in terms of halting curve progression.

The PTD may offer additional specific advantages over the conventional bracing techniques. First, its data-recording capabilities can offer the practitioner a safe way of frequently assessing short-term progress. Second, unlike a brace, it is easily adjustable and thus can keep individuals at the point of best performance. (In fact, a brace may conceivably retard progress, if it is not adjusted frequently enough, and thus, in effect, limits the child.) Third, adjustments of criteria can easily be made by the practitioner in his office, which confers a greater degree of control over all aspects of the therapy of each patient. Fourth, it is now clear that many patients benefit from part-time therapy while they are young adults in their 20s; for example, Salanova (1977) advocated that the mature scoliotic wear a brace at night. Our device provides an inexpensive, more comfortable manner in which to accomplish this.

Finally, compared with other non-surgical alternatives, the PTD is extremely benign. As already discussed, a brace may cause atrophy of truncal musculature, deformation of the rib cage, or skin ulceration and, in some cases, has produced significant gastrointestinal complications. Paraspinal stimulation techniques involve either surgical implantation of electrodes or regular application of transcutaneous electrodes; in either case, the long-term consequences of frequent stimulation with relatively strong electric currents, including the electrochemical effects on skin and deeper structures (some with neurohumoral potential), have not been evaluated.

CONCLUSIONS

In recent years, there has been interest in using learned control of physiological responses as a treatment modality. These techniques, usually referred to as "biofeedback therapies," have typically required cumbersome laboratory-based apparatus for measuring and analyzing the target response. As a consequence, the training time available to each patient has been limited to several hours per week. Under these constraints, only a few biofeedback therapies have produced clearly useful results (Ray, Raczynski, Roger, & Kimball, 1979). Learning affects a reversible equilibrium state. Consequently, a major increase in training time could be expected to increase significantly the effectiveness of certain biofeedback therapies; evaluation of that possibility was what, in part, motivated us to undertake the present study. Thus, aside from its specific function as a treatment for scoliosis, the PTD was more generally intended as a prototype or experimental model for automated portable treatment systems, incorporating the principles of instrumental learning for extended and continuous training of medically desirable responses (Dworkin, 1982; Miller & Dworkin 1982).

The feasibility of the general approach is confirmed by the data and experience described above: 21 patient-years of training in a group of 12 adolescent girls were completed; most patients wore the device 23 hours per day for at least 1 year and adapted satisfactorily to the constant physical presence of the instrument and the artificial reinforcement contingency that it imposed. However, it is also important to note that ontogenetically, scoliosis has certain special characteristics. Beyond an effective shaping strategy, any instrumental learning therapy must sustain the learned behavior throughout the entire pathogenic phase of the disease. When the active pathogenic period is a critical developmental era, correspondingly limited intervention may suffice. The primary progression of mild scoliosis is conveniently restricted to early adolescence, and treatment is necessary only during this period. Subsequently, contingent reinforcement can be removed, allowing the learned postural response to extinguish without danger of relapse.

In addition to developmental diseases of childhood and adolescence, there are other illnesses which can similarly be treated without concern for the occurrence of extinction at the termination of therapy. If the pathogenic mechanism depends on the symptom, then ameliorating the symptom correspondingly reduces the virulence of the pathogenic process. A limited course of instrumental learning therapy may leave the patient free of both symptom and agonist, and therapy can be terminated when symptomatic relief is achieved.

The PTD therapy is different in principle from and should not be confused with a regime of exercises. On the questionable assumption that idiopathic scoliosis is at least partially caused by muscular weakness, a variety of exercise programs to treat scoliosis has been proposed and tested. These programs have met with little, if any, success (Collins & Ponseti, 1969; Ponseti & Friedman, 1950). Although the PTD depends on the patient's own muscular effort to correct spinal curvature, the continuous automated evaluation of the actual physiological effect of that effort distinguishes this method from simple exercise, which is performed without moment-to-moment feedback.

Nevertheless, our device does not employ radically new principles for treatment of scoliosis. To the extent that a brace works by enhancing the patient's perception of incorrect posture and encouraging her to correct the position of her spine, the therapeutic mechanism of the PTD is more explicit, but resembles that of a brace; similarly, the PTD shares with the paraspinal stimulator the activation of specific groups of the patient's muscles to correct scoliotic curvature. However, the PTD develops learned muscle control through the patient's own nervous system rather than forcing contraction with strong extrinsic electric currents.

The PTD is safer than paraspinal stimulation and more comfortable and cosmetically acceptable than bracing. Thus, if more extensive clinical trials confirm the results of our study and of the recently completed collaborative European study, the device may have the potential for replacing conventional nonsurgical therapy for the treatment of idiopathic scoliosis and certain types of kyphosis.

REFERENCES

Azrin, N., Rubin, H., O'Brien, F., Ayllon, T., & Roll, D. (1968). Behavioral engineering: Postural control by a portable operant apparatus. *Journal of Applied Behavior Analysis, 1*, 99-108.

Blount, W. P., & Moe, J. H (1980). *The Milwaukee brace*. Baltimore: Willliams & Wilkins.

Collins, D. K., & Ponseti, I. V. (1969). Long term follow-up of patients with idiopathic scoliosis not treated surgically. *Journal of Bone and Joint Surgery American Volume, 51*, 425-445.

Dworkin, B. (1982). Instrumental learning for the treatment of disease. *Health Psychology, 1*, 45-59.

Edmonson, A. S., Morris, J. T. (1977). Follow-up study of Milwaukee brace treatment in patients with idiopathic scoliosis. *Clinical Orthopaedics and Related Research, 126*, 58-61.

James, J. I. P. (1967). *Scoliosis*. Edinburgh: Livingston.

Kane, W. J. (1977). Scoliosis prevalence: A call for a statement of terms. *Clinical Orthopaedics and Related Research, 126*, 43-46.

Keiser, R. P., & Shufflebarger, H. L. (1978). The Milwaukee brace in idiopathic scoliosis : Evaluation of 123 completed cases. *Clinical Orthopaedics and Related Research, 118*, 19-24.

Miller, N. E., & Dworkin, B. R. (1982). Potentialities of automation and of continuous recording and training in life. In R. S. Surwit, R. B. Williams, A. Steptoe, & R. Biersner (Eds.), *Behavioral treatment of disease* (pp. 245-258). New York: Plenum Press.

Ponseti, I. V., & Friedman, B. (1950). Prognosis in idiopathic scoliosis. *Journal of Bone and Joint Surgery American Volume, 32*, 381-395.

Ray, W. J., Raczynski, J. M., Roger, T., & Kimball, W. H. (1979). *Evaluation of clinical biofeedback*. New York: Plenum Press.

Rogala, E. J., Drummond, D. S., & Gurr, J. (1978). Scoliosis: Incidence and natural history. *Journal of Bone and Joint Surgery American Volume, 60*, 173-176.

Salanova, C. (1977). Les resultats lointain du corset de Milwaukee: Les indications. *Acta Orthopaedica Belgica, 43*, 606-615.

Sevastikoglou, J. A., & Karlman, P. (1973). Conservative treatment of idiopathic scoliosis with the Milwaukee Brace. *Acta Orthopaedica Scandinavica, 44*, 99.

Wickers, F. C., Bunch, W. H., & Barnett, P. M. (1977). Psychological factors in failure to wear the Milwaukee Brace for treatment of idiopathic scoliosis. *Clinical Orthopaedics and Related Research, 126*, 62-66.

5
RELAXATION TRAINING IN ESSENTIAL HYPERTENSION: PROSPECTS AND PROBLEMS

W. Stewart Agras
Stanford University School of Medicine

Because there have been a number of excellent reviews of this area in the past few years (Jacob, Kraemer, & Agras, 1977; Seer, 1982; Shapiro & Goldstein, 1982; Wadden, Laborskey, Greer, & Crits-Christoph, 1984), the major focus of this chapter will be on emergent issues concerning the use of relaxation training and closely related procedures, such as meditation, in the management of essential hypertension. It is, in some ways, a paradox that we should be considering the use of a nonpharmacologic approach to the treatment of essential hypertension at a time when the use of drugs in this condition is so well developed. In addition, large-scale trials have demonstrated the effectiveness of such drugs in reducing morbidity and mortality rates in essential hypertension, including blood pressures between 90 and 105 mmHg considered to be in the mild hypertensive range (Hypertension, 1975; Management Committee, 1980). Yet, despite these successes, there is some disquiet over the prolonged use of medication, particularly when the long-term efects of such medication are unknown (Oliver, 1982). Among the known deleterious effects of antihypertensive medications are impaired glucose tolerance, increases in LDL cholesterol and serium triglyceride levels, and impotence in the case of beta-blocking drugs, and recent evidence, sparked by the findings of the MRFIT trial (Multiple Risk, 1982), that diuretic agents may increase mortality in hypertensive patients with abnormal electrocardiographic findings.

Adding to the extent of the problem are the side effects of antihypertensive medication which seem to lead to a marked reduction in the quality of life. In one study of 75 patients with essential hypertension, physicians regarded 100% as improved, while only 48% of the patients rated themselves as feeling better. Relatives seemed to be least impressed with the results of treatment, rating 75%

of the patients as being worse, mentioning declines in energy, changes in mood or memory, and reduced sexual interest as problems (Jachuck, Brierley, & Jachuck, 1982). It seems that in the lower ranges of blood-pressure elevations, the cost-to-benefit ratio for the use of medication is markedly increased.

These considerations have led to an increasing interest in the use of nonpharmacologic procedures in the management of essential hypertension. Luckily, at the same time, the research literature in this area has expanded in such a way as to bring at least some initial hope that nonpharmacologic approaches may be of value. As might be expected, due to the relative brevity of interest in nonpharmacologic approaches, the development of such research is relatively primitive compared to that for pharmacologic agents. A critical issue addressed in this chapter is the delineation of the role of relaxation training in the management of essential hypertension. To address this issue, further questions must be posed, including the effectiveness of relaxation training in lowering blood pressure; the degree to which blood pressure lowering to effect can be specifically attributed to such training; the generalization and persistence of blood-pressure lowering induced by relaxation training; and the characteristics of patients in which relaxation training might be most beneficial. During this inquiry, gaps in our knowledge will emerge, and areas in need of further research inquiry will be highlighted.

Stemming as it does from a use in religious practices throughout the centuries, meditation and its stripped-down cousin relaxation training, unlike other behavior therapies, are not based on psychological theory. Thus, not only are we faced with determining the specific effects of relaxation training, but also with fitting those effects into a suitable theoretical framework.

Relaxation therapy might exert its effects in several ways. One way would be by reducing central nervous system (CNS) activity, particularly that of the sympathetic nervous system (SNS). Such physiologic effects might in turn produce behavior changes augmenting the blood-pressure lowering effects, reducing, for example, faulty coping behavior leading to affective arousal. Other processes by which relaxation training might exert its effects are equally plausible. Thus, relaxation training might alter the perceived valence of a challenging situation, thereby decreasing CNS arousal. Or, again, relaxation training might directly reduce faulty coping behavior or the affective response to poor coping. Then again, relaxation training might allow the hypertensive to detach himself from environmental events that would ordinarily lead to blood-pressure elevation. It is, of course, most probable that interaction between some or all of these processes leads to blood-pressure reduction. Evidence for each of these processes will be reviewed briefly before we turn to consider the effects of relaxation training on high blood pressure.

PHYSIOLOGIC EFFECTS

Most of the work relevant to the role of relaxation and related procedures, such as meditation, in altering physiological parameters has been carried out in normal individuals, often student populations, rather than in hypertensive individuals, and hence may not be generalizable to the latter population. Carefully controlled studies suggest that relaxation training or meditation produces a hypometabolic state different from that associated with sitting down or resting comfortably in control periods, which is accompanied by reduced oxygen consumption, carbon dioxide production, and blood lactate levels, as well as reduction in galvanic skin response (Wallace, Benson, & Wilson, 1971; Jevning & O'Halloran, 1984). Such changes are not large but have been confirmed in a number of studies. Other studies have shown small reductions in plasma cortisol levels during meditation, and a recent investigation found a marked decline in red-cell glycolysis rate during periods of meditation which were alternated with rest, a further indication of reduction in metabolic rate (Jevning, Wilson, Pirkle, O'Halloran, & Walsh, 1983).

In a study of six patients with implanted tantalum myocardial markers who had been trained in the technique of relaxation, differences in a number of cardiovascular parameters were found between relaxation and resting periods while these patients were undergoing cardiac catheterization (Davidson, Winchester, Taylor, Alderman, & Ingels, 1979). Plasma norepinephrine levels decreased during the relaxation periods, and these decreases were correlated with changes in heart rate and blood pressure, consistent with reduction of sympathetic tone. In addition, there was decreased myocardial circumferential shortening velocity, stroke volume, and ejection fraction, again compatible with decreased sympathetic arousal.

While decreases in plasma norephinephrine levels as a consequence of relaxation training have been found in other studies (Jevning et al., 1984), some workers have reported no changes in such levels. In a recent controlled study (Hoffman et al., 1982), plasma norepinephrine levels collected during a stress test were found to increase in a group of students practicing relaxation, but not in a control group. Blood pressure and heart rate did not increase in either the relaxation or control groups. The authors suggested that these results were most consistent with reduced norepinephrine end-organ responsivity as a consequence of relaxation training. In contrast to these general results, it should be noted that some studies have found experienced meditators to be autonomically aroused during meditation, particularly during intense meditative experiences (Corby, Walton, Zarcone, & Kopell, 1978).

Turning to studies of patients with essential hypertension, Stone and DeLeo (1976) reported reductions in plasma dopamine-beta-hydroxylase activity and furosemide-stimulated renin activity in hypertensive patients practicing relaxation as compared with a control group. These findings suggest that reduction in peripheral adrenergic activity and in the renin-angiotensin system were responsible for the blood-pressure lowering observed in this study. A later, larger-scale study reported by Patel and her coworkers (Patel, Marmot, & Terry, 1981) also found reductions in plasma renin activity and plasma aldosterone levels in the relaxation goup as compared with the control group receiving only health education, again suggesting reduction in SNS activity consequent upon relaxation training. In another study, both plasma aldosterone and urinary cortisol levels were significantly reduced in patients receiving relaxation training as compared with control subjects (McGrady, Tan, Fine, & Woerner, 1981). These results were further confirmed in a recent controlled study of mild hypertensive patients where those receiving relaxation training showed a significant decrease in plasma epinephrine levels as compared with controls (Cottier, Shapiro, Julius, 1984). Thus, in studies of hypertensive patients, there is consistent evidence of decreased SNS activity as a result of the practice of relaxation or biofeedback procedures, findings that are generally consistent with studies of normal volunteers during relaxation or meditation.

EFFECTS ON PERCEPTION AND AFFECT

In general, experienced meditators note the development of an underlying "calm and nonreactive equanimity" and an ability to distance themselves from disturbing experiences by assuming the role of "calm observer" (Walsh, 1979). Whether or not such a state can be reached by less experienced persons practicing relaxation techniques is not clear, although clinical reports suggest that many patients feel better able to handle stressful situations without undue emotional arousal folllowing relaxation training. Changes in objective measures of perceptual sensitivity in the context of controlled experiments of relaxation and meditation have also been reported. These include enhanced reaction times, increased ability to perceive auditory or visual cues, and decreases in field dependency (Davidson, Goleman, & Schwartz, 1976; Linden, 1984). There have been no studies of alterations in perception in the hypertensive individual, an area of neglect that should be remedied.

Affective changes have also been noted as a result of meditation or relaxation training. A number of controlled studies with normal individuals have demonstrated that measures of anxiety decline as a result of relaxation or meditation training. In one such study in children randomly allocated to meditation, to guidance, or to a no-treatment condition, only those receiving meditation training showed a decrement in measures of anxiety (Linden, 1984). However, in other studies, no differences were found in decrement of anxiety scores between meditation and a control condition consisting of sitting still for two periods each day but not using meditative techniques (Smith, 1976). In a recent study, patients with either generalized anxiety or panic disorder were randomly allocated to a waiting-list control condition or to relaxation training (Barlow et al., 1984). Those receiving active treatment showed significantly greater reductions in self-reported anxiety, heart rate, and in electromyographic (EMG) potentials at rest and during a stress test than did those in the control group. Although this study suggests that relaxation training may decrease severe anxiety, no placebo control condition was used, thus the improvements may have been due to nonspecific effects of therapy rather than to relaxation training itself.

In studies involving hypertensive patients, decrements have been reported in both anxiety and depression consequent on relaxation training. Bali (1979) reported a randomized comparison of relaxation training and supportive psychotherapy. Those receiving relaxation training showed significantly larger decreases in anxiety than did those receiving psychotherapy, changes which persisted at one-year follow-up. No correlation was found between these changes and changes in blood pressure. Other studies have generally confirmed that anxiety is reduced in hypertensives as a result of relaxation training (Luborsky, et al., 1982; Wadden, 1983).

BEHAVIOR CHANGES

Less striking effects on various behaviors have been reported for meditation and relaxation training in the context of controlled studies both of normal volunteers and clinical populations. In one study involving social drinkers randomly allocated to meditation, progressive relaxation, and attention-placebo control (two periods of quiet reading each day), and no treatment, reports of alcohol consumption decreased for all three experimental groups as compared with the control condition, thus providing no evidence of a specific effect of meditation on alcohol consumption (Marlatt, Pagano, Rose, & Marques, 1984). In another study conducted at a work site, participants were allocated at random to relaxation training, sitting quietly, or no treatment (Peters, Benson, & Porter, 1977). Those receiving relaxation training showed improvements in work performance and an index of sociability, and decreases in reported symptoms and days absent from work as compared with the control group. Once more, however, there were no differences between relaxation training and sitting quietly. It should also be emphasized that in both of these studies, all measures of behavior change were self-reported.

More extensive work has been carried out in the area of the Type A behavior pattern, although the therapeutic procedures used have often been more complex than relaxation training alone. Although Type A behavior has shown significant reductions in almost all of the studies reported as compared with waiting-list control groups, there has, for the most part, been little advantage for relaxation training as compared with either individual or group psychotherapy control conditions, again questioning the specificity of effect of relaxation training (Thoresen, Telch, & Eagleston, 1981).

In general, these studies suggest that relaxation training or meditation with either normal or hypertensive subjects leads, apart from reductions in blood pressure, to physiologic changes suggestive of reduction in SNS activity and to accompanying affective changes, particularly anxiety. Some perceptual and behavior changes have also been reported consequent on relaxation therapy, but little investigation of either perceptual or behavioral changes accompanying relaxation training has been carried out in the hypertensive patient. The physiologic, perceptual, affective, and behavioral changes accompanying relaxation training required more thorough attention than they have received to date in the use of relaxation therapy in hypertension.

It should also be noted that a pervasive theme emerges from a review of this literature; namely, that the benefits consequent on relaxation training or meditation may also be produced by control conditions, including sitting quietly and psychotherapy, although not by inactive control conditions such as waiting-list control groups. A recent group of studies with normal volunteers clarifies some of the potential confounds in this type of research (Cuthbert, Kristeller, Simons, Hodes, & Lang, 1981). The major outcome variable in this set of studies was lowering of heart rate. A simple meditation procedure was found to be more successful in lowering heart rate than either biofeedback or instructions to lower heart rate. This superiority was, however, dependent on the type of experimenter-subject interaction and knowledge of results. When the experimenter demonstrated interest in the subject (a high-involvement condition), heart rate was lower than in a low-involvement condition. In addition, knowledge of results also influenced outcome in a positive direction. These results demonstrate the difficulty of performing experiments aimed at reducing physiologic arousal since differences in experimenter-subject interaction, a variable rarely controlled in such experiments, could markedly affect outcome. This is undoubtedly one reason why similar experiments produce different results.

Very few deleterious effects of relaxation or meditation have been reported, although evidence of physiologic arousal during intense meditative experiences has been demonstrated. It is unlikely, however, that such effects would be seen during relaxation training as it is used in this country since the exercises are, for the most part, divorced from the intellectual and religious aspects of meditation. We can conclude that the most appropriate theoretical model to approach relaxation from is one of lowered sympathetic arousal, and we must admit that the role of perception, affect, and behavior change remain unclear. Such changes could well be secondary to lowered physiologic arousal or might be primary and lead to decrements in arousal. The psychological mechanisms by which relaxation training produces its effects are completely unknown at the present time. It is possible, however, that relaxation training beneficially affects an individual's perception of control of the environment and, hence, reduces cardiovascular responsivity.

EVIDENCE FOR EFFICACY IN ESSENTIAL HYPERTENSION

Dropout Rate

Dropouts from studies involving relaxation training have not been small. In the

Lockheed Hypertension Study (Agras, Southam, & Taylor, 1983; Agras, Schneider, & Taylor, 1984; Taylor, Agras, Schneider, & Allen, 1983), a randomized controlled work-site trial of relaxation training in essential hypertension, 10.3% of participants dropped out during the initial series of treatment sessions, compared with 5.9% in the monitoring-only condition; 12.6% at one-year follow-up, compared with 8.2% of control subjects; and 21.8% at 18-month follow-up, compared with 15.2% of control subjects. Similar, or even larger, drop-out rates have been reported in other studies (Taylor, Farquhar, Nelson, & Agras, 1977; Brauer, Horlick, Nelson, Farquhar, & Agras, 1979). Thus, while there is little evidence for deleterious side effects of relaxation training—although this area requires a more through examination than it has received to date, focusing, for example, on the effect of relaxation training on quality of life—dropout rates suggest that many people find the daily practice of the relaxation procedure too onerous.

Blood-Pressure Lowering

Numerous reviews of the available research studies have concluded that relaxation training is effective in lowering blood pressure in both the untreated hypertensive and in the hypertensive being treated with pharmacologic therapy (Jacob et al., 1977; Seer, 1979; Shapiro & Goldstein, 1982; Wadden et al., 1984). To summarize the research findings on the efficacy of relaxation training in essential hypertension, studies of the use of relaxation training, hypnosis, or biofeedback which used a control procedure (e.g., no treatment, psychotherapy, or other form of placebo control) and which provided sufficient information concerning in-clinic blood-pressure changes were examined. The data for systolic and diastolic blood-pressure changes for the treatment and control group in each of these studies were plotted against baseline blood-pressure values in Figures 5.1 and 5.2. As can be

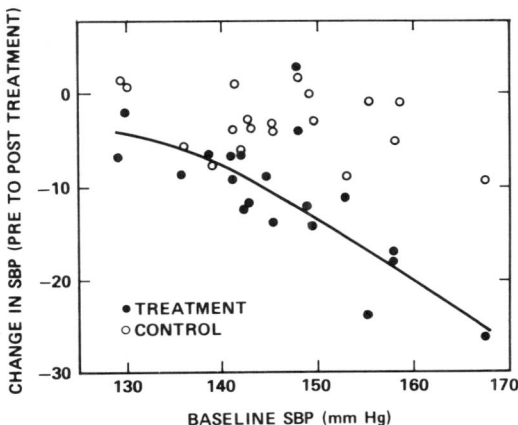

FIGURE 5.1 Systolic blood pressure changes for relaxation training and control groups in selected studies.

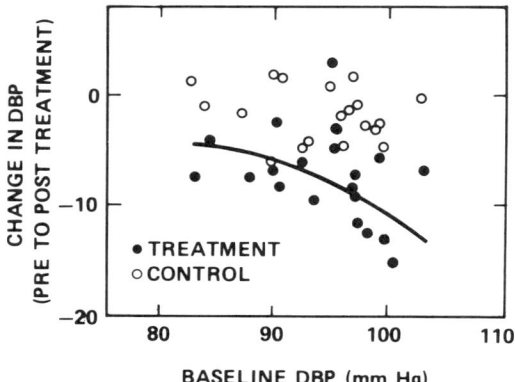

FIGURE 5.2 Diastolic blood pressure changes for relaxation training and control groups in selected studies.

seen, blood-pressure changes tend to be larger as initial blood-pressure levels increase ($r = 0.68$, $p < .005$, systolic; $r = 0.43$, $p < .05$, diastolic). No such relationship exists in the control groups. Active treatment produces a superior lowering for both systolic and diastolic pressures at all starting levels. The range of blood-pressure change for the active treatment groups across studies is from +3 to −27 mmHg systolic and from +3 to −15 mmHg diastolic, while the comparable changes for the control conditions are +3 to −9 mmHg systolic and +2 to −6 mmHg diastolic. Much of the variance in outcome between studies can be accounted for by initial levels of blood pressure, and there is no evidence, at this level of analysis, for the superiority of any one type of treatment. It is interesting to note that the blood-pressure changes in the placebo group of the Australian therapeutic trial in mild hypertension (Management Committee, 1980) fall within the range for the control groups from nonpharmacologic studies shown in Figures 5.1 and 5.2.

The relationship between initial blood-pressure levels and change in blood pressure is also evident within studies. In Figure 5.3, diastolic blood pressures for participants receiving relaxation training in the Lockheed Hypertension Study are displayed by starting value. In this study, 172 participants who had been receiving medical treatment for an average of five years whose diastolic blood pressures were above 90 mmHg after repeated measurement were randomly allocated to either blood-pressure monitoring (with positive expectancy for blood-pressure lowering) or to monitoring plus relaxation training. The majority of these participants were receiving antihypertensive medication. As shown in Figure 5.3, blood-pressure lowering is greater for participants who were most out of control at randomization. Significant differences in blood-pressure lowering were found between those receiving relaxation training and those receiving blood-pressure monitoring up to a 24-month follow-up.

BLOOD PRESSURE LOWERING WITH RELAXATION TRAINING

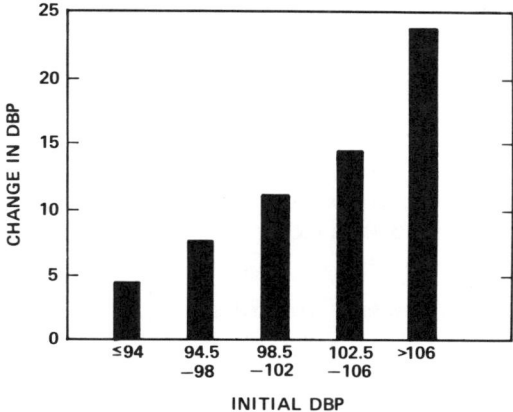

FIGURE 5.3 Systolic blood pressure changes resulting from relaxation training in 172 participants in a controlled study.

Follow-up of subjects treated with relaxation therapy usually reveals that the blood-pressure lowering observed during initial treatment is maintained over time. Participants in controlled studies have usually been followed between 6 and 18 months after completing therapy; however, a recent study reported a four-year follow-up in which the differences between the relaxation and control groups were maintained. Moreover, the relaxation group appeared to have suffered significantly fewer cardiovascular complications, measured by both self-report and objective indices, than did the control group. We can conclude that the initial benefits consequent on relaxation therapy are likely to be reasonably well maintained. The reason for such maintenance is, however, unclear, because there is little evidence to suggest that relaxation is diligently practiced by the majority of subjects following the end of treatment.

Effects On Blood-Pressure Variability

Although it is not entirely clear that variability as well as absolute level of blood pressure is a risk factor for cardiovascular or cerebreovascular disease, a large body of research evidence points in the direction of implicating blood-pressure variability as a risk factor (Krantz & Manuck, 1984). Two studies of the effect of relaxation training on blood-pressure response to exercise and the cold-pressor test in patients with essential hypertension found that relaxation training reduced both recovery time and the blood-pressure response (Datey, 1980; Krantz & Manuck, 1984). In one study, the differences between the groups from before to after treatment for the cold-pressor test were −9.1/−4.0 mmHg for relaxation training as compared with +3.3/+2.1 mmHg for the control group (Datey, 1980). The second study reported comparable changes (Agrawal, Dikshit, Maheshwari, Bose, & Bisariya, 1977).

To test whether such effects might be detectable in the natural environment, 8-hour work-day recordings taken before and after treatment in the Lockheed study were analyzed. The blood-pressure values at the 90th percentile were compared pre- and post-treatment for the two groups. There was a marked reduction in this value in the treatment group ($-11.6/-6.4$ mmHg) but not in the control group ($-0.9/-0.5$ mmHg). These differences were statistically significant. Thus, it seems that not only does relaxation training lower blood pressure, it also reduces blood-pressure variability both in the laboratory and in the natural environment.

Compliance with Treatment Procedures

A subsample of participants in the Lockheed study was given a tape recorder on which to play their practice tapes which contained a microprocessor able to recognize when the relaxation tape (as distinct from other tapes) was being played and which recorded the date and time of onset and offset of tape playing (Taylor et al., 1983). Participants were not aware of the presence of this small device, located in the battery compartment of the recorder, nor of its function. Participants' self-monitoring suggested a relaxation practice rate of 5.9 times per week, with 71% of subjects adhering accurately to instructions. On the other hand, the computer determined that the practice rate was 4.6 times per week, with only 39% of subjects adhering accurately. There was also a steady decline in the rate of practice from the first to the eighth week of practice, 6.9 to 4.2 times per week for self-reported practice, and 6.1 to 2.5 for computer-monitored practice. In another study using similar technology, the investigators reported similar results (Hoelscher, Lichstein, & Rosenthal, in press). Group-based relaxation training appeared to produce slightly better compliance than did individual treament. Adding contingency contracting for adherence to the group-based treatment appeared to have a deleterious effect on compliance with relaxation practice instructions. Wadden (1983) examined self-reported compliance with relaxation training provided either individually or with the spouse. Hypertensive subjects who practiced with their spouse reported higher rates of practice than did those who practiced alone.

It seems that self-reported adherence to a nonpharmacologic therapy, like that to pharmacologic therapy, is a good deal higher than more objectively determined adherence (Dunbar & Agras, 1980). Patients tend to overestimate their compliance with therapeutic instructions. Nonetheless, participants were still practicing with the relaxation tape between two and three times a week, on the average, in the last week of therapy. In the Lockheed study (Taylor et al., 1983), no relationship was found between the rate of practice and blood-pressure lowering ($r = .12$ systolic, $r = -.06$ diastolic). Similar low correlations between practice frequency and blood-pressure lowering were reported in another study using a somewhat different objective measure of relaxation practice (Jacob, Beidel, & Shapiro, 1984). It is possible that subjects were practicing above a critical threshold and that continued practice of the relaxation exercises is not necessary for successful blood-pressure lowering. On the other hand, a significant correlation between amount of practice and change in systolic blood pressure ($r = 0.32$) but not diastolic pressure was found in one of the studies described above (Hoelscher et al., in press), and a significant relationship between practice and both systolic and diastolic pressure was found in another study (Wadden, 1983). The relationship between amount of practice and blood-pressure lowering requires further investigation in experimental rather than correlational studies from a theoretical viewpoint: Is there a dose-response relationship between amount of practice and blood-pressure lowering? And what is the optimal practice schedule for relaxation training? If the optimal amount of practice was found to be less than currently prescribed, then adherence of patients to the therapeutic regimen might be enhanced.

In a further substudy from the Lockheed project (Agras et al., 1984), 22 participants whose blood pressures had returned toward baseline values were randomly allocated to either a second course of relaxation training together with special attention to adherence to practice or to routine care involving a relaxation booster session every two months. No differences in blood-pressure lowering were found either postraining or 6 months after retraining. Practice frequency monitored unobtrusively in a subsample of the retrained group averaged 6.2 times per week for the first 4 weeks of retraining. It seems likely that the reasons for the return of these subjects' blood pressures toward baseline after successful initial treatment had little to do with poor adherence to relaxation training. Most likely, intercurrent stressors were responsible for this phenomenon and with the passage of time, the stressors were alleviated.

Who Responds to Treatment?

Identification of the characteristics of those who respond to relaxation training is a most important task since, as we have seen, the degree of blood-pressure lowering both within and between studies is extremely variable. While procedural differences may explain some of this variance, it is also likely that participant differences are important. As we have seen, initial levels of blood pressure predict outcome both within and between studies, suggesting that participants with higher starting values will demonstrate the largest reductions in blood pressure. Among other participant characteristics predicting outcome, aspects of the Type A behavior pattern, including hard-driving style, have been found in two studies to be negatively associated with blood-pressure lowering (Multiple Risk, 1982; Wadden, 1983). Other studies, however, have failed to find an association between Type A behavior and blood-pressure lowering (Luborsky et al., 1982). Moreover, an attempt at pooling data from several studies of relaxation training with hypertensive patients found no consistent predictors of outcome (Wadden et al., 1984).

Because of the widespread prevalence of mild and borderline essential hypertension and the relatively poor results of relaxation training in these patients, it is particularly important to identify characteristics of mild hypertensives who respond well to treatment. (Cottier et al., 1984) found that mild hypertensives responding to relaxation training showed significantly higher baseline heart rates and norepinephrine levels than nonresponders. In addition, responders reported higher anxiety levels. This suggests that a subgroup of hypertensives with increased sympathetic tone may be particularly responsive to relaxation training. Larger-scale studies seeking to identify characteristics of responders to relaxation training are clearly needed. The possibility that indices of SNS responding may predict outcome is an attractive hypothesis that needs further testing.

Generalization of Blood-Pressure Lowering

Although relaxation training appears to have acute effects on blood pressure measured in the laboratory or in the clinic, does it, like medication, have effects that persist over the 24-hour period? It is possible that individuals simply learn to relax when their blood pressure is being measured. Another possibility is that the effects of relaxation training are situationally specific. In early studies, blood pressures tended to be measured either within treatment sessions or following relaxation therapy in the treatment situation, providing no information on persistence of blood-pressure lowering beyond treament. In later studies, blood pressures were measured in the clinic, often at a time remote from relaxation training sessions. With a very few exceptions, blood-pressure lowering was found to persist in the clinical situation, providing some evidence that the blood-pressure lowering was not situationally specific.

More recently, however, two teams of investigators reported studies in which participants received home-based relaxation training, coupled with self-monitoring of blood pressure, in which differences found between groups in self-reported blood pressures were not found when measures were taken in the clinic by professional personnel (Glasgow, Gaarder, & Engel, 1982; Goldstein, Shapiro, & Thananopavaran, 1984). In one of these studies, the investigators noted that when blood pressures were professionally determined, "the behaviorally treated patients did not differ from the controls in either BP level or BP trend" (Glasgow et al., 1982, p. 164). In the other study, the investigators noted that "the effects of the relaxation technique were less apparent in the laboratory, where reductions in blood pressure from baseline to the end of treatment, although significant, were not as great and were not differentiated between (experimental) groups" (Goldstein et al., 1984, p. 412). These findings are disturbing from a number of viewpoints. First, it is possible that the results of home-based training using self-monitoring of blood pressure do not persist beyond the training situation—in this case, the home (i.e., blood-pressure lowering is limited to the stimulus conditions surrounding training). Second, it is possible that self-reported blood pressures are unreliable and are subject to experimenter demand, thus the differences between experimental conditions reported in these studies may have been spurious.

In fact, the most reliable way to assess the persistence of blood-pressure changes induced by relaxation training is by using ambulatory monitoring or frequent blood-pressure measurements obtained in an inpatient setting. Few studies of this type have appeared to date. In one study, a small number of hypertensive patients, who were unable to tolerate medication, were admitted to a clinical research unit (Agras, Taylor, Kraemer, Allen, & Schneider, 1980). Salt intake was maintained at a slightly higher level than usual for each of these patients, and a positive sodium balance was confirmed by measuring sodium excretion. Blood pressures were frequently taken during the entire 24 hours. Following 2 baseline days, three sessions of relaxation training were provided to these patients for 3 days; and during the final experimental day, no training was given. Blood-pressure lowering was found to persist beyond the training sessions, and systolic blood pressure was significantly lower during relaxation training days and nights than during the days on which no training occurred. Blood pressures taken during sleep revealed sizable differences between training and non-training days, strongly suggesting that the blood-pressure lowering consequent on relaxation training could not be due to active practice of the relaxation procedure.

Although this study provided initial evidence of the persistence of blood-pressure lowering attributable to relaxation training, it did not provide evidence for persistence outside a hospital situation. Thus, in the Lockheed study, a randomly selected subsample of participants in both the monitoring-only and relaxation-training conditions had their blood pressures measured during the workday by means of an ambulatory recorder at baseline, posttreatment, and at 16 months follow-up. This study revealed significant differences in favor of those receiving relaxation training both immediately posttreatment (Agras et al., 1983) and at follow-up. At present, these data provide the only strong evidence of generalization of the effects of relaxation training to the natural environment. Nevertheless, we can tentatively conclude that the blood-pressure lowering consequent on relaxation training is not situationally specific and that it extends beyond the training situation.

Have the Results of Relaxation Training Become Poorer Over Time?

A possible source of variation in the conduct of studies might be the passage of time. In the initial phase of research, for example, investigators' enthusiasm for relaxation therapy or biofeedback may have been greater than in the later phase of research development. Thus, the systolic blood-pressure lowering for the same group of studies discussed above, arrayed by time of publication, is displayed in Figure 5.4. As can be seen, there is no trend toward either worsening or improvement of outcome over the decade represented by this group of studies. Thus,

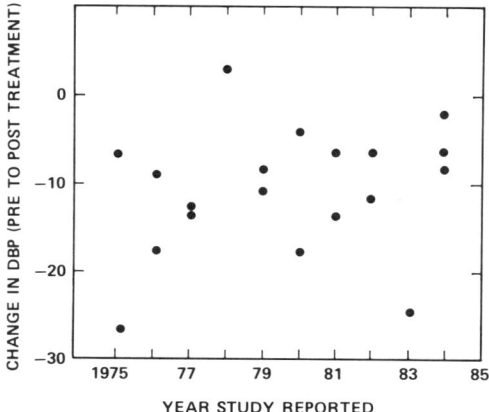

FIGURE 5.4 Changes in diastolic blood pressures for selected studies reported between 1975 and 1984.

we may conclude that relaxation therapy and related procedures are effective in lowering blood pressure in the hypertensive patient and that the results persist around the clock and over time, but next we must inquire whether these effects can be attributed to a specific aspect of treatment or to nonspecific effects of treatment.

EVIDENCE FOR SPECIFICITY OF EFFECT

The evidence for or against relaxation training and related procedures having a specific effect on blood pressure rests on the results of seven studies in which some form of active and credible control condition, together with controls for the amount of time spent with the therapist, were used within the context of a randomized experiment (Bali, 1979; Cottier et al., 1984; Brauer et al., 1979; Luborsky et al., 1982; Peters, Benson, & Peter, 1977; Roberts & Forester, 1979; Taylor et al., 1977). As can be seen in Table 5.1, the results are mixed, although it will be recognized that the sample size in some of the studies is small, thus increasing the chance of false negative findings. In addition, blood-pressure lowering in the control group was less than in the treatment condition in all of the studies. Of the seven studies shown in Table 5.1, four were positive in that relaxation training or a related procedure produced a statistically significant superior blood-pressure lowering either at immediate outcome or, in the case of one study, at six months follow-up. In addition, although Cottier et al. (1984) found no differences between treatment and control conditions in terms of blood-pressure changes, there were significant differences between the groups in plasma epinephrine levels as a result of treatment. Thus, only two studies were com-

TABLE 5.1

	Experimental Conditions		Treatment Length	Immediate Results
Taylor et al. (1977)	Relaxation	($n = 10$)]	6 weeks	$-13.6**/-4.9*$
	Psychotherapy	($n = 10$)]	(trained to	$- 2.8/-1.8$
	Medication only	($n = 11$)]	criterion)	$- 1.1/-0.3$
Peters et al. (1977)	Relaxation	($n = 54$)]		$- 4.6**/-3.2**$
	Sitting quietly	($n = 36$)]	8 weeks	$- 1.9/-0.4$
	No treatment	($n = 36$)]		$- 0.5/-1.1$
Brauer et al. (1979)	Relaxation (therapist)	($n = 10$)]		$-11.0/-6.1$
	Relaxation (tape)	($n = 9$)]	10 weeks	$- 5.3-1.0$
	Psychotherapy	($n = 10$)]		$- 8.8/-4.5$
Bali (1979)	Relaxation	($n = 9$)]		$-12.0**/-9.0**$
	Psychotherapy*	]	8 weeks	
	sham feedback	($n = 9$)]		$- 0.0/-1.0$
Roberts et al. (1979)	Meditation	($n = 22$)]		$- 8.3/-4.3$
		]	9 weeks	
	Health education	($n = 19$)]		$- 6.0/-0.4$
Cottier et al. (1984)	Relaxation	($n = 17$)]		$- 2.0/-2.5$
		]	22 weeks	
	Placebo	($n = 9$)]		$+ 1.0/+2.0$

$*p < .1$
$**p < .05$

pletely negative. None of the studies measured either the expectancy of outcome or the credibility associated with the active treatment and control condition, thus we cannot be sure that the differences found reflect differences due to the treatment procedures used or differences in expectancy or credibility between the conditions that would naturally favor the active therapy.

It must be recognized that controlling for the nonspecific effects of a psychotherapeutic procedure is more difficult than controlling for the effects of pharmacologic agents, where a placebo preparation can be used. Parenthetically, it should be noted that many pharmacologic studies do not report data on the integrity of the blind during the course of the study. Differences in the incidence of side effects between the active and placebo medications often result in unblinding of both patient and physician. Such problems encountered in pharmacologic trials are magnified in research with nonpharmacologic treatments. Therapists may be biased in favor of the active treatment condition and may convey this bias to participants by varying their enthusiasm and the amount of attention given to participants between conditions. As we have seen, such variation affects the outcome of relaxation training in laboratory studies (Cuthbert et al., 1981). Participants may also be biased in favor of one or another treatment condition, hence the need to induce similar levels of expectancy and credibility in both active and control conditions and to measure both expectation of outcome and treatment credibility in such studies. One of the best-designed studies in this regard was that of Cottier et al. (1984), who used a placebo preparation in both the relaxation and control conditions (Cottier et al., 1984) and who controlled for time of therapist contact. Unfortunately, only mild hypertensives could be admitted to such a study, thus limiting power since, as shown in Figures 5.1–5.3, the degree of blood-pressure lowering depends, in part, on the initial blood-pressure level.

Overall, there is a reasonable amount of evidence that the blood-pressure lowering associated with relaxation therapy is due to a specific effect of treatment rather than to a nonspecific placebo effect, although we must admit that none of the studies is methodologically perfect, at least by today's standards. Here, then, is another area for further research. What is needed is a study with adequate power to detect differences between groups, a credible and active control condition, and measures of expectancy and credibility.

Component Analyses of Relaxation Training and Related Therapies

If relaxation training does exert a specific therapeutic effect, it should be possible to identify which components of treatment are essential and which are nonessential to outcome by comparing the results of treatment with the full therapeutic package to a condition in which a crucial element of therapy is omitted. Unfortunately, very few studies of this kind have appeared in the literature to date, thus it is not possible to come to any firm conclusions regarding the essential components of treatment. Peters et al. (1977), in a work-site study, compared relaxation training with a condition in which participants were told to practice sitting quietly. Omitted in the latter condition were two key components of treatment—repeating a mantra (in this case, the word "one") and passively avoiding distracting thoughts. The full relaxation package was significantly more effective in lowering both systolic and diastolic pressures than the control condition. It should be noted that measures of the credibility of the control condition were not obtained. Nonetheless, it is quite possible that one or the other of these procedures, repeating a mantra or avoiding distractions, was crucial to the outcome.

In another study bearing on a similar point, the mantra was omitted in one condition while the full procedure was provided in another (Seer & Raeburn, 1980). No differences were found between the groups in terms of blood-pressure lowering. However, in this study, unlike the previous one, subjects in both groups were told to ignore distracting thoughts. It is possible, therefore, that the crucial procedure is not the use of a mantra—after all, many patients who are taught deep muscle relaxation successfully lower their blood pressure without using a mantra—but rather the act of ignoring distracting thoughts. Such a procedure would make a good deal of psychophysiologic sense, at the very least cutting down on the variability of physiologic responding.

Even more problematic to the search for a specific procedure that might underlie the efficacy of relaxation training and related treatments is the study by Luborsky and his colleagues (Luborksy et al., 1982), who compared the effects of metronome-conditioned relaxation with metronome-conditioned exercise, thus omitting the procedure of muscle relaxation. No significant differences were found between these two groups, although the trends were all in favor of the relaxation condition.

Finally, in a laboratory analogue study, the participants' expectancy regarding blood-pressure lowering was experimentally manipulated (Agras, Horner, & Taylor, 1982). Patients with essential hypertension were brought into the laboratory for three sessions of relaxation training conducted over the course of one morning. All of the participants were told that relaxation training would lower their blood pressure; however, a random half was further told that such lowering would begin immediately, while the other half was told that the lowering would occur only after extended training. The participants' expectancies were carefully manipulated, and a check of the expectancy was made before beginning relaxation training. Systolic blood pressure was significantly lower in the group receiving the immediate blood-pressure lowering expectancy than in the control group (-14.6 mmHg versus -2.3 mmHg), although there were no differences in diastolic pressure. This study suggests that not only general expectancy of benefit, but expectancy that blood pressure will be lowered is a critical element of relaxation training. In light of the two studies reported earlier, it is of interest that the group given the expectancy of delayed benefit reported a higher number of distracting thoughts during training than the other group.

Although no firm conclusions can be drawn from this small set of studies that have attempted to dissect out critical elements of the relaxation-training procedure, some tantalizing information emerges. First, there is no clear evidence that training in muscle relaxation or the use of a mantra is essential to the effects of relaxation training. This conclusion is bolstered by the findings from some, but not all, meditation studies, that sitting quietly produces similar physiologic changes to meditation. Second, the procedure of ignoring distracting thoughts may be important to the outcome of relaxation training, although the evidence to date is indirect rather than direct. Further studies aimed at dissecting out the critical therapeutic ingredients of relaxation training are needed if we are to fully understand both the optimal method of training individuals to "relax" and the procedures that are directly connected with the observed physiologic changes.

The Effect of Blood-Pressure Monitoring Alone

One component of treatment present in many investigations of relaxation training and related procedures is blood-pressure monitoring. Most investigators who have used a blood-pressure monitoring control condition have reported blood-pressure declines in such groups. Jacob and his colleagues (Jacob, Fortmann, Kraemer, Farquhar, & Agras, 1985), for example, found that a group of participants not taking antihypertensive medication who were randomly allocated to clinic blood-pressure monitoring lowered their blood pressure by 9.6/3.9 mmHg over a one-year period. The authors concluded that clinic blood-pressure monitoring was as effective as a nonpharmacologic treatment which included relaxation training, weight management, and salt restriction. Although most studies comparing blood-pressure monitoring with relaxation training have found an advantage for relaxation training, at least one other study found no differences between these conditions for blood pressures taken in the laboratory (Goldstein et al., 1984).

In the Lockheed Hypertension Study, both medicated and unmedicated patients allocated to the blood-pressure monitoring condition showed continued declines in blood pressure during the study. At initial randomization, none of those receiving antihypertensive medication had diastolic blood pressures below 90 mmHg. At one year follow-up, 37.2% in the self-monitoring group were now in control, a proportion that continued to increase to the 30-month follow-up visit when 69.2% were in control. Those receiving relaxation training showed significantly larger proportions of participants whose blood pressures were in control.

These findings of sizable blood-pressure reductions brought about by in-clinic or home blood-pressure monitoring confirm the results of earlier research (Laughlin, Fisher, & Sherrard, 1979), and suggest that in both research and clinical practice, blood-pressure monitoring is an active therapeutic ingredient of relaxation training but that relaxation training usually has an effect over and above that of monitoring alone. The reasons for the blood-pressure lowering effects of monitoring are not clear, but it cannot be attributed to better compliance with medication taking since unmedicated patients show similar declines in blood pressure. Nor is it likely that participants are simply becoming less reactive to the blood-pressure measurement procedure since, in the Lockheed study and in several other studies (Benson, Rosner, Marzetta, & Klemchuk, 1974; Brauer et al., 1979; Patel, 1973; Taylor et al., 1983), patients had been in treatment for several years. Jacob and his colleagues (Jacob, 1985) measured weight and salt intake in both the monitoring and nonpharmacologic treatment groups, finding a reduction in salt intake in both groups at two months but a return to baseline levels thereafter. Weight losses were greater in the nonpharmacologic treatment group at six months (despite there being no differences in blood pressure), but there were no such differences at one year follow-up. In the Lockheed study, both groups showed sizable weight gains in the order of 2.6 kg over the course of the study. Thus, it is not possible to attribute the blood-pressure lowering consequent on blood-pressure monitoring to changes in dietary behavior.

Effects of Adding Other Treatment Procedures to Relaxation Therapy

Several investigators have asked the question: Does adding another procedure or procedures to relaxation therapy enhance the effect of therapy? The answer to this question would seem to be "No." Crowther (1983), for example, added a stress-management package to relaxation training. Stress management consisted of identifying each individual's unique reaction to stressful events, altering cognitions accompanying or leading to stress, and teaching coping strategies to better deal with stressful situations. The addition of stress-management training did not enhance the blood-pressure lowering effect of relaxation training, although both the relaxation training alone and the combined treatment produced significantly greater blood-pressure lowering than did a monitoring-only group. Inspection of these data reveal that the relaxation-training group had consistently (but not significantly) lower blood pressures than the group receiving combined treatment.

Other investigators have added various kinds of biofeedback to relaxation therapy and have found no additional benefit for the combined treatment. Neither electromyographic feedback nor blood-pressure feedback enhances the results of relaxation training (Jacob, 1977; Seer, 1979; Shapiro & Goldstein, 1982; Wadden et al., 1984). In one study, however, the combination of relaxation and blood-pressure biofeedback, provided by the use of a sphygmomanometer at home, was superior to either relaxation training or blood-pressure biofeedback used alone (Engel, Glasgow, & Gaarder, 1983; Glasgow et al., 1982). There was also some evidence that when biofeedback preceded relaxation, the results were better than when relaxation training was used first. However, the blood pressures used for this analysis were self-reported, the differences between groups were small, and no such differences between groups were found for blood pressures taken in the clinic.

Similarly, the addition of hypnosis to a biofeedback-assisted relaxation procedure not only did not add anything to the outcome in terms of blood-pressure lowering, but it seemed to have a deleterious effect since the combined group only did as well as the monitoring-only condition (Friedman & Taub, 1977; Lazarus, 1976). We must, therefore, conclude that adding other psychological treatment procedures to relaxation-training produces no additional effect on blood-pressure lowering. Such results may be due to increasing the complexity of treatment since compliance with therapeutic instructions may decline as complexity increases, thus offsetting any potential added therapeutic benefits.

RELAXATION TRAINING IN THE MANAGEMENT OF ESSENTIAL HYPERTENSION

The evidence presented in this chapter suggests that relaxation training may have its main application in the management of patients who respond poorly to pharmacologic treatment, either for reasons of poor adherence or inability to tolerate the side effects of the medication. In such patients, there is evidence that relaxation training leads to lowering of blood pressure, with some two-thirds of such patients showing diastolic blood pressures below 90 mmHg following training. Some studies have also shown that the dosage of antihypertensive medication can be reduced following the completion of relaxation training (Engel et al., 1983;

Patel, 1973). Again, this is a useful effect since the side effects of medication will thus be diminished.

Less certain is the place of relaxation training in the newly diagnosed hypertensive. Since this group of mild hypertensives is large and, as noted earlier, the cost-to-benefit ratio of treatment in such patients is markedly increased, it would be useful if a nonpharmacologic treatment such as relaxation training could form the first step in therapeutic regimen. However, at the present time, most of the evidence suggests that this is the very group in which the least effect of relaxation training will be observed. Cottier et al. (1984) suggested that subsample of these patients, characterized by excessive sympathetic responding, will be responsive to relaxation training.

Given the findings concerning the beneficial effects of repeated monitoring of blood pressure, it seems reasonable that the first step in a nonpharmacologic approach to all patients should be simple monitoring of blood pressure, perhaps supplemented by home blood-pressure monitoring. Such monitoring might be continued over a 6-month period before commencing relaxation training.

The place of relaxation training in the prevention of hypertension is quite unknown at this piont. It would seem important to establish whether relaxation training in the prehypertensive would slow down or halt the development of the disorder. Since there is evidence that stress interacts with a salt load to raise blood pressure in individuals with a family history of hypertension, at least in the laboratory (Friedman & Taub, 1977; Light, Koepke, Obrist, & Willis, 1983), it would seem theoretically possible that relaxation training and related procedures with their stress symptom-reducing properties might slow the development of essential hypertension. Again, research is needed in this area.

RESEARCH QUESTIONS

The first phase of research into the effectiveness of relaxation training in the management of essential hypertension is now over. A growing number of studies, both of the general effects of meditation and relaxation and of relaxation training and closely related techniques applied to hypertensives, suggests that the procedures lower physiologic responsiveness, diminish affective arousal, and lower blood pressure in the hypertensive. Having said this, it is important to acknowledge that several puzzling questions emerge from this body of research—questions that must be answered during the next phase of research.

One of the first questions that needs to be addressed is the nature of the procedure that might produce optimal effects on blood pressure. Almost every aspect of relaxation training has been removed from the procedure, without unduly diminishing the degree of blood-pressure lowering. This suggests that we are dealing with a state that can be reached in a number of different ways. It also suggests that very simple procedures such as Benson's method of inducing the relaxation response are likely to produce as much benefit as very complex methods. Indeed, there is no evidence that adding new elements to the procedure is beneficial. Careful dissection experiments removing one element of therapy at a time are needed to answer this important question. Answers to this question will not only be useful in clinical practice—the simpler the technique, the better the adherence to it—but they may also shed light on the psychological mechanisms underlying the relaxation response. Most studies of relaxation training have used a preset number of training sessions rather than training participants to lower their blood pressures to a preset criterion. The latter method makes more sense from a skills-learning viewpoint and should be investigated more vigorously.

Delineating psychological mechanisms that underlie the relaxation response is also important. We know very little about this area. The dimensions of cognitive, affective, and behavioral changes induced by relaxation training in the hypertensive patient need to be investigated during the next phase of research. Is blood-pressure lowering produced by changing perception of the environment? Or by a distancing of self from the stressful world—the passive observer of meditation? Such training would appear to diminish anxiety and depression, but further work, particularly investigating effects on anger (which seems to be an important affect in cardiovascular disease), is needed. Similarly, it is possible that relaxation training alters behavior in some way, perhaps improving coping behavior. Again, this is a fertile area for further investigation.

Similar questions arise concerning the physiologic mechanisms involved in blood-pressure lowering as a consequence of relaxation training. While most of the research suggests that the SNS is involved in the observed blood-pressure changes, futher work is needed to clarify the exact hormonal responses to relaxation training.

Finally, the place of relaxation training in the management of essential hypertension needs to be clarified. To accomplish this, a large-scale, multicenter clinical trial involving the entire range of hypertensive individuals is probably needed at this point since the requisite sample size cannot be obtained in one center alone. Many of the questions raised above might be addressed within the context of such a trial. Similarly, as indicated earlier, studies aimed at examining the role of relaxation training in preventing essential hypertension are needed. Overall, this area of research has shown a vigorous development during the past few years. We are now in a position to build on these initial findings in our quest for the better management of the hypertensive patient.

REFERENCES

Agras, W. S., Horne, N., & Taylor, C. B. (1982). Expectation and the blood-pressure-lowering effects of relaxation. *Psychosomatic Medicine, 44,* 389–395.

Agras, W. S., Schneider, J. A., & Taylor, C. B. (1984). Relaxation training in essential hypertension: A failure of retraining in relaxation procedures. *Behavior Therapy, 15,* 191–196.

Agras, W. S., Southam, M. A., & Taylor, C. B. (1983). Long-term persistence of relaxation-induced blood pressure lowering during the working day. *Journal of Consulting and Clinical Psychology, 51,* 792-794.

Agras, W. S., Taylor, C. B., Kraemer, H. C., Allen, R. A., & Schneider, J. A. (1980). Relaxation training. *Archives of General Psychiatry, 37,* 859-863.

Agrawal, R. C., Dikshit, N., Maheshwari, R., Bose, S., & Bisariya, B. N. (1977). Effect of shavasan on vascular response to cold pressor test, serum cholesterol level and platelet stickiness in hyper-reactors. *Indian Heart Journal, 29,* 180-185.

Bali, L. R. (1979). Long-term effect of relaxation on blood pressure and anxiety levels of essential hypertension males: A controlled study. *Psychosomatic Medicine, 41,* 637-646.

Barlow, D. H., Cohen, A. S., Waddell, M. T., Vermilyea, B. B., Klosko, J. S., Blanchard, E. B., & Di Nardo, P. A. (1984). Panic and generalized anxiety disorders: Nature and treatment. *Behavior Therapy, 15,* 431-449.

Benson, H., Rosner, B. A., Marzetta, B., & Klemchuk, H. (1974). Decreased blood pressure in pharmacologically treated hypertensive patients who regularly elicited the relaxation response. *Lancet, 11,* 289-294.

Brauer, A. P., Horlick, L., Nelson, E., Farquhar, J. W., & Agras, W. S. (1979). Relaxation therapy for essential hypertension: A Veterans Administration outpatient study. *Journal of Behavioral Medicine, 2,* 21-29.

Corby, J. C., Walton, T. R., Zarcone, V. P., Jr., & Kopell, B. S. (1978). Psychophysiological correlates of the practice of tantric yoga meditation. *Archives of General Psychiatry, 25,* 571-577.

Cottier, C., Shapiro, K., & Julius, S. (1984). Treatment of mild hypertension with progressive muscle relaxation. *Archives of Internal Medicine, 144,* 1954-1958.

Crowther, J. H. (1983). Stress management training and relaxation imagery in the treatment of essential hypertension. *Journal of Behavioral Medicine, 6,* 169-187.

Cuthbert, B., Kristeller, J., Simons, R., Hodes, R., & Long, A. J. (1981). Strategies of arousal control: Biofeedback, meditation, and motivation. *Journal of Experimental Psychology: General, 51,* 792-794.

Datey, K. K. (1980). Role of biofeedback training in hypertension and stress. *Journal of Postgraduate Medicine, 26,* 68-73.

Davidson, D. M., Winchester, M. A., Taylor, C. B., Alderman, E. A., & Ingels, N. B., Jr. (1979). Effects of relaxation therapy on cardiac performance and sympathetic activity in patients with organic heart disease. *Psychosomatic Medicine, 41,* 303-309.

Davidson, R. J., Goleman, D. J., & Schwartz, G. E. (1976). Attentional and affective concomitants of meditation: A cross-sectional study. *Journal of Abnormal Psychology, 85,* 235-238.

Dunbar, J. M., & Agras, W. S. (1980). Compliance with medical instructions. In J. Ferguson & C. B. Taylor (Eds.), *The comprehensive handbook of behavioral medicine* (pp. 115-145). New York: Spectrum Publications.

Engel, B. T., Glasgow, M. S., & Gaarder, K. R. (1983). Behavioral treatment of high blood pressure. III: Follow-up results and treatment recommendations. *Psychosomatic Medicine, 45,* 23-29.

Friedman, H., & Taub, H. A. (1977). The use of hypnosis and biofeedback procedures for essential hypertension. *International Journal of Clinical and Experimental Hypnosis, 25,* 335-347.

Glasgow, M. S., Gaarder, K. R., & Engel, B. T. (1982). Behavioral treatment of high blood pressure. II: Acute and sustained effects of relaxation and systolic blood pressure biofeedback. *Psychosomatic Medicine, 44,* 155-170.

Goldstein, I. B., Shapiro, D., & Thananopavaran, C. (1984). Home relaxation techniques for essential hypertension. *Psychosomatic Medicine, 46,* 398-414.

Hoelscher, T. J., Lichstein, K. L., & Rosenthal, T. L. (in press). Home relaxation in hypertension treatment: Objective assessment and compliance induction. *Journal of Consulting and Clinical Psychology.*

Hoffman, J. W., Benson, H., Arns, P. A., Steinbrook, G. L., Landberg, L. L., Young, J. B., & Gill, A. (1982). Reduced sympathetic nervous system responsivity associated with the relaxation response. *Science, 215,* 190-192.

Hypertension Detection and Follow-up Program Cooperative Group. (1979). Five-year findings of the Hypertension Detection and Follow-up Program. I: Reduction in mortality of persons with high blood pressure, including mild hypertension. *Journal of the American Medical Association, 242*, 2562-2577.

Jachuck, S. J., Brierley, H., & Jachuck, S. (1982). The effect of hypotensive drugs on the quality of life. *Journal of the Royal College of General Practice, 32*, 103-105.

Jacob, R. G., Beidel, D. C., & Shapiro, A. P. (1984). The relaxation word of the day: A simple technique to measure adherence to relaxation. *Behavioral Assessment, 6*, 159-165.

Jacob, R. G., Fortmann, S. P., Kraemer, H. C., Farquhar, J. W., & Agras, W. S. (1985). Combining behavioral treatments to reduce blood pressure. *Behavior Modification, 9*, 32-54.

Jacob, R. G., Kraemer, H. C., & Agras, W. S. (1977). Relaxation therapy in the treatment of hypertension. *Archives of General Psychiatry, 34*, 1417-1427.

Jevning, R. A., & O'Halloran, J. P. (1984). Metabolic effects of transcendental meditation: Toward a new paradigm of neurobiology. In D. H. Shapiro, Jr. & R. N. Walsh (Eds.), *Meditation: Classic and contemporary perspectives* (pp. 465-473). Chicago: Aldine Publishing Company.

Jevning, R. A., Wilson, A. F., Pirkle, H., O'Halloran, J. P., & Walsh, R. N. (1983). Metabolic control in a state of decreased activation: Modulation of red cell metabolism. *American Journal of Physiology, 245* (Cell Physiology 14), C457-C461.

Krantz, D. S., & Manuck, S. B. (1984). Acute psychophysiologic reactivity and risk of cardiovascular disease: A review and methodologic critique. *Psychological Bulletin, 96*, 435-464.

Laughlin, K. D., Fisher, L., & Sherrard, D. J. (1979). Blood pressure reductions during self-recording of home blood pressure. *American Heart Journal, 98*, 629-634.

Lazarus, A. A. (1976). Transcript of relaxation therapy. In M. R. Goldfried & G. C. Davison (Eds.), *Clinical behavior therapy* (pp. 281-287). New York: Holt, Rinehart and Winston.

Light, K. C., Koepke, J. P., Obrist, P. A., & Willis, P. W. (1983). Psychological stress induces sodium and fluid retention in men at high risk for hypertension. *Science, 220*, 429-431.

Linden, W. (1984). Practice of meditation by school children and their levels of field dependence-independence, test anxiety and reading achievement. In D. H. Shapiro, Jr. & R. N. Walsh (Eds.), *Meditation: Classic and contemporary perspectives* (pp. 89-96). Chicago: Aldine Publishing Company.

Luborsky, L., Crits-Christoph, P., Brady, J. P., Kron, R. E., Weiss, T., Cohen, M., & Levy, L. (1982). Behavioral versus pharmacological treatment for essential hypertension—a needed comparison. *Psychosomatic Medicine, 44*, 203-213.

Management Committee. (1980). The Australian therapeutic trial in mild hypertension. *Lancet, 14*, 1261-1267.

Marlatt, C. A., Pagano, R. R., Rose, R. M., & Marques, J. K. (1984). Effects of meditation and relaxation upon alcohol use in male social drinkers. In D. H. Shapiro, Jr. & R. N. Walsh (Eds.), *Meditation: Classic and contemporary perspectives* (pp. 105-120). Chicago: Aldine Publishing Company.

McGrady, A. V., Tan, S. T., Fine, T. H., & Woerner, M. (1981). The effect of biofeedback assisted relaxation training on blood pressure and selected biochemical parameters in patients with essential hypertension. *Biofeedback and Self Regulation, 6*, 343-353.

Multiple Risk Factor Intervention Trial Research Group. (1982). Multiple risk factor intervention trial: Risk factor changes and mortality results. *Journal of the American Medical Association, 248*, 1465-1477.

Oliver, M. F. (1982). Risks of correcting the risks of coronary disease and stroke with drugs. *New England Journal of Medicine, 306*, 297-298.

Patel, C. H. (1973). Yoga and biofeedback in the management of hypertension. *Lancet, 11*, 783-787.

Patel, C., Marmot, M. G., & Terry, D. J. (1981). Controlled trial of biofeedback-aided behavioral methods in reducing mild hypertension. *British Medical Journal, 282*, 2005-2008.

Peters, R. K., Benson, H., & Peter, J. M. (1977). Daily relaxation response breaks in a working population. II: Effects on blood pressure. *American Journal of Public Health, 67*, 954-959.

Peters, R. K., Benson, H., & Porter, D. (1977). Daily relaxation response breaks in a working popula-

tion. I: Effects on self-reported measures of health, performance, and well-being. *American Journal of Public Health, 67,* 946-953.
Roberts, B. W, & Forester, W. E. (1979). Group relaxation—acute and chronic effects on essential hypertension. *Cardiovascular Medicine, 20,* 575-580.
Seer, P. (1979). Psychological control of essential hypertension: Review of the literature and methodological critique. *Psychological Bulletin, 86,* 1015-1043.
Seer, P., & Raeburn, J. M. (1980). Meditation training and essential hypertension: A methodological study. *Journal of Behavioral Medicine, 3,* 59-71.
Shapiro, D., & Goldstein, I. B. (1982). Biobehavioral perspectives on hypertension. *Journal of Consulting and Clinical Psychology, 50,* 841-858.
Smith, J. C. (1976). Psychotherapeutic effects of transcendental meditation with controls for expectation of relief and daily sitting. *Journal of Consulting and Clinical Psychology, 44,* 630-637.
Stone, R. A., & DeLeo, J. (1976). Psychotherapeutic control of hypertension. *New England Journal of Medicine, 294,* 80-84.
Taylor, C. B., Agras, W. S., Schneider, J. A., & Allen, R. A. (1983). Adherence to instructions to practice relaxation exercises. *Journal of Consulting and Clinical Psychology, 51,* 952-953.
Taylor, C. B., Farquhar, J. W., Nelson, E., & Agras, W. S. (1977). Relaxation therapy and high blood pressure. *Archives of General Psychiatry, 34,* 339-342.
Thoresen, C. E., Telch, M. J., & Eagleston, J. R. (1981). Approaches to altering the Type A behavior pattern. *Psychosomatics, 22,* 6-20.
Wadden, T. A. (1983). Predicting treatment response to relaxation therapy for essential hypertension. *Journal of Nervous and Mental Disease, 171,* 683-689.
Wadden, T. A., Luborsky, L., Greer, S., & Crits-Christoph, P. (1984). The behavioral treatment of essential hypertension: An update and comparison with pharmacological treatment. *Clinical Psychology Review, 4,* 403-429.
Wallace, R. K., Benson, J., & Wilson, A. F. (1971). A wakeful hypometabolic physiologic state. *American Journal of Physiology, 221,* 795-799.
Walsh, R. N. (1979). Meditation research: An introduction and review. *Journal of Transpersonal Psychology, 11,* 161-174.

6
THE SYNTHESIS OF MEDICAL AND BEHAVIORAL SCIENCES WITH RESPECT TO BRONCHIAL ASTHMA

Thomas L. Creer
Ohio University

DEFINITION OF ASTHMA

The term *asthma* is derived from the Greek word for *panting*. Descriptions of asthma extend back to Hippocrates, although it was not until the Christian era when Aretaeus and Galen provided the first detailed discussions of the disorder (Creer, 1982; McFadden & Stevens, 1983). In the 12th century, Moses Maimonides wrote an influential treatise that described the clinical features of asthma and suggested that individual differences could be expected in treating the disorder. His recommendations for treatment were somewhat punitive; for example, he suggested that asthmatic patients sleep as little as possible to avoid the occurrence of attacks (Clark, 1985). Many of the early accounts of observers were remarkably accurate, however. Several recent writers (Clark, 1985; McFadden & Stevens, 1983; Sakula, 1984) have discussed the contributions made by Sir John Floyer in the 17th century. In *A Treatise on the Asthma* (1698), Floyer suggested:

> When the Muscles labor much for Inspiration and Expiration thro' some Obstruction and Compression of the Bronchia, etc, we properly call this a Difficulty of the Breath; but if this Difficulty be by the Constriction of the Bronchia, 'tis properly called the Periodic Asthma: And if the constriction is great, it is with Wheezing; but if less, the Wheezing is not evident. (Sakula, 1984, pp. 249–250)

As far as it goes, the description by Sir John Floyer is as accurate today as when he published his account.

Despite a number of accurate descriptions of asthma throughout the years, however, asthma has proven to be almost impossible to define. There are two reasons for this: First, while a definition of asthma in functional terms, proposed in 1959, has been widely accepted, the degree of reversibility required for a diagnosis of asthma has yet to be determined (Fletcher & Pride, 1984). It is agreed that some reversibility of the airway obstruction must occur if asthma is diagnosed, but the precise degree of reversibility is debatable. Second, it has been impossible to arrive at a definition of asthma that would exclude all other types of respiratory disorders. A CIBA study team, charged with the task of resolving the problem, concluded after considerable debate that their definition would include aproximately 25 percent of patients with chronic bronchitis (Porter & Birch, 1971). The fact that reversibility of airway obstruction may be observed in the latter group made it virtually impossible to distinguish between these patients and those with asthma. Other observers (e.g., Bonner, 1984) have also noted that the terms "asthma" and "wheezy bronchitis" refer to the same set of symptoms, although the latter diagnosis may be used because some physicians apparently believe that it is more palatable to patients than is the term "asthma."

Creer (in press) illustrated the differences apparent in defining asthma by comparing three definitions. In his article, Pearlman (1984) defined asthma in the following way:

> Asthma is a disorder of the tracheobronchial tree in which there is recurrent, at least partially reversible generalized obstruction to the airflow. It is commonly manifested by cough and expiratory distress and classically by respiratory wheezing. Overt wheezing does not have to occur, however, and the major manifestation may be cough. (p. 459)

Pearlman's definition points out two important characteristics of the disorder—the intermittent and reversible nature of the airway obstruction. The remainder of his description concentrates on clinical signs of asthma. This definition may be compared with that of Williams (1982):

> Asthma is defined as reversible airway obstruction. It is characterized by hyperirritability of the airway. Substances that have no effect when inhaled by normal people cause bronchoconstriction in patients with asthma. The principal feature of the condition is extreme variability, both from patient to patient and from time to time in the same patient. It ranges from a mild wheeze with respiratory infection in children, which may disappear in later life, to severe, continuous, and even fatal obstruction of the airways. (p. 23)

This definition also describes the reversibility component of asthma; in particular, however, Williams emphasizes the variable nature of the disorder. He also notes that bronchoconstriction is frequently induced by inhaled substances, a statement that emphasizes the allergic component of asthma.

The final definition is the most widely cited description for asthma—the definition proposed by the American Thoracic Society (1962):

Asthma is a disease characterized by an increased responsiveness of the trachea and bronchi to various stimuli and manifested by a widespread narrowing of the airways that changes in severity either spontaneously or as a result of therapy. (p. 763)

Creer (in press) observed that the definition suffers from several weaknesses, including its lack of specificity and the questionable contention that asthma is a disease. However, it does highlight one characteristic of asthma—the responsiveness of the trachea and bronchi can spontaneously change in severity—that was omitted in the other definitions.

These three descriptions point out the diversity that exists in attempting to define asthma. There are three characteristics of the disorder covered by the definitions, however, that merit special consideration: the intermittent, variable, and reversible nature of asthma. Each of these characteristics will be described separately.

Intermittent Nature

This denotes that attacks suffered by most patients occur on an intermittent basis. The frequency of asthmatic episodes varies from patient to patient and, for any given patient, from time to time. Hence, while a patient may experience a burst of attacks over a brief period of time, he may remain free of the disorder for a duration extending over weeks, months, or, in some cases, years. The intermittency of attacks is particularly vexing with those who suffer childhood asthma. Many experts on childhood asthma believe that most asthmatic children outgrow their asthma and improve during their teens. Such a position was recently noted by Rees (1984), although he cautioned that the prognosis depends on the severity of the disease. Other experts are far less certain about the improvement in asthmatic children with age. Pearlman (1984) remarked that outgrowing asthma may be more the exception than the rule with youngsters who have more than a mild form of the disorder. He summarized research on children who supposedly outgrew their asthma and concluded that while some youngsters appear to be symptom free, they do, in fact, have persistent asthma. Furthermore, noted Pearlman, the airway hyperreactivity that is characteristic of asthma can persist in adulthood in the absence of overt symptoms of asthma. A similar point was emphasized by Bonner (1984), who pointed out that while some individuals have asthma from childhood to adult life, the disorder can begin and remit at any age.

The frequency of attacks experienced by patients over time will depend both on the stimuli that trigger the attacks and the hyperreactivity of the airways. Some patients, particularly children, suffer asthma only during certain seasons of the year; airborne pollen, present in the environment, is the major reason for this increase in attacks. A particular patient may suffer an occasional asthmatic episode during other periods of the year because it is triggered by an event such as a viral infection; overall, however, most of the attacks will be confined to a given season. Siegel, Katz, and Rachelefsky (1983) reported that, regardless of where a child lives, asthma attacks generally occur more often and are more severe in the fall of the year. While the reasons for this finding are unclear, suggested explanations include the increased frequency of viral infections, humidity and temperature changes, increased air pollution, and greater exposures to house dust.

Creer (in press) noted that other patients are less fortunate: They have been diagnosed as having perennial asthma in that they experience attacks during all seasons of the year. There must be some reversibility of the condition in order for the diagnosis to be correct, but some patients with perennial asthma suffer almost daily symptoms of the disorder that may include a sensation of tightness in the chest to mild wheezing.

The major reason why some patients experience perennial asthma is their heightened airway responsiveness. As described by Pearlman (1984),

> The lower airways behave as if they were hyperirritable, overresponsive to various chemical mediators of physiologic and inflammatory processes and to a large number of unrelated stimuli, many of which have the capacity to activate or release these substances. (p. 460)

Creer (in press) illustrated this difference by noting that in comparison to those with seasonal asthma, patients with perennial asthma are more likely to be responsive to an array of attack triggers (e.g., viral infections, exercise, cold air, chemicals, and environmental factors). Hence, while exposure to the same stimulus either will fail to trigger an attack or will precipitate an occasional attack in a patient with seasonal asthma, it may trigger what seems to be an endless series of attacks in the patient with perennial asthma.

Renne and Creer (1985) enumerated three problems generated because of the intermittent nature of asthma; all are important to both medical and behavioral scientists. First, there is the difficult task of recruiting a homogeneous population with respect to asthma. Miklich and his coworkers (Miklich et al., 1977) made every conceivable effort to match asthmatic children on such variables as age, sex, and type of asthma. To achieve their goal they recruited only youngsters diagnosed as suffering from perennial asthma. While this aim of the investigation was achieved, the study demonstrated the inherent fallibility in matching patients on even this single dimension of asthma. For example, while all children suffered attacks throughout the year, some experienced more episodes during particular seasons. One youngster, for example, may have been more sensitive to pollens present during autumn; a second child, on the other hand, may have experienced more attacks induced by cold winter air. Changes in the pattern of attacks experienced in individual patients spawned a host of related problems, including changing the medication regimen prescribed for a given youngster. The changes in their asthma, as well as the responses made to such changes, influenced the outcome of the data collected by Miklich and his colleagues in a large-scale study, involving both medical and behavioral scientists, on the use of systematic desensitization by reciprocal inhibition as an adjunct treatment for childhood asthma. The study has been referred to as the most thorough (Steptoe, 1984) and definitive test of systematic desensitization for the treatment of the disorder (Alexander, 1981; Kinsman, Dirks, Jones, & Dahlem, 1980). It merits this recognition but, more importantly, it demonstrates the complex problems that can be expected both in conducting treatment research with asthma and in interpreting outcome data gathered in such investigations (Creer, in press; Renne & Creer, 1985).

Renne and Creer (1985) also noted a second set of problems posed by the intermittent nature of asthma. These center around how long follow-up data should be obtained from patients after an independent variable is introduced (Creer, 1982, 1983a, in press; Creer & Kotses, 1983). The paucity of longitudinal data regarding asthma once prompted Leigh (1953) to suggest that studies be initiated to investigate asthmatic patients for up to 15 years. The suggestion is laudable and, with adults, possible (Creer, Harm, & Marion, in press). With childhood asthma, it would present the insurmountable task of separating any changes induced by the treatment variable from maturational changes that naturally occur with these youngsters (Creer, in press; Renne & Creer, 1985).

The final set of problems described by Renne and Creer (1985) revolves around expectations acquired by patients and their families because of the intermittent nature of asthma. Patients with perennial asthma expect that they can suffer attacks at any time during the year; thus, at the first indication that they are wheezing or experiencing dyspnea, they initiate treatment. Patients with seasonal asthma, however, acquire a different set of expectations toward their attacks. Before initiating treatment, for example, they may escape from the precipitating stimuli with the hope that their response will be all that is required to control the incipient attack. A number of other expectations based on the nature of the asthma, including the likelihood of the patients complying with medication instructions, are further described by Renne and Creer (1985) and Creer et al. (in press).

Variability

This term refers to fluctuations in the severity both of attacks and of asthma per se. Attacks can range from a mild wheeze to fatal occlusion of the airways, predominantly by mucus plugs. Williams (1980) suggested that the reason why asthma has eluded a precise definition is its variable nature. He pointed out that while a conventional definition of variable or reversible airway obstruction is sufficiently broad to embrace all patients with the condition, it necessarily overlaps with other forms of obstructive lung disease.

Attack severity varies from patient to patient and, within the same patient, from episode to episode (Creer, 1982, in press; Renne & Creer, 1985). At one end of the spectrum, there are patients who occasionally suffer mild wheezing. For these individuals, asthma is nothing more than a nuisance; while they may experience some unpleasantness during attacks, the condition does not ordinarily interfere to any extent with their daily lives (Creer, 1982, 1983a; Creer et al., in press). At the other end of the spectrum, however, Jones (1976) described patients who experience asthma characterized more by persistent debilitation than by discrete attacks (although, it must be emphasized, some reversibility of the condition must occur if the diagnosis of asthma is correctly applied). At this extreme, asthma can become a prepotent consideration in dictating the lifestyle of patients and their families (Creer, 1983a).

Other problems are generated by the variable nature of asthma (Creer, in press; Creer et al., in press; Renne & Creer, 1985). One major problem is that there is no standard way of classifying either any given attack as mild, moderate, or severe, or of categorizing a patient as suffering from mild, moderate, or severe asthma. This is is astonishing, considering how frequently the terms are found in the asthma literature. A number of schemes have been suggested to resolve the problem—usually based on the potency, dosage, and schedule of medications taken by patients to control asthma—but none has been widely accepted (Creer, 1982). A valid and reliable solution to the problem was proposed by Renne (1982). Based on two decades of research with asthmatic children, he suggested that severity of asthma be calculated by using a 5×5 matrix anchored by two objective indices: (a) peak expiratory flow rates as they deviate from a patient's predicted norms; and, (b) the potency, schedule, and dosage level of drugs taken to establish control over an attack. Three levels of attack severity were calculated: (a) no asthma or very mild asthma; (b) mild to moderate asthma; and, (c) moderate to severe asthma. With a group of patients, Renne compared attack severity scores, as obtained by this method, to ratings of attack severity as determined both by a group of experienced allergists and a multidisciplinary team composed of nurses, pulmonary technicians, and behavioral scientists, all of whom worked with the sample group of patients. A correlation coefficient calculated on the two sets of data, gathered over a period of time, was $r = .97$. Hence, the procedure proved to be highly reliable at classifying attacks as mild, moderate, or severe. Furthermore, based on the percentage of attacks experienced by a given patient which are categorized as mild, moderate, or severe, it is possible to agree as to whether the patient's asthma should be classified as mild, moderate, or severe (Creer & Winder, 1986).

Renne and Creer (1985) have reported that the expectations of both patients and their families vary as a function of the severity of the former's asthma. If a patient only experiences minor discomfort during an attack, both he and his family are likely to view asthma as little more than a cold. Rest, drinking warm water, and, at the very most, taking a nonprescribed medication will abort most of these attacks. Under such circumstances, the expectations of a patient with mild asthma probably are no different than those of an individual with hay fever. If a patient has perennial asthma, however, he acquires different expectations. He not only relies more on daily maintenance medications to control his asthma, but his day-to-day activities are, to a considerable extent, dictated by his physical condition. Another problem noted by Renne and Creer occurs when there is an unanticipated change in the patient's asthma. Although a patient may suffer a severe attack only once or twice during his lifetime (Williams, 1982), how he perceives the episode is important not only in establishing control over that attack, but in shaping future expectations of the patient and his or her family both toward asthma and how it should be treated. For example, Creer (1974) described how panic exhibited by some asthmatic children was acquired because the youngsters had observed their parents panic during the children's attacks. Although the parents may only have panicked during a single attack, the children later modeled these parental behaviors when they (the children) experienced attacks. On the other hand, many patients, particularly adults, overuse nebulized medications (e.g., Sly, 1985). This is a serious problem because with overuse, patients may gradually require more and more of a particular medication in order to produce bronchodilation and a remission of symptoms. Many patients have explained their behavior by reporting that they once suffered a severe attack and did not wish to experience anything like it in the future; paradoxically, however, this behavior defeats sound medical treatment with respect to the appropriate use of asthma medications (Branscomb, 1984; Chai & Newcomb, 1973).

A final problem presented by the variability of asthma arises in conducting research on the disorder (Creer, in press). The problem is well described by Clark (1977):

> The benchmark of asthma is its variability, and this in itself makes any assessment of treatment most difficult. Trials are usually undertaken in patients who are in a stable state to minimize this problem, but this state is uncharacteristic of the majority of patients who will be requiring the treatment under test and ignores the long-term fluctuations in severity. Variability may itself lead to difficulties in assessing the response to treatment particularly when symptoms are present at night. A combination of diary cards and regular measurements of the peak expiratory flow rate has simplified the problem caused by short-term variability but has not excluded them. The problems of assessing variability are compounded by the fact that any measurement of airway obstruction may not reflect all the variable changes in lung function. (p. 225)

Reversibility

This term denotes the airway obstruction that characterizes asthma reverses either spontaneously or with adequate treatment (Creer, 1982). The reversible component is the *sine qua non* of asthma (McFadden, 1980); it differentiates the condition from other types of respiratory disorders, such as emphysema, where there is no reversibility of physical impairment.

The characteristic of reversibility presents a number of major problems (Creer & Winder, 1986; Renne & Creer, 1985). As noted earlier, asthma is, at best, a relative condition. Thus, while the attacks of many patients completely remit, there are patients in whom the degree of remission is far less clear. A study by Loren et al. (1978), for example, found many asthma patients had reduced airflow which was irreversible with intensive treatment, including the administration of corticosteroids. This illustrates a point made at the outset: It is still debatable as to the degree of reversibility that should occur in order for asthma to be the correct diagnosis.

Another major problem with the characteristic of reversibility is that spontaneous remission adds uncertainty with respect to the outcome of any treatment procedure (Creer et al., in press; Renne & Creer, 1985). As Creer (1978) asked, How do we know if the treatment we applied resulted in any observable changes that may have occurred? The aim is to answer the question under tightly controlled conditions where a functional analysis can be established between the application of the treatment procedure and the remission of asthmatic symptoms. However, even in the laboratory where conditions can be controlled, there is still uncertainty, as Clark (1977) noted, because even here "the response to treatment appears to be influenced by factors independent of the treatment given" (p. 225). The matter of spontaneous remission becomes even more complex when considering the attacks that disrupt the daily lives of some patients. As Creer (1979, 1982) warned, there are a number of studies in the literature where spontaneous remission cannot be ruled out as a possible, perhaps probable, explanation for the treatment outcome observed with asthmatic patients. The characteristic of spontaneous remission simply defies control, even in the best-designed and executed study.

CONCEPTUALIZATIONS OF ASTHMA

The discussion of the characteristics of asthma has, hopefully, conveyed a sense of the complexity of the disorder. Despite references to asthma that date back to the early Greeks, there are times when it appears to be as misunderstood today as it was in ancient times. One misunderstanding has arisen because both medical and behavioral scientists have been guided by different conceptualizations of the disorder. With physicians, the tendency has been to overemphasize the role played by allergies in triggering attacks. The fact that antibodies could mediate disease was first reported during the early part of the century (Pearlman, 1984). Shortly thereafter, it was observed that histamine, believed to be released by an antigen-antibody reaction, could induce an asthma-like reaction in the guinea pig. Pearlman noted the idea that immune or allergic reactions could cause asthma was a natural consequence of these observations. This premise was greatly strengthened by the discovery of a skin-sensitizing antibody-like substance in many persons with asthma and noninfectious rhinitis. Out of this grew the widespread adoption of such terms as "allergic diseases" or "allergic disorder" in the belief that these disorders were, in fact, due to allergy. Pearlman cautions against this conclusion:

> It has been clear for some time, however, that even though a large proportion of patients with asthma, particularly children and young adults, are "allergic" and that allergic factors can be important triggers of their asthma, allergic reactivity is not universally demonstrable in children or adults who have asthma. Moreover, in the vast majority of allergic asthmatics, asthma is provoked also by numerous other factors apparently unrelated to allergy. (Pearlman, 1984, pp. 459–460)

Behavioral scientists, on the other hand, have generally viewed asthma as a psychosomatic disease. This conception, no doubt, arose because of the many anecdotal descriptions of the onset and course of asthma attacks. The problem with the conceptualization is that a psychosomatic basis for asthma has never, under controlled conditions, been demonstrated (Creer, 1979, 1982). The psychosomatic model has not only failed to enhance our knowledge or to provide any benefit to those afflicted with asthma, but, as noted by Creer (1979), "a very strong case could be made that such a model has contributed more to the distress and anguish of patients, especially to nurturing myths about their disease, than to providing them with any enduring benefit" (p. 8). This does not mean, however, that psychological factors are not important with asthma because, as noted by Creer (1982):

> Perhaps more than occurs with other chronic physical conditions, there is a strong psychological component to asthma. This is reflected in a number of ways, extending from the role of emotional behaviors in eliciting attacks to the consequences of the disorder. Because physical and psychological factors are so inextricably interwoven, the investigation of asthma requires frequent collaboration between medicine and psychology. (p. 913)

Considering the problems inherent in a conceptualization based on either an allergy or psychosomatic model, it is obvious that there is need for a model of asthma that could be used by both medical and behavioral scientists. The hope for such a model was that it would stimulate research while providing a structure on which new information could be added. It would not be bound up with theory, but would be oriented toward assimilating each new bit of knowledge, piece by piece, so as to arrive at a comprehensive model that could be referred to by any scientist, no matter his or her training and background. Such a functional model for asthma was recently proposed by Reed and Townley (1978, 1983). As depicted in Table 6.1, they have classified variables involved in the pathogenesis of asthma into three categories—stimuli (S), variables linking stimuli to responses (O), and physical responses (R). This provides a model with components familiar to both behavioral and medical scientists. For every patient, each of the S-O-R factors should be specified as precisely as possible. Reed and Townley convincingly argue

TABLE 6.1
Factors Involved in the Pathogenesis and Classification of Asthma

---

Stimuli
    Irritants
    Exercise and cold air
    Respiratory infections
    Allergens
    Situations and emotional responses
    Aspirin and related substances
Linkage of stimulus to response
    Pathways
        Immunologic
        Neuromuscular
    Factors influencing pathways
        Genetic and familial
        Endocrine
        Nutritional
Response
    Location of obstruction
    Tempo of obstruction
    Smooth-muscle spasm
    Bronchial inflammation
    Mucous glands

Note. Adapted from Reed & Townley, 1983.

that such a multifactorial approach to the classification of asthmatic patients, as well as the events involved in the pathogenesis of their asthma, is not only accurate in that there is no presumption of the causes and mechanisms that may not exist, but that the model provides a firm basis for planning optimal treatment for individual patients.

Since space limitations prohibit a thorough discussion of the model suggested by Reed and Townley (1978, 1983), interested readers are directed to the original sources. However, in order to illustrate how asthma might be perceived by both medical and behavioral scientists, a brief synopsis is provided.

Stimuli

Behavioral scientists are apt to be interested in the stimuli that trigger attacks because they may be involved in developing strategies, in conjunction with asthmatic patients and medical personnel, to control such problems as smoking or unnecessary exposure to known asthma precipitants. The discussion of stimuli involved in the pathogenesis of asthma is based on a description of these variables by Creer et al. (in press).

IRRITANTS. A wide variety of stimuli can irritate the airways and induce attacks in asthmatic patients. There is currently a strong interest in occupational asthma (e.g., Davies, Blainey, & Pepys, 1983) as the list of workplace stimuli causally related to the development of airway disorders, including asthma, increases with each passing year. For example, while Murphy (1976) enumerated over 80 types of occupations where stimuli in the work environment could induce respiratory reactions, there are over 100 occupations today that could fall into this category (Creer et al., in press). These would include environments where an employee has contact with such stimuli as metal salts, wood and vegetable dusts, pharmaceutical agents, biological enzymes, industrial chemicals and plastics, and animal or insect dusts (McFadden, 1984). These stimuli can not only precipitate attacks in the asthmatic worker, but can sometimes be transported by the worker to his or her home, where they may trigger attacks in other family members.

A potentially harmful irritant for precipitating asthma attacks is air pollution. McFadden noted that injurious air pollutants are usually derived from two sources: incomplete combustion of fossil fuels with the subsequent formation of industrial smog, and ultraviolet irradiation from sunlight acting on hydrocarbons or automobile emissions to produce photochemical smog. He cautioned that while there is no question that these irritants can affect the airways, the long- and short-term effects of such pollution on our health remains unknown.

There is more and more concern about the effects of cigarette smoke, even among those who appear to be healthy. Tager et al. (1985) recently conducted a longitudinal study of adolescents between the ages of 15 and 20 who smoked. In the basis of their analysis, Tager and his colleagues found that, on the average, pulmonary functioning was 92% of the predicted values for youngsters who started smoking at 15 and who continued to smoke. The conclusion was that even with relatively small amounts of cigarette use, there was a significant effect on the growth of lung function in these children. Cigarette smoke is considered to be a prominent irritant in asthmatic patients, even for those who do not smoke. In a well-controlled study, Dahms, Bolin, and Slavin (1981) reported a significant decrease in airway function among asthmatic patients exposed to passive smoking. Control subjects who did not have asthma were unaffected by the passive smoke, thereby suggesting that cigarette smoke may be particularly deleterious to the health of asthmatic youngsters. Supportive evidence for this conclusion was voiced by Gortmaker, Walker, Jacobs, and Ruch-Ross (1982) who found, in two surveys that investigated the relationship between parental smoking and childhood asthma, 18% and 34% of the attacks suffered by the youngsters in the two samples, respectively, were attributable to maternal smoking.

EXERCISE. Reed and Townley (1983) pointed out that "most if not all patients will develop bronchoconstriction after sufficiently vigorous exercise of breathing dry, cold air" (p. 813). Exercise-induced asthma is especially prevalent in asthmatic children because of their high level of physical activity. While the condition has been recognized since 1679, there remains a need for better-controlled and quantified studies of exercise-induced asthma (Smith, 1985).

INFECTIONS. Respiratory infections are among the most common stimuli that evoke acute episodes of asthma, particularly severe attacks that require hospitalization (Reed & Townley, 1983). Although it was once thought that bacterial infections were significant in triggering attacks, several well-controlled studies have demonstrated that viruses, not bacteria, are major etiological factors. There is, in fact, no evidence to support the premise that bacterial infections play a role in the pathogenesis of asthma (McFadden, 1984).

ALLERGENS. Table 6.2 lists common allergens thought to trigger asthma attacks. Although the percentage of patients prone to suffer attacks triggered by such stimuli may vary according to a given survey, it has been suggested that a suspected or proven allergic component may be found in from 35% to 55% of asthmatic patients (McFadden, 1984). Most allergens that precipitate attacks enter the body through the air (Reed & Townley, 1983); in order to induce a state of sensitivity, they must be reasonably abundant in the environment for a period of time (McFadden, 1984). Once sensitivity occurs, the patient can exhibit heightened responsivity so that minute amounts of the offending stimulus can provoke hypersensitivity and, as a consequence, asthma attacks. Allergens are more likely to provoke attacks in children than in adults. As noted earlier, however, Pearlman (1984) pointed out that the link between asthma and airway hyperreactivity per se is much stronger than the link between allergy and asthma.

SITUATIONS AND EMOTIONAL RESPONSES. Earlier it was noted that the psychosomatic model is unable to account for asthma. Nevertheless, it is well recognized that emotional factors may be a potential trigger for attacks suffered by some patients (Creer, 1979, 1982). What is important is the response or responses performed by the patient as part of an emotional reaction (Creer, 1979). For example, crying and laughing are two responses apt to induce attacks, particularly in asthmatic children, whereas coughing may be either a precipitator or a symptom of attacks. Furthermore, an entire pattern of emotional responses may, like

TABLE 6.2
A Partial List of Allergens Known to Trigger Asthma Attacks

Tree pollen
Grass pollen
Weed pollen
Animals or feathers
Molds or fungi
Insects (not insect stings)
Occupational dusts
Chemicals (not acting as irritants)
House dust
Foods

Note. Adapted from Reed & Townley, 1983.

exercise-induced asthma, trigger other asthmatic episodes. The pattern may include laughing, crying, hyperventilation, shouting, screaming, or jumping about; either separately or together, these emotionally aroused responses can precipitate asthma.

Pearlman (1984) has suggested that the ease with which emotional factors influence bronchoconstriction is related to the degree of nonspecific bronchial hyperresponsivity in the same way that reactivity to physical factors is heightened as the degree of nonspecific hyperresponsivity is increased. This may account for why the effect of emotional factors varies from patient to patient and, in the same patient, from episode to episode (McFadden, 1984; Reed & Townley, 1983).

ASPIRIN AND RELATED SUBSTANCES. A large number and variety of drugs can produce airway reactions; however, medications most commonly associated with the precipitation of acute episodes of asthma are aspirin and drug or food additives such as tartrazine, a widely used yellow dye. Spector and Farr (1983) list 489 products that contain aspirin; however, they warn that since formula changes and new products are constantly introduced, their listing must be considered as incomplete. Acetaminophen, the principal compound in a number of pain relievers, can also induce bronchoconstriction, but of a lesser severity than aspirin (Fischer et al., 1983); ibuprofen, recently introduced as a nonprescription pain remedy, induces bronchoconstriction to a degree equal to aspirin (Spector & Farr, 1983).

The prevalence of aspirin-sensitive patients is debatable. Although McFadden (1984) described studies where a range of 3% to 19% of the subjects experienced aspirin-induced asthma, Spector and Farr (1983) cited investigations where a range of 0% to 44% of the patients were sensitive to aspirin. Thus, while the percentages may vary in these studies, it is obvious that a sizable percentage of asthmatic patients could experience attacks if exposed to aspirin.

Link of Stimulus to Response

Reed and Townley (1978, 1983) describe two major pathways by which stimuli may induce asthmatic responses: immunological and neuromuscular. These will be considered as separate although, as will be noted, there is interaction between the two types of pathways.

IMMUNOLOGICAL. As described earlier, Pearlman (1984) traced the interest in the immunology of asthma back to the beginning of the century. However, a major breakthrough in the area was the discovery by Ishizawka and Ishizawka (1967) of human IgE, the immunoglobulin thought to be responsible for 95% of allergic reactions, including allergy-induced asthma. The chain of events that occurs can be briefly summarized. As occurs with other systems of the body, defects can occur in our immune system. A particular combination of an antigen with an immune response may lead to hypersensitivity. There are four types, but Type I, also known as anaphylactic or immediate hypersensitivity, is the type that involves asthma. Here, the antigen combines with mast-cell or basophil-fixed IgE, resulting in degranulation of the cells (Feinberg & Jackson, 1983). The latter is characterized by the release of a number of mediators, including histamine, chemotatic factors, prostaglandins, leukotrienes, and platlet-activating factors. The release of these mediators, in turn, can result in the bronchoconstriction that defines asthma.

The discovery of IgE induced a mushrooming of research on the immunological aspects of asthma. Without even attempting to summarize this work—a number of excellent chapters are found in Middleton, Reed, and Ellis (1983)—two areas should be noted. First, knowledge of the immunology of IgE has led to the development of more effective medications to control asthma. As succinctly described by Williams (1982):

> Inhaled or ingested antigen bridges IgE antibodies, coating the surface of mast cells, perhaps within the airway lumen, to cause mediator release. Cromolyn prevents this reaction by stabilizing the membrane of the mast cell. Stimulation of intracellular c-AMP by adrenergic drugs, and indirectly by theophylline, inhibits the release of mediators. These drugs also act directly on smooth muscle in the airways to reduce bronchoconstriction. The mediators released from mast cells, most notably histamine, produce bronchoconstriction to a variety of inhaled agents and local phenomena, such as the heat exchange induced by exercise, to cause reflex bronchoconstriction via the cholinergic arc. This is blocked by anticholinergic drugs, which also inhibit mediator release from mast cells. (p. 24)

Other medications, formulated and tested in the future, will no doubt be concerned with controlling some aspect of the effect of IgE on mast cells.

A second area has been investigated in the role of immunological factors in bronchoconstriction. The latter, resulting from a narrowing of the large and/or small airways, is caused by muscle spasm, swelling of tissue, excessive mucus secretion, dried mucus plugs, or a combination of these factors. The mediators released from the mast cells that may account for these changes were recently summarized by Kaliner (1985). As noted in Table 6.3, considerable research has been directed at this topic. The table not only graphically depicts the complexity of the immunological basis of asthma, but points out the spectrum of mediators currently underoing scrutiny in laboratories around the world. Three mediators in particular—platelet-activating factors, prostaglandins, and leukotrienes—are of interest to investigators at the present time. The latter—leukotrienes C, D, and E—are generally known as the reacting substance of anaphylaxis or SRS-A. An investigation by Griffin et al. (1983) demonstrated that airflow reduction caused by leukotrine D was not only more prolonged (44 minutes) than that which occurred with inhalation of histamine (20 minutes)—a mediator commonly used to challenge asthmatic patients—but was, on the average, 140 times more potent as a bronchoconstrictor than was histamine. The significance of this finding was emphasized by Weissmann (1983):

TABLE 6.3
Possible Mediators of Pathological Changes in Asthma

Feature	Proposed Mediator
Bronchospasm	Histamine (H_1 response)
	SRS-A (LTC_4, LTD_4, LTE_4)
	Prostaglandins and thromboxane A_2
	Platelet-activating factor (PAF)
	Acetylcholine
	Bradykinin
Mucosal edema	Histamine (H_1 response)
	SRS-A (LTC_4, LTD_4, LTE_4)
	PGE
	PAP
	Bradykinin
Cellular infiltration	Eosinophil chemotactic factors
(airway hyperreactivity)	Neutrophil chemotactic factors
	Inflammatory factors of anaphylaxis (IF-A)
	HETEs (Hydroxyelcosatetraenoic acids)
	LTB_4
Mucus secretion	Histamine (H_2 response)
	Acetylcholine
	Alpha-adrenergic agonists
	Prostaglandins
	HETEs
	SRS-A (LTC_4, LTD_4, LTE_4)
	Macrophage mucus secretagogue (MMS)
	Prostaglandin-generating factor of anaphylaxis (PGF-A)
Desquamation	O_2^- H_2Q_2, OH^-
	Proteolytic enzymes
Basement membrane	O_2^- (superoxide anion)
Thickening	Proteolytic enzymes

Note. Adapted from Kaliner, 1985.

Perhaps an analogy can be drawn with the exploration of the New World: The colonists exploring the leukotrienes have laid out the eastern landscape from Plymouth to Savannah; we confidently await reports of the broad Mississippi, the awesome Rockies, and, in due time, the blue Pacific. (p. 455)

NEUROMUSCULAR. In their chapter, Reed and Townley (1983) focus on the role of histamine, vagal reflexes, and beta-adrenergic blockade as neuromuscular pathways. In doing so, they illustrate how both immunological and physical factors are involved in such pathways. The pathways are involved in the precipitation of asthma through action of the stimuli noted in the last section, but the mechanism by which each stimulus may trigger attacks remains, in general, unknown. Exercise-induced asthma, for example, appears to be related to the degree of airway cooling that occurs during exercise. Thus, noted McFadden (1984), "This, in turn, is an immediate function of the magnitude of heat exchanged within the intrathoracic airways" (p. 417). Spector and Farr (1983) offer five hypotheses that have been advanced to account for the role of aspirin as a trigger of asthma; these involve immunological, acetylation, complement-histamine reactions, abnormal carbohydrate and connective tissues, and prostaglandins. Although Spector and Farr marshal available evidence to support each hypothesis, they caution that the exact mechanism involved in aspirin-induced asthma awaits further research.

A number of theories have been put forward to account for how emotions influence asthma (e.g. , Knapp & Mathe, 1985; Miklich, 1977). However, the exact mechanism remains unknown; plausible pathways for the phenomenon include hyperventilation and hypercapnia, vagal constriction, changes in medullary or cortical activity, and endocrine functions (Reed & Townley, 1983). An answer as to the exact role played by emotions vis-à-vis asthma is apt to await the passage of a long period of time. For example, it is believed that there is a respiratory center in the brainstem that would be influenced by, among other stimuli, emotional factors (Zwillich, 1983). However, the elucidation of the nature of this center, as well as how it controls our breathing, requires experimentation that with present techniques would be unethical to conduct (Cherniack & Cherniack, 1983). It is quite likely, as alluded to earlier, that some physiological pathways will be found to mediate both exercise-induced and emotionally triggered asthma attacks.

Reed and Townley (1983) described genetic, endocrine, and nutritional variables that influence neuromotor pathways; since a discussion of these factors is beyond the scope of this chapter, interested readers are referred to these authors. What should be emphasized in concluding this discussion of the link of stimuli to responses is that while considerable investigation must be conducted before the pathways connecting stimuli and responses are clarified, much progress has occurred in recent years. It should be clear to the reader both that evidence is overwhelmingly abundant that asthma is a complicated physical disorder and that there is no known cure for the disorder. The latter should be recalled the next time we, as behavioral scientists, read of yet another psychological "cure" for asthma.

Responses

Reed and Townley (1983) discussed recent evidence regarding the location of obstruction (i.e., large or small airways) and the tempo of obstruction (i.e., whether an asthmatic episode is abrupt and transient or insidious or prolonged). While these topics are of primary interest to practicing physicians, they pose assessment decisions to both medical and behavioral scientists who conduct asthma research. An example would be the selection of a respiratory measure as a dependent variable. It could be that a group of scientists would wish to use a plethysmograph both because the instrument is more sensitive in measuring human respiration and because no effort is required by subjects in order to assess their breathing. However, the plethysmograph is not only an expensive piece of equipment, but it lacks portability. A peak-flow meter, on the other hand, can be used by asthmatic patients in any environment, including their homes; it is also inexpensive. The problem is that it is not only dependent on the effort of patients in blowing into the instrument, but it is incapable of detecting if any small-airway obstruction is present in patients. Thus, the question of tradeoff arises in selecting the best measure for the purposes of the study.

The fact that there is considerable heterogeneity of the bronchial response strongly supports the need to conduct interdisciplinary research on asthma. Behavioral scientists generally lack both the necessary equipment to assess respiratory changes and the expertise to collect and interpret such data. Medical scientists, on the other hand, generally lack knowledge of the psychological or behavioral techniques being used. As will be noted, the assessment of respiration is a solid dependent measure to add to any study of asthma, including that conducted by behavioral scientists.

PSYCHOLOGICAL AND BEHAVIORAL INTERVENTIONS FOR ASTHMA

The descriptions of asthma provided by early observers were sometimes very accurate. As noted, they contain elements embodied in many present-day descriptions. What proved worthless were many of the explanations, as well as the treatments they generated, which were advanced to account for the disorder. The latter statement resulted from scientific investigation which, over the course of time, discarded general explanations in favor of more specific accounts of the factors important in asthma. And, it can be anticipated that the evolution in explanation from the general to the specific will continue in the future; the immunological basis put forward to explain events involved in asthma, as enumerated by Kaliner (1985) in Table 6.3, will, in due time, be considered too general to account for the immunology of the disorder.

A similar evolution of thought exists with respect to accounting for the role of psychological factors and their relationship to asthma. Some early observations of this relationship were accurate. For example, the report by French and Alexander (1941), suggesting that some asthmatic children avoid crying, is accurate; what is erroneous in the explanation by French and Alexander that this avoidance behavior represents a repressed cry on the part of the youngsters for their mothers. It was not until he interviewed asthmatic children as to why they tried not to cry or they cried in a highly controlled manner that Purcell (1963) discovered that the youngsters were only attempting to avoid the irritation that could trigger their attacks.

An evolution of thought also exists in the development and testing of psychological and behavioral intervention strategies designed to alter the responses of asthmatic patients. This evolution extends from the formulation of general tactics, sometimes with little or no actual testing, to the development and assessment of more precise strategies for changing problems experienced by these patients. A number of salient failures have marked this path. For example, in their review, Purcell and Weiss (1970) noted:

> It is probably safe to state that, at one time or another, almost every variety of psychotherapeutic technique, including psychoanalysis, group psychotherapy, environmental manipulation, behavior therapy, hypnosis, and even ECT has been aplied to the treatment of bronchial asthma. With the single exception of ECT, claims of success have been filed in all instances. (p. 613)

Unfortunately, continued Purcell and Weiss, these claims were based on studies that failed to meet one or more of the basic criteria of adequate treatment studies, ranging from unbiased subject selection to gathering sufficient follow-up data.

A discussion of basic criteria for establishing the efficacy of a given psychological or behavioral intervention provides an overview of why past studies have failed. The criteria, presented in Table 7.4, represent an expansion of basic criteria discussed elsewhere (Creer, 1978, 1982, in press; Purcell & Weiss, 1970; Renne & Creer, 1985). These criteria could guide both medical and behavioral scientists. The importance of each criterion, as well as problems that have arisen when a criterion has been disregarded, serves as the basis for discussion. It would be unfair to single out a particular study to illustrate how any given criterion has been ignored: Violations are more the rule, particularly when studies have been designed and conducted mainly by behavioral scientists, than the exception. The

TABLE 6.4
Basic Criteria for Conducting Intervention Research on Asthma

1.	Confirmation of the diagnosis
2.	Application of unbiased selection procedures.
3.	Selection of subjects from similar populations with respect to severity and classification of asthma. Selection of nonsmoking subjects.
4.	Use of appropriate experimental designs and control procedures.
5.	Application of standardized treatment procedures. Use of reliability checks on application of procedures.
6.	Control concurrent independent variables. a. Control medication regimens of patients. b. Assess medication compliance.
7.	Add broad spectrum of dependent variables to investigation. Ensure the validity and reliability of each measure.
8.	Collect sufficient follow-up data to rule out normal fluctuations of asthmatic symptoms.
9.	Recruit large enough samples of subjects to permit appropriate statistical procedures to be applied. Ensure that assumptions of statistical procedures are maintained.
10.	Apply acceptable criteria for the evaluation of treatment effects.
11.	Interpret data in a reasonable and appropriate manner.
12.	Determine clinical significance of findings.

reader should acquire an awareness, however, of the problems he or she is likely to encounter in designing and conducting an investigation of asthma.

1. *Confirmation of the diagnosis of asthma.* This preliminary step would seem to be the *sine qua non* of any study, but it is a rarity in most behavioral investigations of asthma. It is perplexing why this should be the case, since the very investigator who insists on operational definitions to describe the behavioral measures being employed will overlook this essential step. Basically, the problem is that too many behavioral scientists are willing to accept either the word of patients or the clinical symptoms they describe as indicative of asthma. We all know the weaknesses of self-reports, but may not recognize that clinical symptoms, by themselves, may not indicate asthma but some other respiratory disorder. Earlier, difficulties inherent in defining asthma were discussed, and it was pointed out that symptoms of the disorder may be observed in patients with other respiratory disorders (e.g., chronic bronchitis). The question of diagnosis has been further complicated in the past two decades with reports of another phenomenon that, although mimicking asthma, actually represents a learned pattern of respiratory responses. Included here would be reported cases of acquired sneezing, coughing, and wheezing (Renne & Creer, 1985). This phenomenon is important in its own right, particularly since the respiratory behaviors can be dramatically altered through the application of behavioral techniques. However, these symptoms represent another illustration of where a diagnosis of asthma may be incorrectly applied. A thorough medical examination, including gathering a comprehensive history and performing skin testing and/or bronchial challenges, will confirm the diagnosis of asthma; thus far, such examinations have eliminated learned respiratory responses from such a diagnosis.

2. *Application of unbiased selection procedures.* A number of reports have described the use of various psychological or behavioral techniques to supposedly "cure" asthma. A reading of such articles will frequently reveal that few patients were actually involved; furthermore, in the presented data, it usually appears that the patient's asthma had begun a period of remission and was following the natural course of the disorder independent of intervention. Under these circumstances, the only conclusion is that the patients were selected to be studied and presented in the article. Such reports are nothing more than anecdotal information disguised as science.

3. *Selection of subjects from similar populations.* Selecting enough patients from similar populations is, as noted earlier, easier said than done. It was pointed out that although Miklich and his colleagues (1977) made every effort to enroll only patients with perennial asthma for their study, the youngsters showed differing rates of seasonal attacks that, like a template, overlaid the perennial asthma. Similar problems arise in any study where patients with this type of asthma, particularly children, are recruited. However, the purposes of the study frequently dictate that patients who suffer from asthma throughout the year be recruited for

a study. If the aim is to study the effects of a self-management procedure, for example, investigators would enroll these patients so that sufficient follow-up data could be collected. The problem may be irrelevant in a study on the efficacy of a medication where investigators wish to compare an experimental drug against a placebo. Under circumstances where a shorter period of time is required, the goal of the study may be achieved by recruiting patients with seasonal asthma.

The question of severity of asthma has already been addressed. It behooves investigators to use some schema, such as that proposed and tested by Renne (1982), both to select potential subjects for a study and to assess if there are any changes in the severity of a patient's asthma by virtue of applying an intervention procedure.

There are two major reasons for selecting nonsmoking patients for asthma research: First, by smoking, patients may not only trigger more attacks than occur with other subjects, but they are at risk to develop other respiratory conditions in addition to asthma. In the former case, a higher rate of asthma may occur that is impervious to alteration by any intervention procedure. In a long-term study, on the other hand, these patients are at increased risk for developing emphysema; or there may also be less reversibility to their respiratory condition. Second, smoking interferes with the metabolism of some medications, particularly theophylline-based compounds. If changes in these medications serve as a dependent measure of a study, investigators must be aware that there is a half-life to theophylline when the patient smokes. This introduces a variable difficult to control in a study where such commonly prescribed drugs are taken by patients.

4. *Use of an appropriate experimental design.* In many medical investigations, the experimenter may correctly employ what are referred to as either clinical trials or a group design. There may be enough patients fitting the criteria established by the investigator, particularly in studies of pulmonary physiology or immunology, to allow use of this design. The advantages of such designs are that they permit assessment by multiple dependent variables, as well as the statistical analysis of the data by well-developed techniques. In many other investigations, however, it is highly problematic that enough patients can be recruited and matched to satisfy the design of the study. Indeed, one finds reports in the literature where an inadequate number of subjects were recruited, particularly for control conditions.

A number of scientists have suggested that, wherever possible, group designs be eschewed and subjects serve as their own controls (Clark, 1977; Creer, 1979). Clark (1977), in fact, has declared that wherever possible, patients should serve as their own controls and comparisons between subjects should be kept to a minimum. In behavioral research with asthma where the adequacy of the experimental design is more the exception than the rule, this seems to be very sound advice.

The use of appropriate control procedures is also a problem. As noted above, it is frequently the case that fewer subjects are assigned to these groups than occur with intervention groups. In addition, inappropriate control procedures are often used. For example, in most drug research, the experimental medication is first tested against an inert substance—the placebo. If changes are observed in this first-order type of research, the investigators may wish to compare the experimental drug against similar medications. This is, in effect, a second-order type of investigation because the efficacy of the experimental drug has already been established. Such is not the case with a number of behavioral investigations of asthma, however. For example, a recent study of self-management for asthma equated, as a first-order comparison, the self-management program against an educational program. As a result, no significant differences were noted and, in turn, no meaningful interpretations could be made about the study. Do the data mean that the self-management program was ineffective? This could only have been answered had the procedure been compared against an untreated control group. Does it reflect that the educational program was as effective as self-management? This is the only conclusion that can be drawn from the study, although the finding may not be valid.

5. *Application of standardized treatment procedures.* There are any number of studies where psychotherapy, whether individual, family, or group, is applied; at the same time, there is absolutely no evidence that different therapists involved in a particular study apply similar techniques. In fact, the ambiguous descriptions of many of these intervention procedures suggest that the therapists were uncertain about the intervention procedures they applied. As a result, the reader is not only totally confused about what transpired, but would not attempt to replicate the investigation even if he or she wished to do so. And, unlike a drug study where the investigator will make periodic checks to ensure that the experimental drug is being correctly administered, the ambiguity of psychological interventions has precluded the possibility of probing to determine if therapists adhere to similar guidelines throughout a study. If the latter fail to follow any predetermined criteria in applying an intervention technique, there is no possibility that reliability checks can occur throughout the study.

6. *Control concurrent independent variables.* It might seem to be a foregone assumption that investigators would anticipate and control independent variables, but such is not the case. Thus, there are any number of reports where, alongside the application of a behavioral or psychological procedure, it is cited that medications were taken by the patients during the same period. An allergist or chest physician would quickly argue that any changes that occurred would be expected, given the medications taken by the patients; behavioral scientists, unfortunately, voice different conclusions. If, as occurred in a study of family therapy, the patient is provided with both this type of therapy and corticosteroids, any changes were likely attributable to the latter.

Besides controlling concurrent variables at the outset of the study, it is imperative that behavioral scientists work closely with physicians to ensure that no changes are made in the drug regimen of a patient during the course of a study.

This can usually be achieved although, as described by Miklich and his coworkers (1977), a host of questions, including ethical issues, are raised by such a tactic. For example, will medications be withheld from a patient although such drugs may benefit him? These and related questions can be resolved through close cooperation between behavioral and medical scientists.

The problem of compliance with medication regimens has recently been scrutinized with respect to asthma. Depending on the assessment procedure used, anywhere from 2% to 100% of patients have been found to take their asthma drugs as prescribed. If there is an unannounced drawing of blood serum, studies have indicated levels of serum theophylline that show anywhere from 2% to 10% of patients take their drug as directed; if, on the other hand, patients volunteer for studies knowing that their medication levels will be periodically assessed through blood serum, 100% of the patients may be compliant (Baum & Creer, 1986). Since these findings reflect a wide range of asthmatic patients who are compliant with medication instructions, periodic checks must be made of their behavior.

7. *Add broad spectrum of dependent variables to investigation.* In the past, many behavioral studies relied on self-reports of patients as the major dependent variable, with an occasional psychological test, sometimes applied in an inappropriate manner, thrown in. However, this practice has changed in the past two decades as both objective and subjective measures have been included in studies. It is important that both types of indices be included as, over the years, a number of studies have supported the original investigation by Chai, Purcell, Brady, and Falliers (1968) which indicated that there was a low correlation between the two classes of dependent measures. With respect to objective indices, the most commonly used measures are those that assess pulmonary physiology; other indices that measure biochemical or immunological aspects of the patient's responses have only been added in more recent years. At the same time, more refined measures have been developed to assess subjective changes experienced by patients. Included in this category would be the use of daily diaries, reports of asthma attacks, and attitude surveys. When summed together, a wealth of information can be collected from patients; such data, in turn, is of interest to both behavioral and medical scientists.

When different measures are included in a study, it is important that the reliability and validity of each instrument be established beforehand and throughout the study. This may seem redundant to state, but there are too many examples when the advice is ignored. For example, a behavioral scientist who is using peak-flow meters may neglect to periodically calibrate his or her instruments; as a consequence, spurious data may be gathered with the meters. On the other hand, medical scientists show the proclivity to introduce paper-and-pencil instruments into studies without establishing their validity and reliability. When the instruments are administered several times during the course of a study, it proves impossible to interpret the amassed data.

8. *Collect sufficient follow-up data to rule out normal fluctuations of asthmatic symptoms.* The intermittent nature of asthma has been thoroughly described, as well as the need to gather follow-up data for a period of time after application of an intervention procedure. However, there are any number of violations of this basic axiom, particularly in the behavioral literature. The result is that it is difficult to determine if a procedure produced an effect or if the patients' asthma was merely following its natural course. When reading articles where there is no follow-up data included after some sort of dramatic change in the patients' asthma, the most conservative conclusion is that the patient has seasonal asthma which has ameliorated in accordance with a change in seasons.

9. *Recruit large enough samples of subjects to permit approriate statistical procedures to be applied.* This problem is not endemic to asthma, but there are a number of reports where, following a statement that subjects were randomly assigned to the various groups, the reader discovers that a significantly smaller number of patients was assigned to control conditions. There is no doubt that recruiting patients for the latter conditions can be a difficult task, especially when the investigation involves children with asthma. The pressure to immediately enroll these youngsters in intervention conditions comes not only from their parents and physicians, but also because of time limits in that the children are likely to suffer from seasonal asthma. Solutions to the problem are to have children serve as waiting-list controls for as short a period as possible or to have the youngsters serve as their own controls. There are advantages and disadvantages to either strategy (Creer, in press). The problem does not seem to be as important with adults, as they are more apt to suffer perennial asthma than are children.

The lack of equal numbers in each group has led to the creative use of statistical procedures. While a statistician would blanch at what sometimes occurs, it does not bother investigators who somehow manage to publish their results. Part of the problem arises because many scientists working with asthma, particularly physicians, lack a background in statistics. They rely on the expertise of biostatisticians, but there must occasionally be gaps in communication. This could account for a recent article where, after specifically stating that their data violated the assumptions of parametric statistics, the investigators used an amalgamation of statistical procedures, including analysis of covariance, to treat their data.

10. *Apply acceptable criteria for the evaluation of treatment effects.* Basically, this means that both medical and behavioral scientists use the same criteria for evaluating treatment effects. An example from the literature will illustrate this problem. In a well-known study, the experimental procedure resulted in statistically significant changes in the subjects' flow rate and medication usage. At first glance, these are impressive results. However, in reading the article over again, it becomes clear that the base rate of peak-flow values was relatively high; hence, the subjects were most likely in a period of remission during the course of the study. This suggests that two of the major findings that occurred in the study—an increase in peak-flow values and a decrease in prescribed medications—

were a function of the natural course of asthma and not a result of experimental manipulations. The key was the base rates of the dependent variables at the outset of the study. Had they been very low and only slightly improved with the application of the experimental procedure, the findings would have been more relevant and important than the demonstration of statistical significance.

11. *Interpret data in a reasonable and appropriate manner.* The practice of declaring cures for asthma when none exist has long plagued behavioral studies of asthma. However, other data are interpreted in an incorrect and inappropriate manner. For example, in a presentation made recently, a group of medical and behavioral scientists asserted that the mortality of a group of children was due to psychological factors. However, what they failed to note was that there was a lack of self-management skills practiced by the children; such skills, in turn, should have been taught to the patients, but they were not. This is not only a more parsimonious explanation, but it is congruent with a massive amount of data collected as to why there is mortality from asthma among children (e.g., British Thoracic Association, 1982).

12. *Determine clinical significance of findings.* In the one intervention study that adhered to the other criteria—the investigation by Miklich and his colleagues (1977) on the use of systematic desensitization by reciprocal inhibition—statistically significant findings were obtained. However, in looking at the projected costs of applying the procedure versus limited gains likely to accrue, the authors concluded that while systematic desensitization did warrant application to some patients (e.g., those who panic during attacks), it did not warrant the technique being added to the armamentarium of proven medical treatments for asthma. It simply lacked the same clinical significance as other, more readily available and proven techniques. (As will be argued, however, relaxation training can be an essential skill to the self-management of asthma.)

BEHAVIORAL CONTRIBUTIONS TO THE MANAGEMENT AND REHABILITATION OF ASTHMATIC PATIENTS

The preceding discussion outlined criteria for conducting a medical or behavioral intervention study with asthma. It has become increasingly clear over the past two decades that large behavioral and psychological intervention projects have generally been unfruitful. There simply are no psychological or behavioral techniques that promise to take their place beside medical approaches to treating asthma per se. It is, as suggested throughout this chapter, a physical condition that requires medical intervention of some nature; consequently, this intervention will have a biochemical or immunological basis.

Free from the trappings of useless psychological theories, as well as the search for the grand cure for asthma, behavioral scientists have recently begun to focus their knowledge and expertise on other areas. The shift toward the application of behavioral and psychological techniques to both the management and rehabilitation of asthmatic patients has permitted behavioral and medical scientists, as well as patients, to better control asthma. Three basic goals for the management and rehabilitation of asthmatic patients were proposed by Creer, Renne, and Christian (1976).

First, a concerted effort should be made to decrease or eliminate any behavioral excesses exhibited by asthmatic patients, particularly those that interact with and intensify asthma. The emphasis should be on altering asthma-related behaviors rather than on attempting to change the course of asthma per se (although, as a consequence, altering these behaviors may result in changing the course of the latter).

Second, every effort should be made to teach patients to overcome any behavioral deficits they display. Many of these deficits are a consequence of asthma; it is hoped that correction of these behaviors will permit patients and their families to live more full and productive lives.

Finally, Creer and his colleagues suggested that self-monitoring and self-control skills be taught to patients. It was stated that the ultimate responsibility of their asthma rested on the shoulders of the patients. By teaching them what are widely referred to as self-management skills, it was hoped that patients could assume this responsibility.

Besides pursuing these goals during the past decade, two other trends have marked the quest to apply behavioral techniques to benefit asthmatic patients. First, while initial efforts relied heavily on the manipulation of environmental stimuli by behavioral or medical scientists, there is an increasing reliance on teaching patients to manage their asthma. There are problems where self-management procedures are not the techniques of choice; aspects of the patient's behavior require manipulation of relevant variables by behavioral or medical scientists. However, the trend remains to rely more and more on self-management training. Second, there has been a greater synthesis of medical and behavioral skills to develop these approaches. This is true not only for applying a given technique to change a specific problem, but, in particular, for the design and implementation of self-management programs.

The following categories provide a natural division for describing recent research in the area: application of behavioral techniques to change a patient's behavior; and practice of self-management skills by patients.

APPLICATION OF BEHAVIORAL TECHNIQUES TO ALTER PATIENT BEHAVIORS

Table 6.5 depicts attempts to alter behavioral excesses or deficits through the application of behavioral techniques. The list is not exhaustive, but samples the diversity of problems and approaches taken to change them. To further illustrate

TABLE 6.5
Examples of Behavioral Excesses and Deficits Amenable to Change Through
Application of Behavioral Techniques

Prevention of asthma attacks
    Behavioral excesses
        Unnecessary exposure to precipitators
        Overuse of nebulized medications
        Smoking
    Behavioral Deficits
        Medication compliance
Attack management
    Behavioral excesses
        Panic
        Overuse of hospitals
    Behavioral Deficits
        Symptom discrimination
        Medication use
        Relaxation

the variety of problems, they have been classified into two types with respect to the prevention and management of attacks.

Prevention of Attacks

BEHAVIORAL EXCESSES. The best way to prevent attacks is to teach patients to avoid known precipitators of their asthma, if possible. This was a major component of the rehabilitation program provided at the Children's Asthma Research Institute and Hospital (CARIH) in Denver (Creer, et al., 1976). For example, as noted earlier, a common trigger of childhood asthma is exercise. However, it is necessary that everyone, including asthmatic children, exercise in order to maintain their health. The key in training asthmatic youngsters is to teach them to recognize the threshold between healthy exercise and the precipitation of asthma attacks. Since they alone can learn this threshold, it is necessary that they participate in physical activities to acquire this ability. Involving all asthmatic youngsters in some type of activity was a goal of the CARIH rehabilitation program. On an outpatient basis, Baum and Creer (1986) found that, as a result of self-management training, children learned to avoid and escape from the precipitators of their attacks. Before training, 23% reported that they attempted to escape from the trigger of their attack as their initial step in the management of the episode. Following training, however, 73% of participants reported that escaping from a known precipitator was the first step they took to alleviate the distress of an incipient attack. No such changes were noted in a control group.

The overuse of asthma medications, particularly nebulized medications, has always been a source of concern to physicians. Overuse of medications can not only lead to more side effects from the drugs, but a tolerance to many asthma medications may be gradually established (e.g., Sly, 1985). The latter, in turn, can lead to the spiraling cycle of patients taking more and more medications in order to obtain relief. Ways to control this problem have generally involved closer monitoring by physicians of medications prescribed for patients. As Sly pointed out, this remains a recommended method for controlling the overuse of asthma drugs. Since many asthma medications are inhaled—medications dispensed in this manner have a rapid onset of action, require a smaller dose, and produce minimal side effects—they have often been difficult to monitor. A team of medical and behavioral scientists, however, has developed an ingenious device for monitoring such usage. Spector and his colleagues (1983) reported on the application of a chronolog, which houses any standard container of nebulized medication. Each use of the medication activates a microswitch; in turn, a memory unit in tha device stores the date and time of each inhalation of medication within four minutes of the actual usage. Later, the chronolog can be attached to another device so that data on inhaled medications can be obtained. There is no guarantee that patients actually inhaled the medications as instructed, but use of the device, coupled with patient education and close monitoring by physicians, improves the likelihood that overuse of inhaled asthma medications can be curtailed.

As noted earlier, smoking is particularly deleterious to asthmatic patients both because it may precipitate attacks and because it reduces the efficacy of some asthma medications. There have been no specific smoking-cessation programs developed for asthmatic patients per se; however, many such patients become involved with various programs such as those sponsored by the American Lung Association (ALA). There are no data available as to the effectiveness of these programs with asthmatic patients, but these patients are probably as successful as other individuals who attempt to halt smoking via this route. Data collected by the ALA indicate that at the end of one year, 2% of people who approach them, but who do not enter their programs, reportedly achieve abstinence; 12% of smokers who do enter into the ALA's programs, however, achieve the same goal (Davis, Faust, & Ordentlich, 1984). The latter percentage is slightly lower than the percentage reported by Glasgow (1978), who found an abstinence rate of 16% following introduction of self-help manuals; however, the follow-up data were gathered at three months instead of a year, so the results from both Glasgow's study and the investigation by Davis and his colleagues (1984) may have become more comparable with equal time for follow-up.

Lichtenstein (1982) reported that smoking clinics produce one-year abstinence rates of 15% to 20%, with more successful programs showing 30%–40% rates. Lando (1977, 1981) for example, has achieved abstinence rates of 50% or more by application of a broad-spectrum package, including behavioral self-control skills and rapid smoking. This seems to be the most promising approach to take with most individuals who wish to quit smoking; however, rapid smoking would likely cause more harm than good in many asthmatic patients. It is for this reason that a smoking program, tailored specifically for asthmatic patients, must be developed and tested.

BEHAVIORAL DEFICITS. One of the major ways patients can prevent asthma attacks is by taking maintenance medications as instructed. However, they frequently fail to do so, a finding not dissimilar to that found with patients afflicted by other chronic disorders (Haynes, Taylor, & Sackett, 1979). The lack of medication compliance has been documented among both adult and pediatric asthma populations, but most of the studies have been directed toward the latter group. Here, compliance has ranged from 0 to 100%. In an early study, Eney and Goldstein (1976) analyzed serum theophylline levels in a sample of asthmatic children. They detected levels in the therapeutic range in 11% of their sample, less than the therapeutic range in 65%, and no measurable drug in the remaining 24% of the sample. Sublett, Pollard, Kadlec, and Karibo (1979) found an even bleaker picture: By examining theophylline levels in 50 consecutive cases of childhood asthma admitted to a hospital emergency room, they found only one patient with levels in the therapeutic range. More recently, Miller (1982) investigated medication compliance in 21 asthmatic adolescents, aged 12 to 17. Although the theophylline dosages followed established guidelines, only 10% of the patients had serum levels in the therapuetic range. Wood, Casey, Kolski, and McCormick (1985) also analyzed serum theophylline levels in 111 children seen in an emergency room. They found that 66 percent of the youngsters were partially compliant, but 33% were totally noncompliant.

Almost the reverse was discovered in a double-blind study conducted by Baum and Creer (1986). By analyzing the serum theophylline levels of 20 asthmatic children over the course of a study, it was found that the youngsters were 100% percent compliant to medication instructions throughout the investigation. However, these children represented a sample of youngsters, recruited from a pool of 85, who volunteered for the investigation. The conclusion offered by Baum and Creer is that there appear to be differences among those who volunteer for studies with the expectation that their medications will be monitored via serum levels, and those who hold no such expectations, such as was the case in the other studies. These subject characteristics add yet another variable to the assessment of medication compliance in asthmatic patients.

Three approaches have been taken to improve medication compliance, primarily in asthmatic children (Creer et al., in press): increased medical monitoring, self-management training, and patient-generated strategies. Each will be summarized:

1. *Increased medical monitoring.* To improve compliance in the patients they investigated, Eney and Goldstein (1976) divided the youngsters into two groups. In the control group, theophylline levels were assessed, but no monitoring was provided in taking the drugs. In the monitoring group, the measurement of theophylline levels was coupled with close monitoring of the youngsters' asthma. For the latter group, compliance improved so that 47 percent achieved therapeutic levels, 51% were below therapeutic levels, and 6% showed no measurable drug. Weinstein and Cuskey (1985) investigated 39 asthmatic children over a 6-month period. A number of components were added to the intervention, including

telephone reminders and parental monitoring. The latter, coupled with parental encouragement, proved to be the most effective technique in maintaining compliance in 72% of the patients who participated in the study. Finally, while not an intervention study per se, Cluss, Epstein, Galvis, Fireman, and Friday (1984) assessed medication compliance through a riboflavin tracer. The method showed that those who took 80% percent or more of their medications experienced fewer days where they wheezed and less variability in their peak-flow rates than did noncompliant children. The major result of this finding, however, was the use of a less invasive method for detecting medication compliance (i.e., the riboflavin tracer). This has an advantage over drawing blood to assess theophylline levels, a method that seemed to be a factor in dissuading patients to volunteer for the study described by Baum and Creer (1986).

2. *Self-management.* The procedure used at CARIH was developed by Parker, Parker, and Christian (cited in Creer, 1979). Basically, it entailed shaping the youngsters to manage their own medications. Thus, while medications were initially taken when youngsters reported to the nursing station for their scheduled medications, control was gradually transferred to the children. The final step involved the youngsters controlling their medications with only periodic checks made by medical personnel to monitor the children's behavior. Results of the approach showed that the health of most children was maintained long after they returned to their homes (Creer, 1987). Data collected in a large study (Creer et al., 1987) also demonstrated that children could be taught to comply with their medication instructions through the practice of self-management skills.

3. *Self-generated medication compliance.* Schachter (1982) presented data suggesting that many individuals achieve long-term self-cure of smoking, obesity, and drug abuse. As suggested by Baum and Creer (1986), there are asthmatic patients who learned on their own to comply with medication instructions. What motivates their behavior would be of great interest in designing and implementing medication compliance programs for all chronic disorders.

Management of Attacks

BEHAVIORAL EXCESSES. Medical and behavioral scientists have cooperated to manage two types of behavioral excesses displayed by asthmatic patients during their attacks: panic and overuse of hospitals.

1. *Panic.* There are some asthmatic patients who display responses during their attacks that cause them to be labeled as panicking (Creer, 1974, 1979, 1982; Creer et al., 1976; Creer & Renne, 1968; Creer, Renne, & Chai, 1982). The label covers a broad range of responses. At one end of the spectrum, patients complain that they do not receive enough medicine or that it is ineffective. They appear agitated and frightened, a behavior that can be contagious to others

around them (including the attending medical staff). At the other end of the spectrum, there are patients who appear almost opposite to the above description. They remain silent and frozen in their beds; often, they will not signal for help when required, but can quietly lapse into unconsciousness unless monitored carefully.

The assessment of this behavior proved difficult, in part because the term "panic" was used to cover such a gamut of responses. However, reports of the problem disappeared through application of systematic desensitization by reciprocal inhibition (Wolpe, 1958). With this method, children were seen individually both for training in muscle relaxation and to obtain hierarchies of the stimuli they thought provoked the panic. Most of the hierarchies were based on an especially severe attack they had suffered in their homes with their families; in many instances, it was based on a single severe episode. Initially, there was some skepticism about the possibility of their acquiring panic behavior on the basis of one-trial learning, but this is supported by Williams (1982), who noted that many patients are likely to suffer only one particularly severe attack during their lifetimes. It was further supported by what appeared to be a modeling paradigm whereby the youngsters acquired their responses from observing others—usually their parents—panic during the children's attacks.

Following training in muscle relaxation, the youngsters were asked to imagine the fear-arousing scenes they had described which composed the hierarchies. The juxtaposition of relaxation and the anxiety supposedly elicited by the imagined stimuli led to a diminution and extinction of the panic both in hospital and home environments. Thus, systematic desensitization became an important technique in the arsenal of methods to treat panic; as noted earlier, it sometimes has value in assisting in the overall treatment of these patients (Miklich et al., 1977).

2. *Hospital overuse.* Initially, Creer (1970) referred to asthmatic patients who seemingly made an effort to be admitted to or remain in a hospital as "malingering." However, this term has so many other connotations that the label "overusers," suggested by Hochstadt, Shepard, and Lulla (1980), is preferred. The technique to alter the problem was first reported by Creer (1970) and Creer, Weinberg, and Molk (1974). Briefly, baseline data were gathered on both frequency and duration of hospital admissions in children considered to be overusers of the hospital. After this information was collected, the youngsters were exposed to a time-out procedure. This entailed the removal of TV from the children's room, limiting reading materials to school texts, and reducing the opportunities for interacting with peers. The procedure was applied during each hospitalization (Creer, 1970) or on a less frequent, aperiodic schedule (Creer et al., 1974). The results were the same: a reduction in the number and duration of hospitalizations of children thought to overuse the hospital. In the investigation by Hochstadt and his colleagues (1980), for example, this was reflected in a statistically significant reduction in the mean length of stay in the hospital from 18.3 days before treatment to 9.0 days after treatment. At the same time, the mean time between

hospitalizations increased from 48.9 days to 85.3 days as a result of application of the time-out procedure.

BEHAVIORAL DEFICITS. Several types of behavioral deficits can interfere with the management of asthma attacks. Three will be described in this review: symptom discrimination, medication use, and lack of relaxation.

1. *Symptom discrimination.* "Symptom discrimination represents a complex set of events that, when correlated, result in the detection and treatment of an asthmatic episode" (Creer, 1983b, p. 607). The correlation represents a reciprocal interaction among environmental, cognitive, physiological, and behavioral events. Unfortunately, these events may not always be correlated, thus resulting in failures to discriminate the onset of an attack. The result may be, as demonstrated by Rubinfeld and Pain (1976), that patients will report no impediment in their breathing when, at the same time, pulmonary function tests indicate that they are exhaling less than 50% of their predicted values. The reverse may also be true: Patients may claim to experience asthma when there is no indication of respiratory impairment in their pulmonary functioning (Creer et al., 1982).

A classification of the types of errors that occur in symptom discrimination was described by Creer (1983b). These range from the misperception of environmental stimuli as precipitators of attacks to failures in interpreting symptoms of an attack. Three approaches have been taken to correct these errors and to improve the patients' ability to discriminate symptoms:

a. *Predicting attacks.* The use of peak-flow meters, as well as other measures of pulmonary physiology, can assist patients in predicting the likelihood that they will suffer asthma within a specified period of time. The prototypical demonstration was reported by Taplin and Creer (1978). They entered peak-flow rates, obtained from two children, into a conditional probability equation to predict the occurrence of asthma. The base rate (or prior probability) for the occurrence of an attack and a critical peak-flow value which most enhanced the predictability of asthma were determined for each child. Two conditional probabilities were calculated for each subject: the first was the probability of asthma occurring in a 12-hour period following a flow rate less than or equal to the critical value, and the second was the probability of asthma in a 12-hour period following a flow rate greater than the critical value. Using this procedure, Taplin and Creer found an approximate 300% increase over the base rate in predicting asthma attacks in the two children. Harm, Kotses, and Creer (1985) extended the procedure and examined its usefulness with a group of 25 asthmatic youngsters. The children recorded their flow rates daily, as well as the date and the time of each attack. Two conditional posterior probabilities—identical to those described above—and the ratio of hits to misses were computed for each child at successively lower flow rates. The findings were greater than those found by Taplin and Creer (1978): The average improvement in predictability from the prior to the highest posterior probability was 491%. In addition, examination of the posterior probabilities and the ratio of hits to misses at successively lower peak-flow rates revealed another interesting finding; while the posterior probability increased at successively lower flow rates, the ratio of hits to misses, as well as the actual number of episodes predicted, decreased. In other words, more prediction errors (misses) were made, and fewer attacks predicted, at lower flow rates. This suggests that careful consideration must be made in selecting a flow-rate value most helpful for a given child.

To refine the likelihood that a patient could predict an asthma attack, we have conducted a number of studies to compare portable respiratory devices to determine their relationship to one another and to a spirometer (Harm, Kotses, & Creer, 1984; Kotses, Harver, & Creer, 1984; Wigal, Kotses, Creer, Harm, & Tinker, 1986). The results demonstrate that correlations between the instruments are lower than generally assumed; this suggests that data from the array of instruments should not be considered as equivocal, particularly in comparison to spirometric data. However, the introduction of portable spirometers, as well as the greater number of respiratory indices assessed with the instruments, will reduce the use of many of the currently available peak-flow devices. A second area of research has sought to determine how to maximize a patient's performance in using these meters and a spirometer. All of the instruments are effort-dependent in that they rely on cooperation from the patient to obtain reliable and accurate information. Both instructions (Harm, Marion, Creer, & Kotses, 1985) and subject effort (Harm, Marion, Kotses, & Creer, 1984) has been demonstrated to affect the data obtained with the instruments. These factors should be considered in using these very helpful devices.

b. *Teaching patients to attend to and correlate behavioral and physical events.* This approach resulted from the development and implementation of a self-management program for asthma (Creer, Backial, Ullman & Leung, 1986; Creer et al., 1982, 1987). However, the approach can be applied independently of such a program. Basically, the approach involves teaching patients and, in the case of children, their parents to attend to events that occur just prior to or concurrent with the onset of attacks and to correlate these events with decreases in pulmonary measures. Thus, as reported by Creer and his co-workers (Creer et al., 1982, 1987), participants learned what changes in patients signaled the onset of attacks by correlating behavioral and physical changes with decreases in peak-flow rates. After repeatedly observing that such relationships existed, the patients reported that they relied on behavioral changes, idiosyncratic to each patient, as reliable signs of the onset of asthma. Thus, an objective referent assisted the patients to develop and refine the subjective impressions they formed of an impending attack.

c. *Shaping subjective impressions.* Renne, Nau, Dietiker, and Lyon (1976) taught children to match subjective impressions of their asthma with peak-flow data. The training procedure involved classic psychophysiological techniques in that the children learned to correlate the magnitude of one response system (their subjective impressions) to the magnitude of a second response system (their respiratory status as reflected by flow rates). Renne and his colleagues instructed the youngsters to report for symptomatic treatment of their asthma at what, according to a predetermined criteria, the children perceived as increasingly higher peak-flow values. Reinforcement was added by giving the youngsters scrip, exchangeable for inexpensive gifts or the opportunity to chart their progress, when they reported with perceived pulmonary functioning at or above the established criteria. Measurements of peak flow were taken only after the children reported for treatment. Results indicated that the youngsters learned to discriminate asthmatic symptoms earlier in an attack and to report for treatment while the episodes were relatively mild.

2. *Medication use.* Renne and Creer (1976) observed that a number of asthmatic children did not appropriately use equipment designed to dispense medications during attacks. In particular, they focused on the intermittent positive-pressure breathing apparatus (IPPB machine). It was observed that children had to coordinate three responses—diaphragmatic breathing, attending to the apparatus, and inhaling the dispensed medication properly—in order for the IPPB machine to achieve its goal. By employing a multiple baseline design, shaping was carried out on each of these behaviors; training, in most instances, involved a single, 30- to 40-minute session. The results showed that the youngsters not only required less medication to control their attack—there was an 80% improvement in the efficacy of medications taken in this manner—but a procedure was developed that could be readily used by nurses and respiratory therapists to teach patients to correctly use the IPPB apparatus. In a later study, Marion, Creer, and Burns (1983) targeted behaviors required for youngsters to correctly use hand-held nebulizers. By introducing an intervention composed of shaping, modeling, and reinforcement, asthmatic children were taught to correctly use the nebulizer during their attacks. Since many medications are dispensed via this method, the study offers a technique that could be used with any asthmatic patient, no matter his or her age.

3. *Lack of relaxation.* The role of relaxation and asthma is somewhat confusing. On one hand, most physicians suggest that patients relax during their attacks. The basis for this suggestion is that perhaps relaxation will alleviate the distress of the attack. Studies by Alexander, Miklich, and Hershkoff (1972) and Alexander (1972) explored the role of relaxation by having one group of asthmatic children relax, while a second group served as controls. Peak-flow rates, obtained before and after relaxation, served as the dependent measure. The results of the two studies showed that children who had been taught to relax exhibited significant increases in their flow rates over sessions; no changes were observed with the youngsters assigned to the control condition.

More recent reports have been somewhat skeptical of the role of relaxtion and asthma. Alexander, Cropp and Chai (1979) noted that although they could demonstrate statistical significance, their results were not clinically significant. As was noted earlier, however, relaxation does seem to assist those who panic or experience other types of fear and anxiety reactions during asthma attacks. Another article on the role of relaxation, authored by Kinsman et al. (1980), had even harsher criticisms of the role of asthma in arguing against the general application of relaxation procedures to asthmatic patients.

There have always been two problems inherent in relaxation research with asthma, however. First, the studies were conducted when the patients were asymptomatic; under these conditions, their respiration may be little different from that of healthy patients. Thus, it becomes mere speculation as to whether relaxation assists asthmatic patients when there is no actual assessment of such responding during attacks. Second, the arguments of Kinsman and his colleagues (1980) are based on a drive-theory approach to relaxation in that it is averred that while some patients should relax, such a response might be harmful to other patients. The key to this position is that while anxiety should be decreased in some patients, it should be enhanced in others. The argument has some value, but it is basically untestable. What seems most appropriate is to add, when necessary, relaxation component to self-management packages where such a skill may enhance the self-monitoring, self-instruction, and decision-making skills required by patients. This approach eschews interest in either relaxation per se or the theoretical basis for such a practice; rather, as will be noted shortly, it is but one skill that may be used by patients to improve their practice of self-management procedures to control their asthma.

Self-Management of Asthma

More than with other physical disorders, there has recently been a strong push to develop and implement self-management programs for asthma, particularly childhood asthma (Creer & Winder, 1986). Not only have a number of programs been generated, but the results obtained by different groups of investigators have been presented and are available through a conference summary published by the National Institute of Allergy and Infectious Diseases (1981a, 1981b). In addition, several papers which outline significant issues in the self-management of the disorder, written by experts in their areas, as well as responses to the papers by individuals with expertise in creating and implementing such programs, were published in a special issue of the *Journal of Allergy and Clinical Immunology* (Green, Goldstein, & Parker, 1983). These sources provide background material for interested readers.

There are differences between programs developed to teach self-management skills to asthmatic patients. However, the process of self-management should entail many, if not all, of the actions depicted in Table 6.6. A discussion of self-management will rely on this outline.

TABLE 6.6
Process of Self-Management of Asthma

EDUCATION
SELF-MANAGEMENT SKILLS

1. Information gathering
   a. Self-monitoring
   b. Self-recording
2. Information processing and evaluation
3. Decision making
4. Self-instruction
   a. Stimulus change
   b. Response change

COMPETENCIES

1. Experience
2. Coping skills
   a. Reaxation
   b. Rehearsal

ATTITUDES

1. Self-motivation
2. Self-efficacy

PERFORMANCE

EDUCATION. Outside of their focus on childhood asthma, the one commonality shared by self-management programs has been a major educational component. Although the subject matter differs according to the particular program topics covered usually include a discussion of the physiology of breathing, the treatment of asthma (particularly with an emphasis on the medications taken to control the disorder), self-management skills, and the application of such skills to manage asthma. All programs cover the physiology and treatment of asthma; differences between the programs begin to emerge in elucidating self-management skills that should be practiced by participants.

SELF-MANAGEMENT SKILLS. In their review article, Thoresen and Krimil-Gray (1983) concluded that two programs in particular—Living with Asthma (Creer et al., 1986, 1987) and the Family Asthma Project (Cropp & Hindi-Alexander, 1981; Hindi-Alexander & Cropp. 1981, 1984)—"deserve recognition for their comprehensive application of the psychology of self-managed change to asthma" (Thoresen & Kirmil-Gray, 1983, pp. 605–606). Both programs used somewhat different procedures both to teach self-management skills an to assess the effectiveness of applying such training; however, overall they are more similar than dissimilar (Creer, in press). Accordingly, self-management skills taught in the Living with Asthma (LWA) and the Family Asthma Project (FAP) will be described.

1. *Information Gathering.* A major aspect of self-management is gathering information regarding a behavior or physical condition. There are two aspects of information gathering: self-monitoring and self-recording. Self-monitoring refers to participants observing and monitoring any changes that occur in relation to their asthma. This includes observing changes in respiration, as assessed by a peak-flow meter, in LWA, and monitoring the use of asthma medications in FAP.

Both FAP and LWA required participants to record information regarding a youngster's asthma. In LWA, for example, this involved recording four types of information: (a) whether a child suffered an attack during any 24-hour period, as well as his or her impresssion of the severity of the episode; (b) the highest peak-flow value obtained in both the morning and afternoon; (c) how compliant a child was to any medication instructions; and, (d) an estimate of any expenses incurred because of asthma. In addition, children in LWA completed a report of an attack after each asthmatic episode they experienced.

2. *Information processing and evaluation.* This involved participants processing and evaluating information they gathered about themselves. Creer (in press) noted that an acronym for the exact steps involved in information processing and evaluation is "CAPE." This means that participants: (a) *c*ollected information about their condition; (b) continually *a*nalyzed this information; (c) determined if there was a potential *p*roblem that required action on their part; and, (d) *e*valuated the problem with respect to possible solutions they might take. Of particular interest was the fact that the youngsters processed information about their respiration and any deviations from their usual breathing patterns. Any changes, in turn, required evaluation on their part as to whether or not some course of action was necessary.

3. *Decision making.* This required children first to consider potential solutions to the problem they detected and evaluated and then to select the most appropriate solution from among these choices (Creer, 1986, 1987, in press). Both education and experience with asthma were factors influencing the youngsters' decision with respect to a given situation. In addition, strategies worked out jointly by patients and their physicians would have dictated many decisions made by patients.

4. *Self-instruction.* This refers to statements made by oneself to prompt, direct, or maintain behavior (O'Leary & Dubey, 1979). Self-instruction was a skill of self-management taught to participants in both FAP and LWA. Both programs emphasized that youngsters cooperate with their physicians to determine the best strategy to manage an incipient attack. Usually this involved the children performing a sequence of actions (CAPE) to bring an attack under control. The exact sequence varied from child to child; a general example of such steps, however,

has been described (Creer, 1980; Creer et al., 1982, 1985a, 1985b, in press). As noted by Creer and Kotses (1983):

> From the outset, they were taught to conceive of asthma management as a chain of responses. Each link in the response chain occurs in a sequence so that the patient performed one response, then a second, and so on until control was established over the episode. By working in conjunction with the physician, a patient and his or her family could develop a coherent script that could be performed by the patient in the event of an attack. Management of asthma is more readily achieved when a patient follows a predetermined sequence of responses; self-instruction in turn becomes the core of the subsequent recall and performance of such a sequence. (p. 1032)

As noted by Creer (in press), by managing their asthma in such a manner, the patients also mimicked the way experienced physicians treat asthma (i.e., initiate a step, evaluate its effect on asthma, initiate a second step if necessary, etc.).

Self-induced stimulus change and self-induced response change were also used by children to manage their asthma. The former refers to a youngster avoiding, if possible, known precipitators of his or her asthma. As noted by Baum and Creer (1986), children learned to perform self-induced stimulus change. Self-induced response change refers to the ability of patients to alter their responses to either avoid or alleviate an attack. A child learning to alter exercise in order to avoid an attack characterizes the application of self-induced response change (Creer et al., 1976).

COMPETENCIES. These refer to the skills an asthmatic child knows and can perform. They do not reflect as much a static accumulation of knowledge about asthma as they represent the ability to generate, transform, and apply information to solve problems (Creer, in press). Skills pertinent to asthma include the competency, intelligence, and maturity required to manage the disorder; these are required to perform the sequence of behaviors, as described above, to bring an attack under control. There are two major types of coping skills (Creer, 1986, 1987, in press). Relaxation has already been discussed; it is important in self-management because if relaxed, the patient can concentrate on performing the steps required to control asthma. If her or she is not relaxed, there is the likelihood that the patient's asthma will intensify and become more difficult to manage. Rehearsal of self-management skills permits the child to better perform such actions when necessary. In LWA, for example, rehearsal of skills involved everyone in the family, ranging from a child rehearsing actions required to bring his or her attack under control to the parents rehearsing how they would react if more intensive treatment were required (e.g., what to ask the child's physician, the quickest way to the nearest emergency room, etc.).

ATTITUDES. The attitudes of the child, as well as those of the parents, were described by Creer (1986, 1987, in press) as the gas that fuels the entire self-management effort. Two important types of attitudes are important: self-motivation and self-efficacy. Self-motivation refers to the motivation of the patient to make a contribution to the managment of his or her asthma. If he or she so wishes, a patient can have a substantial impact on the overall control of his or her asthma; as will be noted, self-management is effective when applied to asthma. By the same token, however, any asthmatic patient can defeat the best medical advice and instructions if he or she wishes. Merely disregarding medication instructions, as so many do, is certainly apt to lead to the patient's admission to an emergency room for the treatment of his or her attack. Self-motivation depends, to a considerable extent, on how the patient views future outcomes of his or her behavior. If a patient anticipates that certain actions will bring relief, he or she will perform such actions; if he or she expects other outcomes, such performance will not be exhibited. Self-efficacy refers to what we believe ourselves to be capable of doing as strongly influencing the choices and decisions about what we actually do. Again, we have two possibilities: If the patient feels that he or she is capable of performing skills required to control asthma, he or she will persistently expend the effort required to do so. If he or she feels incapable of such performance, he or she may not take any action to bring the attack under control. Thus, self-efficacy can play a major role in affecting decisions, effort, and persistence with respect to self-management and asthma.

PERFORMANCE. If what the patient does proves to be effective, he or she will not only execute the skills required to control an asthma attack, but there will be an increase in the patient's confidence about his or her ability to do so in the future. As depicted in Table 6.6, successful performance of self-management skills provides a feedback loop that strengthens a patient's knowledge about asthma, his or her ability to perform self-management skills, his or her competencies with respect to such performance, and his or her expectations about himself or herself and his or her overall perceptions about managing asthma.

The dependent measures used in studies of the self-management of asthma are depicted in Table 6.7. As noted, a variety of variables have been assessed in these studies; they are appropriate to any behavioral or medical intervention program with asthma.

A. *Mortality data*. Asthma is not a disorder that claims a large number of lives each year. Thus, despite a trend toward an increase in deaths due to childhood asthma in the U.S., the disorder only claimed 104 children in 1982 (*NCHS Monthly Vital Statistics Report*, 1984). However, an analysis of the reasons children die from asthma suggests that a primary factor is that they wait too long to initiate treatment (British Thoracic Association, 1982) and fail to practice self-management skills (Creer, 1985). Thus, if only a few lives were saved each year, it would be an impressive testimony to self-management programs for asthma.

B. *Morbidity data*. By far, the major focus of attention has been directed toward

TABLE 6.7
Dependent Measures Applicable to the Assessment of Self-Management Programs for Asthma

---

A. Mortality data
B. Morbidity data
   1. Paper-and-pencil instruments
      a. Behavioral checklists
      b. Knowledge-of-asthma quizzes
      c. Attitude surveys
      d. Locus-of-control measures
      e. Self-concept measures
      f. Self-efficacy measures
   2. Asthma diaries
   3. Reports of attacks/episodes
   4. Pulmonary function measures
   5. School and hospital data
   6. Medication scores
   7. Economic indices
   8. Family relationship indices

---

assessing changes in morbidity indices that occur as a result of self-management. Here is where the real impact of asthma is experienced by both patients and their families; thus, it seems only appropriate that such dependent variables should be added to studies. The major assessment indices used thus far include:

1. *Paper-and-pencil measures.* A number of paper-and-pencil instruments have been developed for assessing self-management programs with asthma. The strength of such instruments is that they provide considerable information that, unless assessed in such a manner, would be unavailable to the investigator; the weakness of such instruments is that their reliability and validity is rarely established (Creer & Winder, 1986). Hence, data gathered in many of the studies are, at best, equivocal; at worst, they are uninterpretable. However, I will briefly summarize instruments that do have value, as well as any data gathered through use of the paper-and-pencil measures.

    a. *Behavioral checklists.* These are useful instruments because they reveal behaviors that may be targeted for change in a self-management program. An example of such an instrument is the Asthma Problem Behavior Checklist (Creer, Marion, & Creer, 1983). It has demonstrable validity and reliability; besides proving to be useful in targeting behavior potentially amenable to change, it can serve as a pre–post assessment measure in a self-management study.

    b. *Knowledge-of-asthma questionnaires.* All self-management programs have questionnaires to determine whether or not participants acquire knowledge of asthma through their involvement with a self-management program. Both FAP and LWA used valid and reliable knowledge questionnaires; statistically significant changes in knowledge of asthma were reported with the participants in both studies.

c. *Attitude surveys.* LWA used reliable and valid surveys to assess changes in the attitudes of children and their parents as a consequence of their participation in a self-management program. Significant positive changes occurred with both groups. The surveys have also been applied successfully in other asthma self-management programs, particularly the program sponsored by the American Lung Association, *Superstuff* (Weiss, 1981).

d. *Locus-of-control measures.* FAP used two standardized locus-of-control instruments—the Multidimensional Health Locus of Control (Wallston, Wallston, & DeVellis, 1978) and the Children's Health Locus of Control (Parcel & Meyer, 1978). LWA employed the I-E Locus of Control (Rotter, 1966) with parents involved with the program. In both FAP and LWA, statistically significant changes were obtained with the locus-of-control measures as a result of participation in the self-management programs. This indicates that participants shifted their perceptions to believe themselves, not others, to be basically responsible for the health of themselves or their children.

e. *Self-concept measures.* LWA used the Piers-Harris Children's Self-Concept Scale (Piers & Harris, 1966) to determine if there would be any positive changes in the attitudes of children toward themselves as a result of their participating in self-management training. Results indicated that a statistically significant change occurred.

f. *Self-efficacy measures.* Many of the self-management programs were designed and implemented before Bandura (1977) introduced his concept of self-efficacy. However, valid and reliable measures to assess self-efficacy, described in the last section, in asthmatic patients have since been developed (Tobin, Wigal, Winder, Holroyd, & Creer, 1987). Such instruments should prove to be useful in future self-management programs.

2. *Asthma diaries.* Patient self-reports represent the best and the worst data gathered in self-management studies for asthma (Creer & Winder, 1986). In both FAP and LWA, a wealth of data were gathered via asthma diaries. To increase the accuracy of self-reports, certain procedures were followed. In LWA, children were taught to complete the diaries while their parents served as reliability checks. This improved the reliability of the collected information. In both LWA and FAP, external checks of the data were made by comparing the information against that collected by schools, hospitals, physicians, and so forth. This, too, improved the overall reliability of diary data.

A mass of data was collected in both studies through the use of asthma diaries (for example, data from over 10,000 days were recorded by participants in LWA). A number of statistically significant findings emerged from both studies. In FAP, for example, the acquisition and practice of self-management skills resulted in a significant increase in total activity and a significant decrease in both health-care visits and school absenteeism. This, as well as other data, will be described further later. In LWA, major findings included significant improvements in the pulmonary physiology of participants and a reduction in the number of asthma attacks suffered by children involved in the project. In the year prior to their acquisition of self-management skills, the children averaged five attacks per month, or more than an attack per week. In the year following their participation in LWA, however, they reportedly experienced an average of only one attack per month. Other information, particularly as concerned compliance to medication instructions, was gathered with the asthma diary in LWA.

3. *Reports of attacks/episodes.* In LWA, a rich vein of information was gathered by having children complete a report of an attack following each asthmatic episode they experienced (Creer, in press). This not only indicated the sequence of steps taken by the youngsters to bring their attacks under control, but data as to the precipitators of their attacks. The same report format later proved invaluable in the study by Baum and Creer (1986) in assessing changes in steps taken to manage attacks that occurred as a result of self-management training.

4. *Pulmonary function measures.* In LWA, each child was given a Mini-Wright Peak Flow meter and asked to record the highest of three peak-flow values taken both in the morning and the evening. The results gathered from this data permitted us to calculate the conditional probabilities used to improve the ability of the instrument to predict the likelihood of future attacks (Harm, Kotses, & Creer, 1985; Taplin & Creer, 1978). With the emergence of more and less expensive pulmonary instruments, it can be confidently stated that measures of pulmonary physiology will be added to most future studies on the self-management of asthma.

5. *School and hospital data.* Asthmatic children miss a considerable amount of school each year. In 1963, Schiffer and Hunt reported that asthma was a leading cause of school absenteeism by accounting for nearly one fourth of days lost from school because of chronic illness conditions. Two decades later, the disorder still ranks as a leading cause of school absenteeism; for example, a review of recent school absenteeism data from across the U.S. found that an average of 18 days were lost each year because of childhood asthma.

Significant changes were reported by both FAP and LWA as a result of the acquisition and practice of self-management skills. Hindi-Alexander and Cropp (1984) found that an almost 50% decrease in school absenteeism occurred as a result of FAP. An even greater reduction in school absenteeism was reported by Creer (in press) and Creer et al. (1987); the mean number of days absent from school was 17.5 in the year prior to the youngsters' involvement with LWA. This decreased to an average of 6.4 days in the year after the children received self-management training, a 273 percent decrease in emergency room visits, and a 44% reduction in hospital admissions of the youngsters involved with FAP. These were highly significant changes. Hospital admissions were not assessed in LWA—many of the children lived in rural areas and were rarely admitted to hospitals for any reason. However, using a condensed adaptation of LWA, Winder (1984) found significant decreases in both physician visits and the use of hospital emergency rooms. Thus, where it can be obtained, hospital data are another highly useful dependent index to be incorporated into a self-management program.

6. *Medication scores*. Where it can be collected, medication data are also a valuable addition to a self-management program. Hindi-Alexander and Cropp (1984) found that there was a 10% reduction in the medication score they used—indicating that the patients required less medicine—as a result of FAP. In LWA, however, we were unable to assess medication scores because the subjects were recruited from a number of physicians who subscribed to different philosophies as to the prescription of medications for the treatment of asthma. For this and other reasons described by Creer and Winder (1986), medication scores are sometimes difficult to obtain. However, as occurred in FAP, reducing the amount of medications taken by patients through the acquisition and practice of self-management skills is certainly a worthy outcome.

7. *Economic indices*. Both FAP and LWA found that self-management was a highly economical approach to the treatment of asthma. A reduction in the costs of hospitalization and medicine, as occurred in FAP, represent significant savings to families, health-insurance companies, and, in the end, all of us. In LWA, a concerted attempt was made to gather economic data with respect to asthma. Based on the receipts furnished by families who paid for the costs of their children's asthma but who were later reimbursed by insurance companies, it was found that there was a 66% savings in health-care expenditures for asthma as a result of LWA. The decrease in health-care expenses is even geater when indirect costs are entered into the total equation. According to data reported by Marion, Creer, and Reynolds (1985), the latter represented more of an economic burden to participants in LWA than did the direct costs of asthma. Little more need to be added except, in calculating cost-benefit analyses of such programs, they are indeed economical.

8. *Family relationship indices*. In a 12-year study, Renne and Creer (1985) conducted a large study to investigate the interactions of families where there was a child with asthma. This analysis involved following a complex observation described by Renne and Creer, the details of which are not relevant to the current discussion. What is important is that application of components of LWA proved to be invaluable in reducing the friction between family members where there was a child with asthma. Although this is a tangential finding in the overall puzzle of asthmatic children and their families, it does suggest that self-management training can improve the significant area of family relationships.

SUMMARY

Three general themes have been interwoven into this chapter. First, the respiratory condition of asthma has been described. This included not only discussing characteristics of the disorder, but providing a description of both stimuli that trigger attacks and possible mechanisms involved in asthma. Second, a conceptual schema with potential relevance to both behavioral and medical scientists has been outlined. The purpose here was to offer a method for improving the integration of medical and behavioral efforts with respect to asthma. Finally, behavioral contributions to asthma have been briefly sketched by emphasizing how knowledge from medicine and behavioral science can be synthesized to promote the development of more effective ways to treat asthmatic patients.

It is imperative that even greater integration of medical and behavioral knowledge occur in the future. Asthma is increasingly becoming a health problem of significant concern to all segments of society. This is reflected in several crucial indices. For example, the percentage of children with chronic illnesses, including asthma, more than doubled between 1958 and 1981 (Creer, & Kotses, in press). This means that thousands more youngsters and, eventually, adults will suffer from asthma in the decades ahead. Costs for the disorder continue to escalate. Reed (1985) reported that approximately $382 million was spent in the United States in 1983 for medications taken to treat airway disease, especially asthma. A similar trend has been reported in world surveys (Mitchell, 1985). Furthermore, the number of patients hospitalized for asthma is surprisingly high: Not ony is asthma the leading reason for pediatric hospitalization in the U.S. (Reed, 1985), but a similar tendency has been observed in a number of countries around the world (Mitchell, 1985). These ominous signs indicate that more attention must be directed at solving the riddle of asthma, a disorder that will require greater medical and behavioral knowledge, plus cooperation between these disciplines, before it will be conquered.

REFERENCES

Alexander, A. B. (1972). Systematic relaxation and flow rates in asthmatic children: Relationship to emotional precipitants and anxiety. *Journal of Psychosomatic Research, 16,* 405–410.

Alexander, A. B. (1981). Behavioral approaches in the treatment of bronchial asthma. In C. F. Prokop & L. A. Bradley (Eds.), *Medical psychology: Contributions to behavioral medicine* (pp. 373–394. New York: Academic Press.

Alexander, A. B., Cropp, G. J. A., & Chai, H. (1979). Effects of relaxation training in children with asthma. *Journal of Applied Behavior Analysis, 12,* 27–35.

Alexander, A. B., Miklich, D. R., & Hershkoff, H. (1972). The immediate effects of systematic relaxation on peak expiratory flow rates in asthmatic children. *Psychosomatic Medicine, 34,* 388–394.

American Thoracic Society Committee on Diagnostic Standards for Nontuberculous Diseases. (1962). Definitions and classification of chronic bronchitis, asthma, and pulmonary emphysema. *American Review of Respiratory Disease, 85,* 762–768.

Bandura, A. (1977). Self-efficacy: Toward a unifying theory of behavioral change. *Psychological Review, 84,* 191–215.

Baum, D., & Creer, T. L. (1986). Medication compliance in children with asthma. *Journal of Asthma, 23,* 49–59.

Bonner, J. R. (1984). The epidemiology and natural history of asthma. *Clinics in Chest Medicine, 5*, 557-565.
Branscomb, B. V. (1984). The difficult asthmatic. *Clinics in Chest Medicine, 5*, 695-713.
British Thoracic Association (1982). Death from asthma in two regions of England. *British Medical Journal, 285*, 1251-1255.
Chai, H., & Newcomb, R. W. (1973). Pharmacologic management of childhood asthma. *American Journal of Diseases of Children, 125*, 757-765.
Chai, H., Purcell, K., & Falliers, C. J. (1968). Therapeutic and investigational evaluation of asthmatic children. *Journal of Allergy, 41*, 23-46.
Cherniack, R. M., & Cherniack, L. (1983). *Respiration in health and disease* (3rd ed.) Philadelphia: W. B. Saunders.
Clark, T. J. H. (1977). Definition of asthma for chinical trials. In J. E. Stark, & J. V. Collins (Eds.), Methods in clinical trials in asthma. *British Journal of Diseases of the Chest,71*, 225-226.
Clark, T. J. H. (1985). The Philip Ellman lecture: The circadian rhythm of asthma. *British Journal of Diseases of the Chest, 79*, 115-124.
Cluss, P. A., Epstein, L. H., Galvis, S. A., Fireman, P., & Friday, G. (1984). Effects of compliance for chronic asthmatic children. *Journal of Consulting and Clinical Psychology, 52*, 909-910.
Creer, T. L. (1970). The use of a time-out from positive reinforcement procedure with asthmatic children. *Journal of Psychosomatic Research, 14*, 117-120.
Creer, T. L. (1974). Biofeedback and asthma. *Advances in Asthma and Allergy, 1*, 6-11.
Creer, T. L. (1978). Asthma: Psychologic aspects and management. In E. Middleton, Jr., C. E. Reed, & E. F. Ellis (Eds.), *Allergy: Principles and practice* (pp. 796-811). St. Louis: C. V. Mosby Co.
Creer, T. L. (1979). *Asthma therapy: A behavioral health care system for respiratory disorders.* New York: Springer.
Creer, T. L. (1980). Self-management behavioral strategies for asthmatics. *Behavioral Medicine, 7*, 14-24.
Creer, T. L. (1982). Asthma. *Journal of Consulting and Clinical Psychology, 50*, 912-921.
Creer, T. L. (1983a). Respiratory disorders. In T. G. Burish & L. A. Bradley (Eds.), *Coping with chronic diseases: Research and applications* (pp. 316-336). New York: Academic Press.
Creer, T. L. (1983b). Response: Self-management psychology and the treatment of childhood asthma. *Journal of Allergy and Clinical Immunology, 72* (Part 2), 607-610.
Creer, T. L. (1985). Reflections on residential treatment centers for childhood asthma. *Pediatrics of Japan, 26*, 951-956.
Creer, T. L. (1986). Is your asthmatic patient his own worst enemy? *Journal of Respiratory Diseases,* 27-32.
Creer, T. L. (1987). Psychological and neurophysiological aspects of childhood asthma. In D. G. Tinkelman, C. J. Falliers, & C. K. Naspitz (Eds.), *Childhood asthma: Pathophysiology and treatment* (pp. 341-371). New York: Marcel Dekker, Inc.
Creer, T. L. (in press). Asthma. In W. Linden (Eds.), *Biological barriers in behavioral medicine.* New York: Plenum Press.
Creer, T. L., Backial, M., Ullman, S., & Leung, P. (1986). *Living with asthma* (NIH Publication No. 86-2364). Washington: U.S. Department of Health and Human Services.
Creer, T. L., Backial, M., Burns, K. L., Leung, P., Marion, R. J., Miklich, D. R., Taplin, P. S., & Ullman, S. (1987). *The evolution and development of Living with Asthma.* Manuscript submitted for publication.
Creer, T. L., Harm, D. L., & Marion, R. J. (in press). Asthma. In D. K. Routh (Ed.), *Handbook of pediatiric psychology.* New York: Guilford Press.
Creer, T. L., & Kotses, H. (1983). Asthma: Psychological aspects and management. In E. Middleton, Jr., C. E. Reed, & E. F. Ellis (Eds.) *Allergy: principles and practice* (2nd ed., pp. 1015-1036). St. Louis: C. V. Mosby.

Creer, T. L., & Kotses, H. (in press). Asthma. In T. H. Ollendick & M. Herson (Eds.), *Handbook of child psychopathology (second editon).* New York: Plenum Press.
Creer, T. L., Marion, R. J., & Creer, P. P. (1983). The Asthma Problem Behavior Checklist: Parental perceptions of the behavior of asthmatic children. *Journal of Asthma, 20,* 97-104.
Creer, T. L., & Renne, C. M. (1968). *Panic in asthmatic children.* Unpublished manuscript, Children's Asthma Research Institute and Hospital.
Creer, T. L., Renne, C. M., & Chai, H. (1982). The application of behavior techniques to childhood asthma. In D. C. Russo & J. W. Varni (Eds.), *Behavioral pediatrics: Research and practice* (pp. 27-66). New York: Plenum.
Creer, T. L., Renne, C. M., & Christian, W. P. (1976). Behavioral contributions to rehabilitation and childhood asthma. *Rehabilitation Literature, 37,* 226-232, 247.
Creer, T. L., Weinberg, E., & Molk, L. (1974). Managing a problem hospital behavior: Malingering. *Journal of Behavior Therapy and Experimental Psychiatry, 5,* 259-262.
Creer, T. L., & Winder, J. A. (1986). The self-management of asthma. In K. A. Holroyd & T. L. Creer (Eds.), *Self-management in health psychology and behavioral medicine* (pp. 268-303). New York: Academic Press.
Cropp, G., & Hindi-Alexander, M. (1981). Program at Children's Hospital in Buffalo. In *Self-management educational programs for childhood asthma. Volume II: Manuscripts* (pp. 245-256). Bethesda, MD: National Institute of Allergy and Infectious Diseases.
Dahms, T. E., Bolin, J. F., & Slavin, R. G. (1981). Passive smoking: Effects on bronchial asthma. *Chest, 80,* 530-534.
Davies, R. J., Blainey, A. D., & Pepys, J. (1983). Occupational asthma. In E. Middleton, Jr., C. E. Reed, & E. F. Ellis (Eds.), *Allergy: Principles and practice* (2nd ed. pp. 1037-1065). St Louis: C. V. Mosby Co.
Davis, A. L., Faust, R., & Ordentilich, M. (1984). Self-help smoking cessation and maintenance program: a comparative study with 12-month follow-up by the American Lung Association. *American Journal of Public Health, 14,* 1212-1217.
Eney, R. D., & Goldstein, E. O. (1976). Compliance of chronic asthmatics with oral administration of theophylline as measured by serum and salivary levels. *Pediatrics, 57,* 513-517.
Feinberg, G., & Jackson, M. A. (1983). *The chain of immunology.* Oxford, England: Blackwell Scientific Publications.
Fischer, T. J., Guilfoile, T. D., Kesarwala, H. H., Winant, J. G., Jr., Kearns, G. L., Gartside, P. S., & Moomaw, C. J. (1983). Adverse pulmonary responses to aspirin and acetaminophen in chronic childhood asthma. *Pediatrics, 71,* 313-318.
Fletcher, C. M., & Pride, N. B. (1984). Definitions of emphysema, chronic bronchitis, asthma, and airflow obstruction: 25 years on from the CIBA symposium. *Thorax, 39,* 81-85.
French, T. M., & Alexander, F. (1941). Psychogenic factors in bronchial asthma. *Psychosomatic Medicine Monographs,* No. 4.
Glasgow, R. E. (1978). Effects of a self-control manual, rapid smoking, and amount of therapist contact in smoking reduction. *Journal of Consulting and Clinical Psychology, 46,* 1439-1447.
Gortmaker, S. L., Walker, D. K. Jacobs, F. H., & Ruch-Ross, H. (1982). Parental smoking and the risk of childhood asthma. *American Journal of Public Health, 72,* 574-579.
Green, L. W., Goldstein, R., & Parker, S. R. (Eds.). (1983). Workshop proceedings on self-management of childhood asthma. *Journal of Allergy and Clinical Immunology, 72* (Part 2).
Griffin, M., Weiss, J. W., Leitch, A. G., McFadden, E. R., Jr., Corey, E. J., Austen, K. F., & Drazen. J. M. (1983). Effects of Leukotriene D on the airways in asthma. *New England Journal of Medicine, 30,* 436-439.
Harm, D. L., Kotses, H., & Creer, T. L. (1984). Portable peak flow meters: Intrasubject comparisons. *Journal of Asthma, 21,* 9-13.
Harm, D. L., Kotses, H., & Creer, T. L. (1985). Improving the ability of peak flow rates to predict asthma. *Journal of Allergy and Clinical Immunology, 76,* 688-694.

Harm, D. L., Marion, R. J., Creer, T. L., & Kotses, H. (1985). Effects of instructions on performing forced expiratory maneuvers on pulmonary function measures. *Journal of Asthma, 22,* 289-294.
Harm, D. L., Marion, R. J., Kotses, H., & Creer, T. L. (1984). Effect of subject effort on pulmonary function measures. *Journal of Asthma, 21,* 295-298.
Haynes, R. B., Taylor, D. W., & Sackett, D. L. (Eds.). (1979). *Compliance with therapeutic regimens.* Baltimore: Johns Hopkins University Press.
Hindi-Alexander, M., & Cropp, G. J. A. (1981). Community and family programs for children with asthma. *Annals of Allergy, 46,* 143-148.
Hindi-Alexander, M. C., & Cropp, G. J. A. (1984). Evaluation of a family asthma program. *Journal of Allergy and Clinical Immunology, 74,* 505-510.
Hochstadt, N., Shepard, J., & Lulla, S. H. (1980). Reducing hospitalizations of children with asthma. *Journal of Pediatrics, 97,* 1012-1015.
Ishizawka, K., & Ishizawka, T. (1967). Identification of IgE antibodies as a carrier of reaginic activity. *Journal of Immunology, 99,* 1187-1198.
Jones, R. S. (1976). *Asthma in children.* Acton, MA: Publishing Sciences Group.
Kaliner, M. (1985). Mast cell mediators and asthma. *Chest, 87,* 25-55.
Kinsman, R. A., Dirks, J. F., Jones, N. F., & Dahlem, N. W. (1980). Anxiety reduction in asthma: Four catches to general application. *Psychosomatic Medicine, 42,* 397-405.
Knapp, P. H., & Mathe, A. A. (1985). Pyschophysiologic aspects of bronchial asthma. In E. B. Weiss, M. S. Segal, & M. Stein (Eds.), *Bronchial asthma: Mechanisms and therapeutics (2nd ed.,* pp. 914-931).
Kotses, H., Harver, A., & Creer, T. L. (1984). An intraindividual comparison of standard and mini-Wright scores. *Annals of Allergy, 52,* 419-422.
Lando, H. (1977). Successful treatment of smokers with a broad-spectrum behavioral approach. *Journal of Consulting and Clinical Psychology, 45,* 361-366.
Lando, H. A. (1981). Effects on preparation, experimenter contact, and a maintained reduction alternative on a broad-spectrum program for eliminating smoking. *Addictive Behavior, 6,* 123-135.
Leigh, D. (1953). Asthma and the psychiatrist: A critical review. *International Archives of allergy and Applied Immunology, 4,* 227-246.
Lichtenstein, E. (1982). The smoking problem: A behavioral perspective. *Journal of Consulting and Clinical Psychology, 50,* 804-819.
Loren, M. L., Leung, P. K., Cooley, R. L., Chai, H., Bell, T. D., & Buck, V. M. (1978). Irreversibility of obstructive changes in severe asthma in children, *Chest, 74,* 126-129.
Marion, R. J., Creer, T. L., & Burns, K. L. (1983). Training asthmatic children to use a nebulizer correctly. *Journal of Asthma, 20,* 183-188.
Marion, R. J., Creer, T. L., & Reynolds, R. V. C. (1985). Direct and indirect costs associated with the management of childhood asthma. *Annals of Allergy, 54,* 1-4.
McFadden, E. R., Jr. (1980). Asthma: Pathophysiology. *Seminars in Respiratory Medicine, 1,* 297-303.
McFadden, E. R., Jr. (1984). Pathogenesis of asthma. *Journal of Allergy and Clinical Immunology, 73,* 413-424.
McFadden, E. R., Jr., & Stevens, J. B. (1983). A history of asthma. In E. Middleton, Jr., C. E. Reed, & E. F. Ellis (Eds.), *Allergy: Principles and practice* (2nd ed, pp. 805-809). St. Louis: C. V. Mosby Co.
Middleton, E., Jr., Reed, C. E., & Ellis, E. F. (Eds.). (1983). *Allergy: Principles and practice (2nd ed.).* St. Louis: C. V. Mosby Co.
Miklich, D. R. (1977). Chronic homeostatic vagal efferent activity turndown: A theory of asthma. *Medical Hypotheses, 3,* 226-234.
Miklich, D. R., Renne, C. M., Creer, T. L., Alexander, A. B., Chai, H., Davis, M. H., Hoffman, A., & Danker-Brown, P. (1977). The clinical utility of behavior therapy as an adjunctive treatment for asthma. *Journal of Allergy and Clinical Immunology, 60,* 285-294.
Miller, K. A. (1982). Theophylline compliance in adolescent patients with chronic asthma. *Journal of Adolescent Health Care, 3,* 177-179.

Mitchell, E. A. (1985). International trends in hospital admission rates for asthma. *Archives of Disease in Childhood, 60,* 376-378.

Murphy, R. H., Jr. (1976). Industrial disease with asthma. In E. B. Weiss & M. S. Segal (Eds.), *Bronchial asthma: Mechanisms and therapeutics* (pp. 517-536). Boston: Little, Brown & Co.

National Institute of Allergy and Infectious Diseases. (1981a). *Self-management educational programs for childhood asthma. Volume I: Conference summary.* Bethesda, MD: NIAID.

National Institute of Allergy and Infectious Diseases. (1981b). *Self-management educational programs for childhood asthma. Volume II: Manuscripts.* Bethesda, MD: NIAID.

NCHS Monthly Vital Statistics Report. (1984, December 20). *Advance report of final mortality statistics, 1982, 33.* Washington, D. C.: U.S. Department of Health and Human Services.

O'Leary, S. G., & Dubey, D. R. (1979). Applications of self-control procedures by children: A review. *Journal of Applied Behavior Analysis, 12,* 449-465.

Parcel, G. S. & Meyer, M. P. (1978). Development of an instrument to measure children's health locus of control. *Health Education Monographs, 6,* 149-159.

Pearlman, D. S. (1984). Bronchial asthma: A perspective from childhood to adulthood. *American Journal of Diseases of Children, 138,* 459-466.

Piers, E. V., & Harris, D. B. (1966). Age and other correlates of self-concept in children. *Journal of Educational Psychology, 55,* 91-95.

Porter, R., & Birch, J. (Eds.). (1971). Report of the working group on the definition of asthma. *Identification of asthma.* London: Churchill Livingston.

Purcell, K. (1963). Distinctions between subgroups of asthmatic children: Children's perceptions of events associated with asthma. *Pediatrics,* 486-494.

Purcell, K., & Weiss, J. H. (1970). Asthma. In C. C. Costello (Ed.), *Symptoms of psychopathology* (pp. 597-623). New York: John Wiley & Sons, Inc.

Reed, C. E. (1985, April). *New therapeutic approaches in asthma.* Paper presented at the 41st Annual Meeting of the American Academy of Allergy and Immunology, New York, NY.

Reed, C. E., & Townley, R. G. (1978). Asthma: Classification and pathogenesis. In E. Middleton, Jr., C. E. Reed, & E. F. Ellis (Eds.), *Allergy: Principles and practice* (pp. 659-677). St. Louis: C. V. Mosby Co.

Reed, C. E., & Townley, R. G. (1983). Asthma: Classification and pathogenesis. In E. Middleton, Jr., C. E. Reed, & E. F. Ellis (Eds.), *Allergy: Principles and practice* (2nd ed., pp. 811-831). St. Louis: C. V. Mosby Co.

Rees, J. (1984). ABC of asthma: Clinical course. *British Medical Journal, 288,* 1441-1442.

Renne, C. M. (1982). *Asthma in families: Behavioral analysis and treatment* (Final Report Grant No. RO1-HL 22021). Bethesda, MD: National Heart, Lung, and Blood Institute.

Renne, C. M., & Creer, T. L. (1976). The effects of training on the use of inhalation therapy equipment by children with asthma. *Journal of Applied Behavior Analysis, 9,* 1-11.

Renne, C. M., & Creer, T. L. (1981). [The rehabilitation of children with chronic asthma]. Unpublished raw data.

Renne, C. M., & Creer T. L. (1985). Asthmatic children and their families. In M. L. Walraich & D. K. Routh (Eds.), *Advances in developmental and behavioral pediatrics* (pp. 41-81). Greenwich, CT: Jai Press.

Renne, C. M., Nau, E., Dietiker, K. E., & Lyon, R. (1976, December). *Latency in seeking asthma treatment as a function of achieving successively higher flow rate criteria.* Paper presented at 10th Annual Convention of the Association for the Advancement of Behavior Therapy, New York, N.Y.

Rotter, J. B. (1966). Generalized expectancies for internal versus external control of reinforcement. *Psychological Monographs, 80* (1, Whole No. 609).

Rubinfeld, A. R., & Pain, M. C. F. (1976, April 24). Perception of asthma. *The Lancet,* 882-884.

Sakula, A. (1984). Sir John Floyer's *A Treatise of the Asthma. Thorax, 39,* 248-254.

Schachter, S. (1982). Recidivism and self-cure of smoking and obesity. *American Psychologist, 37,* 436-444.

Schiffer, C. G., & Hunt, E. P. (1963). *Illness among children* (Children's Bureau Publication No. 405). Washington, DC: U.S. Goverment Printing Office.

Siegel, S. C., Katz, R. M., & Rachelefsky, G. S. (1983). Asthma in infancy and childhood. In E. Middleton, Jr., C. E. Reed, & E. F. Ellis (Eds.), *Allergy: Principles and practice (2nd ed.*, pp. 863–900). St. Louis: C. V. Mosby.

Sly, R. M. (1985). Adverse effects and complications of treatment with beta-adrenergic agonist drugs. *Journal of Allergy and Clinical Immunology, 75*, 443–449.

Smith, S. B. (1985). Excercise-induced asthma. *Postgraduate Medicine, 77*, 42–50.

Spector, S. L., & Farr, R. S. (1983). Aspirin idiosyncrasy: Asthma and urticaria. In E. Middleton, Jr., C. E. Reed, & E. F. Ellis (Eds.), *Allergy: Principles and practice* (pp. 1249–1273). St. Louis: C. V. Mosby Co.

Spector, S. L., Katz, R., Siegel, S., Rachelefsky, O., Fitzgerald, J., Hardick, H., Kinsman, R., & Dirks, R. (1983). The use of the nebulizer chronolog as a monitoring device for compliance. *Annals of Allergy, 50*, 359.

Steptoe, A. (1984). Psychological aspects of bronchial asthma. In S. Rachman (Ed.), *Contributions to medical psychology* Vol. 3, pp. 7–30). Oxford, England: Pergamon Press.

Sublett, J. L., Pollard, S. J., Kadlec, G. J., & Karibo, J. M. (1979). Non-compliance in asthmatic children: A study of theophylline levels in a pediatric emergency room population. *Annals of Allergy, 43*, 95–97.

Tager, I. B., Munoz, A., Rosner, B., Weiss, S. T., Carey, V., & Speizer, F. E. (1985). Effects of cigarette smoking on the pulmonary function of children and adolescents. *American Review of Respiratory Disease, 131*, 752–759.

Taplin, P. S., & Creer, T. L. (1978). A procedure for using peak expiratory flow rate data to increase the predictability of asthma episodes. *Journal of Asthma Research, 16*, 15–19.

Thoresen, C. E., & Kirmil-Gray, K. (1983). Self-management psychology and the treatment of childhood asthma. *Journal of Allergy and Clinical Immunology, 72*, 596–606 (Part 2).

Tobin, D. L., Wigal, J. K., Winder, J. A., Holroyd, K. A., & Creer, T. L. (1987). The asthma self-efficacy scale. *Annals of Allergy, 59*, 273–277.

Wallston, K. A., Wallston, B. S., & De Vellis, R. (1978). Development of the multidimensional health locus of control (MHLC) scales. *Health Education Monographs, 6*, 160–170.

Weinstein, A. G., & Cuskey, W. (1985). Theophylline compliance in asthmatic children. *Annals of Allergy, 54*, 19–24.

Weiss, J. H. (1981). Superstuff. *Self-management educational programs for childhood asthma. Volume II: Manuscripts* (pp. 273–293). Bethesda, MD: National Institute of Allergy & Infectious Diseases.

Weissmann, G. (1983). The eicosanoids of asthma. *New England Journal of Medicine, 308*, 454–456.

Wigal, J. L., Kotses, H., Creer, T. L., Harm, D. L., & Tinker, T. R. (1986). Total respiratory resistance and peak expiratory flow rate: An intrasubject comparison. *Journal of Asthma, 23*, 11–13.

Williams, M. H., Jr. (1980). Clinical features. *Seminars in Respiratory Medicine, 1*, 304–314.

Williams, M. H., Jr. (1982). *Essentials of pulmonary medicine*. Philadelphia: W. B. Saunders Co.

Winder, J. A. (1984, January). Keep asthma patients in your practice and out of the ER. *Practice/84*, 19–25.

Wolpe, J. (1958). *Psychotherapy by reciprocal inhibition*. Stanford, CA: Stanford University Press.

Wood, P. R., Casey, R., Koski, G. B., & McCormick, M. C. (1985). Compliance with oral theophylline therapy in asthmatic children. *Annals of Allergy, 54*, 400–404.

Zwillich. C. (1983). The control of breathing in clinical practice: Its significance and assessment. *Seminars in Respiratory Medicine, 4*, 247–257.

7
STRESS, BEHAVIOR, AND GLUCOSE CONTROL IN DIABETES MELLITUS

Richard S. Surwit
Duke University Medical Center

There is currently renewed interest in behavioral aspects of diabetes mellitus and its treatment (Fisher, Delamater, Bertelson, & Kirkley, 1982; Surwit, Feinglos, & Scovern, 1983; Surwit, Scovern, & Feinglos, 1982). The thrust of such efforts has been to encourage a biobehavioral model of diabetes mellitus, a disease which may affect as many as 14 million Americans *(National Diabetes Data Group,* 1985). In this chapter we review existing research that suggests that direct physiological effects of stress can influence metabolic homeostasis in diabetes. Diabetes mellitus was one of the first diseases to be described by ancient physicians. Yet, diabetes still has no cure. Today it remains one of the most common chronic diseases.

Diabetes is characterized by a defect in insulin secretion or action. Insulin acts to make cell membranes permeable to glucose—a process that is essential for normal metabolism. In diabetes, because of an absolute or relative lack of insulin, glucose cannot be readily utilized by the cells of the body and, hence, it accumulates in the bloodstream. Some is excreted in the urine, causing an osmotic diuresis. Because glucose is not available to them, the cells, instead, metabolize glycogen, fat, and protein, depleting the body's energy reserves. This process, if unchecked, is accompanied by fatigue, weight loss, and dehydration, leading to either hyperosmolar coma or ketoacidosis, and, ultimately, death. With proper medical treatment, the consequences of severe hyperglycemia can be avoided and life can be prolonged. However, moderately elevated blood glucose levels over a long period may be related to the eventual appearance of the "long-term" complications of diabetes. It is widely believed that the control of hyperglycemia is the key factor in preventing the development of retinopathy, neuropathy, and nephropathy (Davidson, 1981). Furthermore, intensive treatment regimes designed to reduce hyperglycemia have had favorable effects on risk factors such as lipid abnormalities, which may be important in the development of atherosclerosis (Schade, Santiago, Skyler, & Rizza, 1983).

Two types of diabetes are commonly recognized. Insulin-dependent diabetes mellitus (IDDM) is often referred to as "juvenile" diabetes because of its frequent appearance during childhood. In this condition, the beta (or insulin-producing) cells of the pancreatic islets of Langerhans secrete little or no insulin. The patient, therefore, must continuously be treated with single or multiple daily insulin injections. In contrast, patients with non-insulin-dependent diabetes mellitus (NIDDM), which is often referred to as "adult-onset" diabetes, retain significant beta cell function. However, high somatic resistance to insulin (often exacerbated by obesity) puts increased demands on the insulin-secretory capacity of these patients, who suffer from an inability to secrete enough insulin to meet these demands. In such cases, diet, or oral hypoglycemic agents that increase the effectiveness of endogenous insulin, can be used for treatment, although a few patients do require additional insulin. One million diabetics in the United States are classified in the first category, five million in the second. Eight million additional people not presently diagnosed are estimated to have the disease as it is currently defined (National Diabetes Data Group, 1985).

DIABETES AND STRESS

It is widely known that diverse stressors, when of sufficient intensity, lead to an alarm response, which includes sympathetic discharge and elevations in circulating levels of catecholamines, glucocorticoids, and growth hormone. Common to these responses are their energy-mobilizing and insulin-inhibiting effects (Davidson, 1981). In that glucoregulation is compromised in diabetic individuals, the energy-mobilizing effects of stress can be deleterious to the control of blood glucose in a diabetic patient (Surwit et al., 1983, 1982). Therefore, the extent to which environmental stress and other behavioral variables contribute to blood glucose control is theoretically important in the clinical management of this disorder.

The autonomic nervous system (ANS) is intimately involved in the regulation of carbohydrate metabolism. The effects of the ANS on insulin action are both facilitatory and inhibitory. Branches of the right vagus nerve innervate the pancreatic islets, and stimulation of the right vagus nerve causes increased insulin secretion. Stimulation of pancreatic islets, beta-adrenergic receptors also facilitates insulin secretion. However, insulin secretion is inhibited by stimulation of the sympathetic nerves of the pancreas through the activation of alpha-adrenergic receptors. This sympathetic and parasympathetic innervation of the pancreas may modulate insulin and the normal regulation of carbohydrate metabolism. In addition to its effects on the pancreas, the ANS has other metabolic effects. Beta-adrenergic stimulation facilitates conversion of glycogen to glucose in the liver as well as fat to free fatty acids in adipose tissue. Free fatty acids are further metabolized to ketoacids in the liver. Neurogenic (as well as humoral) stimulation of the adrenal cortex leads to the secretion of cortisol, which elevates blood glucose and impairs glucose tolerance. Thus, the hypothalamic pituitary adrenocortical and adrenomedullary systems and the ANS have both direct and indirect hormonal control pathways in the regulation of glucose metabolism.

Animal Studies

Despite the fact that numerous physiologic mechanisms by which stress might disrupt glucose metabolism in diabetes are known, there are few studies on how stress and behavior actually interact with the development or expression of diabetes in animals. Although Cannon (1941) described stress-induced hyperglycemia in normal animals a half century ago, the effects of stress on diabetic animals have not been systematically studied.

Two existing reports of the effects of stress on the development of experimentally induced IDDM in animals appear, at first glance, to contradict one another. Capponi, Kawada, Varela, and Vargas (1980) studied the effect of repeated restraint stress on rats that had been partially pancreatectomized. Although few of these animals develop diabetes spontaneously, restraint stress produced permanent diabetes in a significant percentage of pancreatectomized animals. In contrast to this result, another recent study (Huang, Plout, Taylor, & Wareheim, 1981) found that light-shock stimulation could inhibit the development of streptozotocin-induced diabetes (chemical pancreatectomy) in young mice receiving a single dose of streptozotocin. Although the mechanism of this effect was not defined, other investigators (Roudier, Portha, & Picon, 1980) have found that administration of exogenous steroids can inhibit the development of another streptozotocin-induced model of diabetes. It is therefore possible that the protective effect of shock on the development of diabetes observed in animals treated with a single dose of streptozotocin may have been mediated through the adrenal corticotropic effects of stress. These two reports highlight the complex nature of the relationship between environmental stimulation and the development of diabetes in animals rendered susceptible to the disease. However, they do not provide insight into how stress affects animals with established diabetes.

One of the first observations that stress could contribute to the expression of hyperglycemia in an animal model of spontaneously occurring NIDDM was made during metabolic studies of the sand rat (psammomys obesus). The sand rat is a North African rodent that eats an exclusively low-calorie diet of succulent plants in its natural habitat. Animals that are newly captured or maintained on a low-calorie, low-carbohydrate diet do not develop diabetes. However, when they are fed laboratory chow and allowed to become obese, a significant percentage of the animals develop an analogue of NIDDM.

Mikat, Hackel, Cruz, and Lebovitz (1972) have shown that stress, as well as diet and obesity may play a role in the expression of hyperglycemia in these animals. Sand rats between 7 and 14 months of age were maintained on a low-calorie, low-carbohydrate diet of vegetables and saline so that they remained euglycemic. Glucose or saline was administered to rats either through an esophageal tube or intraperitoneally by injection. Similar procedures were carried out on a group of Sprague-Dawley rats. Blood samples were drawn on all animals at 30 and 120 minutes and analyzed for glucose and insulin. Sand rats receiving glucose via an intraperitoneal injection showed normal glucose tolerance values. However, sand rats receiving glucose through esophageal intubation showed a clearly abnormal glucose tolerance, typical of diabetes. In contrast, route of administration did not alter the normal glucose tolerance values which were observed in the Sprague-Dawley rats. Thus, it appears that the stress of intubation can precipitate glucose intolerance in sand rats genetically predisposed toward developing diabetes mellitus—even in their lean, euglycemic state.

We have studied the effects of stress on hyperglycemia in the genetically obese mouse (C57BL/6Job/ob), another commonly used model of NIDDM (Surwit, Feinglos, Livingston, Kuhn, & McCubbin, 1984). It is characterized by a syndrome of obesity, hyperinsulinemia, insulin-resistance hyperglycemia, and glucose intolerance. These animals also display hyperadrenocorticism, hypogonadotropism, and other endocrine abnormalities. The obese mouse tends to have mild diabetes, and it can survive for a long time. There has been some controversy over the degree to which the obese mouse is hyperglycemic. Different laboratories have reported "resting" plasma glucose levels ranging from 130 mg/dl to over 300 mg/dl. We have shown that the degree to which this animal is hyperglycemic is dependent, in part, on whether it is exposed to stressful stimuli.

In one experiment, blood samples were drawn from obese and lean mice following either a rest period or exposure to stress. Stress consisted of restraint in a wire-mesh cage for 60 minutes punctuated by a 5-minute period of shaking. Stress produced an increase in plasma glucose in both lean and obese animals. However, the effects were significantly greater in the obese animals than in their lean litter mates. Similarly, although plasma insulin decreased in all animals following stress, the decrease was significantly greater in obese animals.

A second experiment was conducted to assess the effects of epinephrine on plasma glucose and insulin in both lean and obese animals. Epinephrine bitartrate was injected into both lean and obese mice. Control animals were injected with an equal volume of saline. Blood samples were drawn one hour following injection. The effects of epinephrine were analogous to those of stress. Epinephrine produced an increase in plasma glucose in all animals, with obese mice showing a greater response than their lean litter mates. Epinephrine decreased plasma insulin only in obese mice. These data demonstrate that the expression of hyperglycemia in obese mice is, to some degree, dependent on the stress the animals experience in their environment. Furthermore, it appears that the differential responsivity of the obese animals to stress may be related to a heightened sensitivity of the obese animals to adrenergic stimulation.

We have also gathered some preliminary evidence that suggests that social stimulation may be an effective hyperglycemic stimulus in animals genetically predisposed to develop NIDDM. Although most forms of diabetes become more severe with age, the hyperglycemia of the obese mouse has been reported to improve with age. One possible explanation for this effect is that these animals habituate to the laboratory environment and handling procedures over time and therefore show less stress hyperglycemia. If this were the case, the course of hyperglycemia over time in these animals should be affected by different rearing environments. Using a chronic social stress situation, 4-week-old obese mice were group housed with animals from two other strains. Specifically, five obese mice were housed with five C576Job/? lean mice, and five Swiss Webster male and five Swiss Webster female mice in each of three group cages. Every week, the groups of obese, C57 lean Swiss Webster male and Swiss Webster female mice were randomly rotated among the three group cages to force the animals to reestablish dominance orders. Control animals were housed in regular-sized cages with four animals of the same strain to each cage. Each month, blood samples were drawn by retro-orbital sinus puncture and analyzed for plasma glucose. At the end of three months, animals in the social stress condition were moved into small group cages as used for the controls. All animals were then followed for two additional months after which they were sacrificed. Histologic examination was performed and data collected on pancreas size, islet size and number, and beta cell size and number. All animals had similar plasma glucose levels at the beginning of the study. However, by month three, obese animals reared under stressful conditions had significantly higher plasma glucose levels than animals reared under control conditions. Lean animals showed no analogous effect of social stress. Furthermore, when stress was removed, obese animals returned to baseline levels which were not different from those of lean animals. Examination of mouse pancreata revealed that, as expected, obese animals had larger and more numerous islets than lean animals. However, obese animals exposed to stress showed exaggerated hyperplagia of the insulin secreting beta cells as compared to animals not receiving stress. These data support the hypothesis that the course of hyperglycemia in the obese mouse is environmentally dependent, underscoring the importance of behavioral variables in understanding this animal model of diabetes.

That environmental stimulation can have a direct effect on the expression of diabetes in animals raises the possibility of indirect environmental (psychologic) effects occurring through learning and conditioning. Indeed, there is much literature on the classical conditioning of blood glucose responses in both animals and humans (see Woods & Kulkosky, 1976 for review). In the majority of these studies, large doses of insulin were used to produce an unconditioned hypoglycemic response (blood glucose from 30-50 mg/dl). If this procedure was repeated numerous times in the presence of the specific environmental stimuli, these stimuli developed the capacity to elicit a conditioned decrease in blood glucose. Statistically significant conditioned decreases in blood glucose ranging from 10 to 25 mg/dl have been observed. Similar conditioned decreases in blood glucose have also been demonstrated using tolbutamide as the unconditioned stimulus (US) (Woods, Alexander, & Porte, 1972). Although the mechanism of this effect has not been systematically delineated, conditioned decreases in blood glucose are not observed in animals in which vagal input to the pancreas has been severed (Woods, 1972) or in which pancreatic B cells have been destroyed with streptozotocin (Woods, Hutton, & Makous, 1970). This suggests that conditioned decreases in blood glucose may be mediated through vagal stimulation of insulin release.

Another series of studies demonstrated that when glucose (Woods & Shogren, 1972) or glucagon (Siegel, 1972) are used as unconditioned stimuli, small but significant conditioned decreases in blood glucose can be obtained. However, attempts to produce conditioned decreases in blood glucose following administration of epinephrine have not been successful (Savchenko, 1940). Although the sheer number of studies reporting conditioned changes in blood glucose argue persuasively for the existence of this phenomenon, in only one report was insulin assayed, and the effects of these conditioning paradigms on counter-regulatory hormones have not been systematically studied. Furthermore, these studies do not determine what role classical conditioning of blood glucose may play in hyperglycemia in normal or diabetic animals.

We have recently demonstrated that by pairing a stressful stimulus known to produce hyperglycemia (shaking) with a previously neutral stimulus (a metronome), ob/ob mice could be trained to show classically conditioned hyperglycemia (Surwit, McCubbin, Livingston, & Feinglos, 1985). Shaking was used as an US and the sound of a metronome was used as a conditioned stimulus (CS). To determine the effects of the unconditioned stimulus alone, six obese and six lean mice were individually placed in small foam padded chambers placed on top of a mechanical shaker. Following a 10-minute pre-stimulus interval, animals were shaken for 10 minutes at 200 strokes per minute with a 6-cm excursion. Immediately after the shaking procedure, blood samples were obtained by retro-orbital sinus puncture, and the animals were returned to their home cages. Blood samples were immediately centrifuged and plasma was frozen until assayed for glucose (Beckman Autoanalyzer II) and insulin (radioimmunoassay, Cambridge Medical Diagnostics). To determine if the hyperglycemic response to shaking could be conditioned, 12 obese mice and 12 lean litter mates were placed in a mechanical shaker as previously described. A metronome was activated at 120 beats/minute for 10 minutes prior to and during the 10 minutes of shaking. The metronome and the shaking were then stopped simultaneously, and the animals were returned to their home cages. Two control groups were used. In control group I, animals were exposed to 20 minutes of the metronome alone while remaining otherwise undisturbed in their home cages. Control group II received exposure to the metronome in their home cages and shaking in another room at another time (noncontingent control). Conditioning trials, exposure to the metronome alone or the noncontingently presented metronome and shaking, were repeated 7 times over 3 days. On the fourth day, both control and experimental animals were tested for conditioning of stress-induced hyperglycemia by exposure to the metronome alone for 20 minutes while remaining in their home cages. Blood samples were obtained immediately following this last metronome exposure and analyzed as described above.

The training procedure produced acquisition of conditioned hyperglycemia in obese animals only, despite the fact that both lean and obese animals showed a significant rise in plasma glucose as an unconditioned response to shaking. Obese animals showed a significantly greater rise in plasma glucose in response to shaking than lean animals. There was no significant change in plasma insulin in either obese or lean animals following any of the experimental manipulations. It is not immediately clear why the obese mouse demonstrates conditioned hyperglycemia and the lean mouse does not. In this study, as in earlier studies, the obese mouse showed a significantly greater unconditioned response (UR) than the lean mouse. Because a strong US must be present for classical conditioning to occur, this animal's tendency to show large hyperglycemic responses to stress may make it more susceptible to classically conditioned hyperglycemia. Regardless of mechanism, however, this phenomenon clearly demonstrates that a purely behavioral or psychologic manipulation such as conditioning can play a major role in the expression of hyperglycemia in at least one animal model of diabetes.

Finally, there is also evidence that anxiolytic pharmacotherapy can be used to attenuate the effects of stress on hyperglycemia in the obese mouse. We gave lean and obese animals injections of either 5mg/kg of alprazolam, a triazolobenzodiazepine, or vehicle alone prior to exposure to restraint and shaking stress or to a no-stress control period each lasting 60 minutes (Surwit, McCubbin, Gerstenfeld, McGee, & Feinglos, 1986). Blood samples were drawn and then analyzed for glucose, insulin, and corticosterone. Alprazolam significantly lowered plasma glucose in obese mice during stress, but it had no effect on plasma glucose in lean mice or in obese mice at rest. Alprazolam also appeared to reduce plasma corticosterone more in obese mice than in lean mice.

Human Studies

The investigation of the effects of psychologic stress on glucose metabolism in diabetic patients was first undertaken by Hinkle and his co-workers (Hinkle, Evans, & Wolf, 1951a; Hinkle, Evans & Wolfe, l95lb; Hinkle & Wolfe, 1952). Their studies demonstrated increases in blood glucose and ketones following stressful psychiatric interviews in diabetic patients. However, their work is poorly controlled and difficult to interpret. Vandenbergh, Sussman, and Titus (1966) examined the impact of hypnotically-induced emotion on predominantly IDDM subjects in a controlled fashion. Coincident with non-significant increases in plasma free fatty acids, they observed blood glucose decreases. These findings were replicated in a subsequent study (Vanderbergh, Sussman, & Vaughan, 1967). However, these investigators did not fully document whether or not their subjects had endogenous insulin reserves.

McLesky, Lewis, and Woodruff (1978) found a clear hyperglycemic response in patients with both IDDM and NIDDM during a surgical stress. Furthermore, insulin-dependent diabetic children have been shown to demonstrate elevated blood glucose and more rapid ketone release following epinephrine infusion compared to normal children (Baker, Kaye, & Haque, 1967). More recently, Bradley (1982) reported that noise stress increased blood glucose in initially hyperglycemic diabetic subjects and decreased blood glucose in initially hypoglycemic diabetic subjects. Others have found that mental arithmetic can produce both increases or decreases in blood glucose (Carter, Gonder-Frederick, Cox, Clarke, & Scott, 1985) in patients with IDDM, and that the direction of blood glucose change is idiosyncratic. Finally, low-dose epinephrine infusions have been shown to impair glucose tolerance in normal human subjects (Hamburg, Hendler, & Sherwin, 1980). Thus, some of the studies investigating the impact of psychologic stress on blood glucose in human diabetes report that stress has a hyperglycemic effect, whereas others find the opposite response. There are several explanations for these apparently contradictory results. First, the term "stress" is itself a cause of confusion. "Stress" is used to describe an enormous variety of both experimental stimuli (e.g., noise) as well as responses (e.g., mental arithmetic). In the studies just cited, no two groups of investigators used the same stress and, hence, the disparity of results is not surprising. Furthermore, many of the above studies did not carefully describe the nature of their subjects' diabetes. The effects of a given environmental stimulus on a patient with some endogenous insulin could be quite different than if applied to a patient without endogenous insulin. Because none of these investigations examined the mechanisms of the observed stress-induced effects, the question of how stress interacts with blood glucose in human diabetes remains open.

Therapeutic approaches aimed at reducing the stress response and its metabolic effects in diabetic patients have included intensive family therapy (Minuchin, Rosman, & Baker, 1978) and long-term beta blockade (Baker, Barcai, Kaye, & Haque, 1969). However, psychotherapeutic approaches lack cost effectiveness, and long-term beta blockade may directly alter pancreatic islet cell physiology in NIDDM. It can possibly increase the risk of unheralded hypoglycemia and interfere with the recovery from a hypoglycemic event in patients with IDDM. Relaxation techniques offer a potential alternative. They have been employed in the treatment of a variety of autonomically mediated illnesses (Shapiro & Surwit, 1979), and they appear to decrease adrenocortical activity (DeGood & Redgate, 1982; Jevning, Wilson, & Davison, 1978). Consequently, relaxation therapy might serve to moderate some of the negative effects of the stress response on metabolic control in diabetic patients without undue adverse effects caused by adrenergic blockade. Growing literature supports this notion. Fowler, Budzynski, and Vandenbergh (1976) reported that intensive relaxation training and EMG biofeedback lowered the insulin requirements and reduced the frequency of ketoacidosis in one patient with IDDM but they failed to provide outcome data. Seeburg and DeBoer (1980) reported the treatment of a similar case of IDDM. Although relaxation training appeared to produce a significant reduction in the patient's insulin requirement, the patient began to experience frequent hypoglycemia and training had to be discontinued.

Rosenbaum (1983) reported the use of EMG biofeedback and relaxation training combined as a comprehensive stress-management program with four IDDM patients and two NIDDM patients who were being treated with insulin. Three of the patients with IDDM reduced their insulin requirement, and one of the patients with NIDDM was taken off insulin entirely. Finally, Lammers, Naliboff, and Straatmeyer (1984), using a multiple-baseline within-subject design, demonstrated that relaxation produced significantly lower blood glucose levels in four insulin-requiring patients during discrete treatment periods.

Although these studies provide suggestive evidence for the utility of relaxation training in the control of plasma glucose in diabetes, they have been relatively uncontrolled, and the patient populations reported on have been poorly defined. There have been three recent reports of the application of relaxation training to patients with clearly documented IDDM. Landis et al. (1984) trained six patients with IDDM who were being closely followed and intensively treated. All patients received 15 weekly sessions of biofeedback-assisted relaxation training and three monthly follow-ups. Although absolute glucose levels, glycohemoglobin, and insulin requirements did not change significantly following training, patients did appear to experience an improvement in plasma glucose control as measured by the daily range in blood glucose levels divided by the daily insulin dose. Bradley, Moses, Gamsu, Knight, and Ward (1985), compared conventional insulin treatment, insulin treatment with a continuous subcutaneous insulin infusion, conventional insulin treatment plus relaxation training, and conventional treatment plus biofeedback-assisted relaxation training. No differences among the four treatment groups were found on daily measures of blood glucose or glycohemoglobin, although individual differences within groups were considerable.

We have studied the acute effects of relaxation training on glucose tolerance in a carefully defined population of patients with NIDDM (Surwit & Feinglos, 1983) and IDDM (Feinglos, Hastedt, & Surwit, 1987). In the first study, nine male and three female patients with NIDDM in poor control (2 hour postprandial glucose greater than 200 mg/dl) who were not using insulin were admitted to the clinical research unit of Duke University and placed on a weight-maintenance diabetic diet. The day after admission, a 3-hour oral glucose tolerance test (GTT) was performed on each patient using 100 grams of glucose. Blood was sampled every 30 minutes for measurement of plasma glucose, insulin, cortisol, and catecholamines. The following day, an intravenous insulin tolerance test was performed on all patients using 0.1 U of regular port insulin per kilogram of body weight, and plasma glucose was measured at 5 minute intervals for 30 minutes. Half of the patients (2 men, 4 women) were then assigned to receive instruction in a modified version of progressive relaxation, which was prerecorded on a cassette and practiced by the patient in his or her hospital room 2 times per day for 5 days. In addition, all patients in the relaxation group were given 5 50-minute EMG biofeedback sessions. During these sessions, patients received continuous information about muscle tone from an audio analogue of EMG recorded from surface electrodes placed over the frontalis muscle. The other 6 patients (1 man, 5 women) remained in the hospital under identical conditions but did not receive relaxation training. At the end of the week, the glucose and insulin tolerance tests were repeated, and patients receiving relaxation training practiced the technique with the aid of the cassette tape.

Glucose tolerance was estimated by calculation of the incremental glucose area (area of the glucose tolerance curve above the fasting glucose) (Feinglos & Lebovitz, 1980). Glucose-stimulated insulin secretory activity was estimated by calculation of the incremental insulin area from values obtained during the GTT (Feinglos & Lebovitz, 1980). Insulin sensitivity was assessed by measuring the decrement in plasma glucose with time in response to a dose (0.1 U/kg) of intravenous insulin. The glucose disposal constant in response to insulin, KI (% plasma glucose fall/min), was derived by multiplying by 100 the slope of the initial, linear portion of the regression line of log in plasma glucose versus time (Lebovitz & Feinglos, 1980).

Relaxation therapy produced a significant reduction in incremental glucose area in treated subjects compared with untreated controls. These effects were independent of weight change. Although fasting glucose improved for all subjects with hospitalization, 2-hour postprandial blood glucose values improved significantly only in treated patients. The improvement in glucose tolerance was not accompanied by a change in insulin sensitivity as measured by KI. Changes in glucose-stimulated insulin secretory activity were variable, and not significantly different, in both groups of patients. Plasma cortisol and catecholamines were measured immediately prior to the first and second GTT. Cortisol and catecholamine levels during the first test were subtracted from those of the second to yield a difference score. Subjects receiving relaxation showed a decrease in plasma cortisol of 96 ug/ml between the first and second glucose tolerance tests, whereas control subjects showed an increase of 36 ug/ml over the same period (Surwit & Feinglos, 1984). These differences were significant. Plasma catecholamines decreased in both groups from the first to the second test. Differences between the groups were not significant.

Feinglos, Hastedt and Surwit (1987) investigated whether this same relaxation program would effect glycemic control in 20 patients with IDDM who reported stress-induced elevations of blood glucose. Patients in the treatment group were given 5 50-minute biofeedback sessions and instructions to practice twice daily during a 1-week hospitalization period and at home following discharge. They were also instructed to practice relaxation for 30–60 seconds 10–20 times per day without a tape. Those in the control group did not receive any relaxation training but received a similar amount of therapist contact while in hospital. In contrast to the earlier study with patients with NIDDM, relaxation did not significantly improve glucose tolerance in treated patients. Furthermore, there were no differences between treatment and control groups in mean daily blood glucose, required insulin dose, or other measures of chronic control.

There are numerous reasons why relaxation training may have had a differential effect on NIDDM and IDDM. First, because NIDDM is by far the more common disease, and may be confused with IDDM when the patient requires insulin (as sometimes occurs in NIDDM), early reports of relaxation improving control in IDDM may have been due to improper diagnoses. Second, patients with IDDM may be a more heterogeneous population in terms of their response to stress than patients with NIDDM. Several studies have shown that patients with IDDM can show either increases or decreases in blood glucose in response to stress and that these differences appear to be idiosyncratic. The effects of relaxation may then depend upon the nature of the subject's response to stress. Third, glycemic control tends to be more labile in patient with IDDM, with greater fluctuations resulting from the effects of diet, insulin, exercise, and nonpsychological stressors such as illness. This variable baseline may make it more difficult to evaluate the response of blood glucose to stress or relaxation than in patient with NIDDM.

Finally, the direct physiologic effects of stress on glucose metabolism may be more profound in NIDDM than in IDDM. There is substantial evidence to support the notion that increased alpha adrenergic sensitivity is a characteristic of NIDDM. For example, Kuhn, Cochrane, Feinglos, and Surwit (1987) investigated the contribution of altered peripheral sympathetic function to the exaggerated glycemic response of ob/ob mice to stress. Obese mice and their lean littermates were injected with one of three doses of epinephrine bitartrate or phentolamine mesylate. Epinephrine administration resulted in a dose related increase in plasma glucose in lean animals in the dose range from 1–5 ug/10 g body weight, while plasma glucose responses were maximal at the lowest dose of epinephrine tested in the obese mice, suggesting that the dose response relationship is altered in obese animals. Moreover, phentolamine, alpha-adrenergic antagonist, produced a greater increase in plasma insulin in ob/ob mice than the lean litter mates, suggesting that this increased sensitivity to catecholamines may be largely alpha-adrenergic. Altered peripheral responses to sympathetic stimuli are therefore important in the exaggerated glycemic responses of ob/ob mice to stress and may be an etiologic factor in the development of diabetes in these animals.

Fujimoto, Sakaguchi, and Ui (1981) observed a similar exaggerated sensitivity to epinephrine in the KK mouse, another animal model of NIDDM. Furthermore, they also observed that alpha-adrenergic blockade with phentolamine could provoke an exaggerated insulin response in KK mice compared to control mice, suggesting that KK, like ob/ob mice, have altered adrenergic sensitivity.

There is also evidence of altered adrenergic sensitivity and responsibility in patients with NIDDM. Linde and Deckert (1973) and Robertson, Halter, and Porte (1976) observed that alpha-adrenergic blockade with phentolamine increased glucose-stimulated insulin secretion in patients with NIDDM, the latter group showing that this increase is five times greater in diabetic patients than in normal controls. This suggests that alpha-adrenergic stimulation may be having a greater effect on insulin release in diabetic patients than in normals. Robertson, et. al. (1976) also reported that patients with NIDDM also show increased levels of circulating catecholamines both at rest and following glucose infusion compared to controls, implying greater responsibility of the sympathetic nervous system in these patients as well. Most recently, Kashiwagi et al. (1986) demonstrated that selective blockade of alpha-2 receptors increased both insulin secretion and glucose disposal rate following a mixed meal. Finally, it has been reported that glyburide, one of the sulfonylurea oral agents used to treat NIDDM, binds to alpha-2 receptors in the pancreas, suggesting that one effect of this drug on insulin secretion may be due to antagonism of adrenergic activity (Cherksey & Altszaler, 1984). These findings suggest that environmental stress, which activates the sympathetic nervous system, may be particularly deleterious to patients with NIDDM and that methods to reduce the effects of stress may have some clinical utility in this disease.

SUMMARY AND CONCLUSIONS

Within the last ten years, there has been renewed interest in the problem of stress and glycemic control in diabetes. Recent research has provided some empirical evidence for the clinical observations made over the past 300 years that stress can adversely affect glucose control. Research has also provided new insights into the role of both behavior and the central nervous system in various forms of diabetes. Although initial interest in the role of behavior in diabetes focused on IDDM, studies on the effects of stress on glucose control in this disease have been contradictory. There have been few animal studies of how stress affects the development and course of IDDM and human studies have yielded somewhat confusing results. Some investigators have reported that stress produces hyperglycemia in patients with IDDM, but others have reported the opposite.

There is, perhaps, somewhat better data on how stress affects glycemic control in NIDDM. Numerous animal studies exist that suggest stress can adversely affect glycemic control in this form of diabetes. Furthermore, there is evidence from both animals and humans that suggest that individuals with NIDDM have altered adrenergic sensitivity in the pancreas (and perhaps other sites as well), which could make them particularly sensitive to stressful environmental stimulation. However, although there is substantial data showing the importance of stress in understanding hyperglycemia in animal models of NIDDM, there is no direct evidence that stress plays a role in the expression or control of the human disease. Indirect support for the hypothesis that stress is important in NIDDM is provided by several studies that show that relaxation can attenuate hyperglycemia in patients. This is in contrast to three studies which failed to find that similar relaxation procedures had any effect on patients with IDDM.

In summary, although the role of stress in the development and course of IDDM is unclear, there is mounting evidence of autonomic nervous system abnormalities in NIDDM. This has lead us to speculate that the resultant exaggeration of sympathetic nervous system effects would impair insulin secretion and glucose utilization, the pathophysiologic hallmarks of the disease (Surwit & Feinglos, 1988). This hypothesis does not require the presence of unusual psychologic stress for metabolic dysregulation to occur for the metabolic effects of even normals NS activity appear to be exaggerated. Thus, NIDDM may be, in part, a problem of neurally regulated homeostasis in which stress and the autonomic nervous system interact in contributing to the development and course of the disease.

ACKNOWLEDGMENT

Preparation of this manuscript was supported by Research Scientist Development Award No. KO2-MH-00303 from the National Institute of Mental Health.

REFERENCES

Baker, L., Barcai, A., Kaye, R., & Haque, N. (1969). Beta adrenergic blockade in juvenile diabetes: Acute studies and long-term therapeutic trial. *Journal of Pediatrics, 75*, 19-29.
Baker, L., Kaye, R., & Haque, N. (1967). Studies on metabolic homeostasis in juvenile diabetes mellitus II: Role of catecholamines. *Diabetes, 16*, 504-505.
Bradley, C. (1982). Psychophysiological aspects of the management of diabetes mellitus. *International Journal of Mental Health, 11*, 117-132.
Bradley, C., Moses, J. L., Gamsu, D. S., Knight, G., & Ward, J. D. (1985). The effects of relaxation on metabolic control in type I diabetes: A matched control study. *Diabetes, 34*, 17A.
Cannon, W. B. (1941). *Bodily changes in pain, hunger, fear and rage.* New York: MacMillan.
Capponi, R., Kawada, M. E., Varela, C., & Vargas, L. (1980). Diabetes mellitus by repeated stress in rats bearing chemical diabetes. *Hormone and Metabolic Research, 12*, 411-412.
Carter, W. R., Gonder-Frederick, L. A., Cox, D. J., Clarke, W. L., & Scott, D. (1985). Effects of stress on blood glucose in IDDM. *Diabetes Care, 8*, 411-412.
Cherksey, B., & Altszuler, N. (1984). Tolbutamide and glyburide differ in effectiveness to displace alpha- and beta-adrenergic radioligands in pancreatic islet cells and membranes. *Diabetes, 33*, 499-503.
Davidson, M. B. (1981). *Diabetes mellitus: Diagnosis and treatment.* New York: Wiley.
DeGood, D. E., & Redgate, E. S. (1982). Interrelationship of plasma cortisol and other activation indexes during EMG bio-feedback training. *Journal of Behavioral Medicine, 5*, 213-224.

Feinglos, M. N., Hastedt, P., & Surwit, R. S. (1987). The effects of relaxation therapy on patients with Type I diabetes mellitus. *Diabetes Care, 10*, 72-75.

Feinglos, M. N., & Lebovitz, H. E. (1980). Sulfonylurea treatment of insulin independent diabetes mellitus. *Metabolism 29*, 488-494.

Fisher, E. B., Jr., Delamater, A. M., Bertelson, A. D., & Kirkley, B. G. (1982). Psychological factors in diabetes and its treatment. *Journal of Clinical and Consulting Psychology, 50*, 993-1003.

Fowler, J E., Budzynski, T. H., & Vandenbergh, R. L. (1976). Effects of an EMG biofeedback relaxation program on the control of diabetes. *Biofeedback and Self-Regulation, 1*, 105-112.

Fujimoto, K., Sakaguchi, T., & Ui, M. (1981). Adrenergic mechanisms in the hyperglycaemia and hyperinsulinaemia of diabetic KK mice. *Diabetologia, 20*, 568-572.

Hamburg, S., Hendler, R., & Sherwin, R. S. (1980). Influence of small increments of epinephrine on glucose tolerance in normal humans. *Annals of Internal Medicine, 93*, 566-568.

Hinkle, L. E., Jr., Evans, F. M., & Wolf, S. (1951a). Studies in diabetes mellitus III: Life history of three persons with labile diabetes, and the relation of significant experiences in their lives to the onset and course of their disease. *Psychosomatic Medicine, 13*, 160-183.

Hinkle, L. E., Jr., Evans, F. M., & Wolf, S. (1951b). Studies in diabetes mellitus IV: Life history of three persons with relatively mild, stable diabetes, and relation of significant experiences in their lives to the onset and course of the disease. *Psychosomatic Medicine, 13*, 184-202.

Hinkle, L. E., Jr., & Wolf, S. (1952). Importance of life stress in course and management of diabetes mellitus. *Journal of the American Medical Association, 148*, 513-520.

Huang, S. W., Plout, S. M., Taylor, G., & Wareheim, B. A. (1981). Effect of stressful stimulation on the incidence of streptozotocin-induced diabetes in mice. *Psychosomatic Medicine, 43*, 431-437.

Jevning, R., Wilson, A. F., & Davidson, J. M. (1978). Adrenocortical activity during meditation. *Hormones and Behavior, 10*, 54-60.

Kashiwagi, A., Harano, Y., Suzuki, M., Kojima, H., Harada, M., Nishio, Y., & Shigeta, Y. (1986). New alpha-2 adrenergic blocker(DG-5128) improves insulin secretion and in vivo glucose disposal in NIDDM patients. *Diabetes, 35*, 1085-1089.

Kuhn, C. M., Cochrane, C., Feinglos, M. N., & Surwit, R. S. (1987). Exaggerated peripheral responsivity to catecholamines contributes to stress-induced hyperglycemia in the ob/ob mouse. *Physiology, Biochemistry and Behavior, 26*, 491-495.

Lammers, C. A., Naliboff, B. D., & Straatmeyer, A. J. (1984). The effects of progressive relaxation on stress and diabetic control. *Behavior Research and Therapy, 22*, 641-650.

Landis, B., Javonic, L., Landis E., Peterson, C. M., Groshen, S., Johnson, K., & Miller, N. E. (1984). Stress reduction program reduces glycemia excursions 9% to 40% from baselines without raising insulin needs. *Diabetes, 33*, 69A.

Lebovitz, H. E. & Feinglos, M. N. (1980). Therapy of insulin independent diabetes mellitus: General conditioning. *Metabolism, 29*, 474-481.

Linde, J., & Deckert, T. (1973). Increase of insulin concentration in maturity-onset diabetics by phentolamine (Regitine) infusion. *Hormone and Metabolic Research, 5*, 391-395.

McLesky, C. H., Lewis, S. B., & Woodruff, R. E. (1978). Glucagon levels during anesthesia and surgery in normal and diabetic patients. *Diabetes, 27*, 492.

Mikat, E. M., Hackel, D. B., Cruz, P. T., & Lebovitz, H. E. (1972). Lowered glucose tolerance in the sand rat (psammonys obesus) resulting from esophageal intubation. *Proceedings of the Society for Experimental Biology and Medicine, 139*, 1390-1391.

Minuchin, S., Rosman, B., & Baker, L. (1978). *Psychosomatic families*. Cambridge: Harvard University Press.

National Diabetes Data Group (1985). *Diabetes in America*, Bethesda, U. S. Department of Health and Human Service. Publication No. 85-1468.

Report of the National Commission on Diabetes, 197S.

Robertson, P. R., Halter, J. B., & Porte, D. (1975). A role for alpha-adrenergic receptors in abnormal insulin secretion in diabetes mellitus. *The Journal of Clinical Investigation, 57*, 791-795.

Rosenbaum, L. (1983). Biofeedback assisted stress management for insulin-treated diabetes mellitus. *Biofeedback and Self-Regulation*, 8, 519-532.

Roudier, M., Portha, B., & Picon, L. (1980). Glucocorticoid-induced recovery from streptozotocin diabetes in the adult rat. *Diabetes*, 29, 201-205.

Savchenko, V. A. (1940). Conditioned reflex hypoglycemia, gluycosuria and hyperglycemia. *Bull Biol Med Exp*, 9, 361-363.

Schade, D. S., Santiago, J. V., Skyler, J. S., & Rizza, R. A. (1983). *Intensive insulin therapy*. Princeton: Exerpta Medica.

Seeburg, K. N., & DeBoer, K. F. (1980). Effects of EMG biofeedback on diabetes. *Biofeedback and Self-regulation*, 5, 289-293.

Shapiro, D., & Surwit, R. S. (1979). Biofeedback. In O. F. Pomerleau and J. P. Brady (Eds.), *Behavioral medicine: Theory and practice* (pp. 45-73). Baltimore: Williams & Wilkins, Co.

Siegel, S. (1972). Conditioning of insulin-induced glycemia. *J. Comp. Physiol. Psychol.*, 78, 233-241.

Surwit, R. S., & Feinglos, M. N. (1988). The effects of relaxation on glucose tolerance in non-insulin dependent diabetes mellitus. *Diabetes Care*, 7, 203-204.

Surwit, R. S., & Feinglos, M. N. (1984). Relaxation-induced improvement in glucose tolerance is associated with decreased plasma cortisol. *Diabetes Care*, 7, 203-204.

Surwit, R. S., & Feinglos, M. N. (1988). Stress and the autonomic nervous system in type II diabetes mellitus: An hypothesis. *Diabetes Care*, 11, 83-85.

Surwit, R. S., Feinglos, M. N., Livingston, E. G., Kuhn, C. M., & McCubbin, J. A. (1984). Behavioral manipulation of the diabetic phenotype in ob/ob mice. *Diabetes*, 33, 616-618.

Surwit, R. S., Feinglos, M. N., & Scovern, A. W. (1983). Diabetes and behavior: A paradigm for health psychology. *American Psychologist*, 38, 255-262.

Surwit, R. S., McCubbin, J. A., Gerstenfeld, D. A., McGee, D. J., & Feinglos, M. N. (1986). Alprazolam reduces hyperglycemia in ob/ob mice. *Psychosomatic Medicine*, 48, 278-282.

Surwit, R. S., McCubbin, J.A., Livingston, E. G., & Feinglos, M. N. (1985). Classically conditioned hyperglycemia in the obese mouse. *Psychosomatic Medicine*, 47, 565-568.

Surwit, R. S., Scovern, A. W., & Feinglos, M. N. (1982). The role of behavior in diabetes care. *Diabetes Care*, 26, 467-468.

Vandenbergh, R. L., Sussman, K. E., & Titus, C. C. (1966). Effects of hypnotically induced acute emotional stress on carbohydrate and lipid metabolism in patients with diabetes mellitus. *Psychosomatic Medicine*, 28, 382-390.

Vandenbergh, R. L., Sussman, K. E., & Vaughan, G. D. (1967). Effects of combined physical-anticipatory stress on carbohydrate-lipid metabolism in patients with diabetes mellitus. *Psychosomatics*. 8, 16-19.

Woods, S. C. (1972). Conditioned hypoglycemia effect of vagotomy and pharmacological blockade. *American Journal of Physiology*, 223, 1424-1427.

Woods, S. C., Alexander, K. R., Porte, D., Jr. (1972). Conditioned insulin secretion and hypoglycemia following repeated injections of tolbutamide in rats. *Endocrinology*, 90, 227-231.

Woods, S. C., Hutton, R. A., Makous, W. (1970). Conditioned insulin secretion in the albino rat. *Proceedings of the Society for Experimental Biology and Medicine*, 133, 964-968.

Woods, S. C., & Kulkosky, P. J. (1976). Classically conditioned changes of blood glucose level. *Psychosomatic Medicine*, 38, 201-219.

Woods, S. C., & Shogren, R. E. (1972) Glycemic responses following conditioning with different doses of insulin in rats. *Journal of Comparative and Physiological Psychology*, 81, 220-225.

8
A PROPOSAL FOR A CURRICULUM IN BEHAVIORAL BIOLOGY AND MEDICINE IN MEDICAL SCHOOLS

Herbert Weiner
Behavioral Medicine, Neuropsychiatric Institute
University of California, Los Angeles

The flurry of recent publications on medical education (Association of American Medical Colleges, 1984; Committee on Medical Education, 1984; Eichna, 1983; Institute of Medicine, 1983; Josiah Macy, Jr. Foundation, 1980; Seldin, 1981) attests to a recurrent crisis with a 10-15 year cycle, manifested by conference reports. A comparison of the present and past reports inclines one to the view that nothing much has changed or is likely to do so. But how could it? The political and academic structure of medical schools is invariant, the teaching of medical students is a low priority in academic medicine (Chin, Hopkins, Melman, & Holman, 1985), and little thought is given to educating (rather than teaching) students how to think as doctors.

Medicine continues to be defined as a mysterious brew of "compassion and reductionism." A recent symposium entitled, "On the Training of Tomorrow's Physicians" (Committee on Medical Education, 1984) says nothing coherent about the bureaucratic and mechanized tomorrow that is already here today—the impact that for-profit hospitals, DRGs, and computerized diagnoses, and so on, already have and will have in the future on medical education and practice. And yet, the multiple tensions and contradictions that abound in academic medicine paralyze any attempt to change the education of students.

The education of medical students is also tied to the incoherence of a system by which they are selected—by a reliance on grades and MCAT scores (when it is already known that these are, in part, obtained by dishonesty (Sierles, Hendrick, & Circle, 1980)—a fact with the consequence of misconduct on the part of physicians (Sharpiro & Charrow, 1985)). It is also determined in large part by the content of National Board examinations. Students, in short, are picked to pass exams, not for those qualities which make for good physicians.

Additionally, the process of educating students is not guided by an overall theory or goal except in the most general terms. In operation, it is splintered into special areas of study (Committee on Medical Education, 1984) which are defended to the death by specialists who consider their field as preeminent for the student's education. The student never gets an overview of medicine and how it fits into the scheme of things—of nature and society. Students receive piecemeal information—they are not taught a unified theory of health, illness, and disease or a patient-oriented rather than a disease-oriented theory of disease. They remain uninstructed about the nature and kind of ubiquitous complaints for which most patients seek help. Most patients they will see are ill (e.g., are anxious, have headaches, etc.) (Patient's, 1977-1978) or they are pregnant. They do not have diseases. Yet, most of medical education is narrowly focused on searching out the nonexistent molecular and cellular basis for their ill health, as if it were invariably the product of disease when it is not. The recognition of illness without disease is not taught. Nor are students taught what questions to ask so that they can elicit a history of such illnesses—they are wholly innocent about a "medicine without signs," in Lloyd's (1983) phrase.

Not to know how to ask the right question, and then to seek out the correct answer, based on existing knowledge, begins at the very start of medical school. The preclinical curriculum (taught so frequently by nonclinicians), in addition to being fragmented, exists in a vacuum. Students complain that they have no idea of the reasons for being taught an unending array of detailed facts. They see only dimly the relevance of immunology, endocrinology, virology, metabolism, biochemical genetics, and molecular biology to diseases about which they do not yet have any knowledge. What is the question, they ask, to which the answers are provided? In fact, they do not see patients until after they learn details, soon forgotten, and are taught by different departments and at different times in their careers.

No attempt is made to integrate these scattered facts into an overall scheme already touched upon or alternatively integrated around the concept of the central role of the brain in regulating and monitoring every bodily organ and its functions. But the brain also receives and processes inputs from the environment and responds to them with the appropriate behaviors. [In fact, the medical curriculum is structured in such a manner that the outside observer would get the impression that behavioral and organismic biology did not exist as one of the two main pillars of modern biology (the other being molecular biology), and, hence, of medicine.]

Therefore, one proposal would be to introduce behavioral biology into the curriculum, around which much of the material of the first year could be integrated. By behavioral biology, I mean the biology of those vital functions that allow the organism to survive in its environment. These functions are disturbed in ill health and in disease. Such a course integrates material from many disciplines—it is not designed to supplant them.

THE FIRST YEAR

Specifically, the content of the first-year curriculum should be:

I. The Biology of Food and Water Intake: Medical Significance
   A. The biological significance of food intake—Short-term and long-term requirements
   B. Feeding—not only a matter of ingestion: food seeking, predation, food gathering, storing, eating
   C. Roles of odors, taste, and sight
      (Aversive learning—the psychic phase)
   D. Peripheral mechanisms—the infant rat
      1. Attachment and feeding
      2. Sucking
      3. Milk let-down
   E. Mechanisms of satiety and feeding
      1. Neural, humoral, and peripheral mechanisms
      2. Medullary, pontine, and midbrain relays
      3. The hypothalamus
         a. Integration
         b. Effects of VMH and LH lesions.
            (1) Immediate and long-lasting effects on behavior and body.
            (2) Recovery
         c. Catecholamines and monoamines
            (1) Peptides (CCK, bombesin, Substance P, TRH, somatostatin, enkephalins, and endorphins)
            (2) Amino acids
            (3) Fatty acids
            (4) GABA
            (5) Insulin
            (6) Sex hormones
         d. Regulation of carbohydrate intake
         e. Role of amygdala and septum
         f. Models of obesity and of anorexia
   F. The biological significance of water intake
      1. Thirst and drinking behavior
      2. Osmotic pressure: The role of sodium
      3. Osmoreception and osmoreceptors
      4. Cellular dehydration
         a. Hypovolemia
         b. Angiotensin II (AII)
      5. Relative roles of osmoreceptors and AII
      6. Vasopressin
      7. Water intoxication
      8. Mechanisms of drinking behavior
         a. Physiology
         b. Social factors
         c. Alcohol intake
II. The Biology of Sleep and Waking

A. Relevance for medicine
   B. The waking EEG
      1. Alpha rhythms
      2. Alpha blocking
      3. Delirium, stupor, and coma
   C. The sleeping EEG
      1. Sleep stages: Ontogenesis
      2. REM periods
      3. Dreaming
      4. Mechanisms
   D. Physiological correlates of sleep
      1. Spinal mechanisms
      2. Temperature
      3. Hormonal rhythms
         a. Melatonin
         b. Catecholamines
         c. Sex hormones
         d. Prolactin
         e. Cortisol
   E. Sleep deprivation: Effects
   F. Jet lag: Effects on behavior and physiology
   G. Circadian rhythms
      1. Role of oscillators
      2. "Zeitgeibers"
III. The Biology of Sexual Behavior, Including Mating
   A. Relevance for medicine
   B. Sexual differentiation
      1. Genetic factors
      2. Anatomical factors
      3. Hormonal factors
      4. Social fctors—learning
      5. Rearing
         a. Heterosexual
         b. Isosexual
   C. Sexual dimorphism: Hermaphroditism
   D. Puberty—hormonal factors
      1. Secondary sexual characteristics
      2. Pheromones—olfaction
         a. Tactile stimulation
         b. Temperature and light
      3. Lordosis behavior—hormonal factors
      4. Mating behavior
         a. Neural mechanisms
         b. Hormonal mechanisms
         c. Neuromuscular mechanisms
      5. Estrus and menstrual cycle regulation
IV. The Biology of Emotional Behavior
   A. Relevance to medicine
   B. The tripartite characteristics of the emotions
   C. The specificity and integrated nature of emotional behavior
   D. The communication of emotion

E. The psychobiology of emotion
      1. Autonomic components
      2. Endocrine components
      3. Immune components
   F. The neurobiology of emotional behavior
      1. Pontine mechanisms
      2. Midbrain mechanisms
      3. Hypothalamic mechanisms
      4. Limbic mechanisms
         a. Septum
         b. Amygdala
         c. Cingulate gyrus
   G. The integration of behavior and physiology—Role of brain peptides
V. The Biology of Learning and Memory
   A. Relevance for medicine
   B. Types of learning
      1. Simple: Habituation and sensitization—neurobiology
      2. Associative: Classical, operant, one-trial (aversive)
         a. Neurobiology
         b. Psychobiology—conditioning of visceral responses
      3. Complex: Imprinting, latent, vicarious
   C. Memory
      1. Neurobiology: Synaptic mechanisms
      2. New connections
      3. Peptides
      4. The hippocampus

THE SECOND YEAR

In the second year, the student's view of medicine is biased further toward pathological anatomy and physiology—the classical topics of medicine which we owe to Morgagni, Bichat, Pasteur, and Virchow. The student's concepts of pathogenesis and etiology (frequently not differentiated) are directed toward their (outdated) unicausal nature in virology, bacteriology, and genetics. A complex interactive model is rarely taught—one that incorporates the fact, for example, that the time of day a bacterium is injected into an animal determines the outcome. And, the immune system is taught as if it were a "Ding an Sich"—as if it operated in a vacuum, independent of the rest of the body.

But, most seriously, the student never learns that there is a "medicine without signs," or that the greatest cause of morbidity and mortality in adolescence is the consequence of violence, alcohol ingestion, and human error. To exemplify, figures on the reasons for physician visits in the United States in 1977-1978 indicate the following: headache (9×10^6), weight gain (6.2×10^6), anxiety and nervousness (6×10^6), low back pain (4.8×10^6), depression (4.5×10^6), and tiredness and exhaustion (4×10^6). These are complaints that are most unlikely to have a pathological anatomy. Their diagnostic relevance and understanding are not taught—certainly not in the pathology laboratory or in any course in the behavioral sciences or psychiatry that I know of. Should these data not be brought to the attention of the student immediately and tied to knowledge about behavior and the impact of experience on human beings? I would suggest that this information be brought to the attention of students at a time when they are learning pathology, to counteract the impression that all illness is only due to disease. Such a course might have the following content:

I. Medicine Without Signs
   A. A conceptual framework for health, illness, and disease
   B. The nature of illness
   C. The epidemiology of illness
II. The antecedents of Illness
   A. Natural disasters and danger
   B. Manmade disasters
   C. Bereavement
   D. Unemployment
   E. Retirement
III. Selective Pressures on Man
IV. Their Consequences and Their Psychobiology
   A. The post-traumatic syndromes
   B. Grief and its consequences
   C. Responses to danger
V. Illness Behaviors and Their Consequences
   A. Alterations in food intake—obesity and anorexia
   B. Alterations of liquid intake
      1. Water intoxification
      2. Alcoholism
      3. Diabetes insipidus
   C. Drug abuse
   D. Alterations in sleep patterns
      1. Fatigue
      2. Fibromyalgias
      3. Cardiovascular consequences
   E. Alterations of cardiorespiratory function
      1. Hyperventilation syndrome
      2. Anxiety syndromes
   F. Alterations in bowel function
   G. Alterations in growth
   H. Headache
   I. Other pain syndromes
   J. Disturbances of action
   K. Alterations in reproductive function
VI. Prevention, Intervention and Treatment
   A. Support, self-help groups
   B. Relaxation
   C. Meditation
   D. Biofeedback in the specific illnesses—epilepsy, hypertension, headaches, bowel disorders, hyperventilation, etc.

THE CLINICAL YEARS

Clinical teaching has a very low priority in medical schools (Swanson, 1984). A great deal of the teaching of students is left to the least experienced physicians—interns, residents, or fellows. Furthermore, in most major university centers, there has been a radical shift in the patient population: Only the terminally ill have ready access—those with AIDS; malignancies (in the end stages or several at the same time); multiple-system diseases; end-stage brain, renal, or pulmonary disease; or exotically rare diseases. An atmosphere of therapeutic pessimism and hopelessness thus pervades the wards. Additionally, little attention is paid to the anxieties, discomforts, pains, griefs, and hopelessness of patients and their families. Over and over again, because students and young physicians feel they cannot "do" anything—that is, "cure" mortal diseases—they turn away from patients. Their own grief, dimly recognized, is defended against by annoyance at and/or hardening of attitudes toward patients. I submit that no number of courses on ethics will teach students to be involved in the care of their severely ill or dying patients. Negative attitudes should be negatively reinforced immediately. And, the skills of recognizing grief, helplessness, etc. in themselves and in their patients should be taught. No amount of reading and lecturing substitutes for proper role modeling and focused teaching. Nor can compassion be left to chance—the skills that make compassionate physicians *can* be taught.

The early exposure of students to mortal, physical disease forces the student to embrace a narrow conceptual model of medicine—espoused by Seldin, "...the relief of pain, the prevention of disability and the postponement of death..." (Seldin, 1981, pp. xxxiii). Nothing in this definition of medicine is said about health maintenance, the prevention of illness and disease, rehabilitation, or helping patients to cope with disease or to die gracefully.

The care of patients as people and the recognition and tolerance of their distress requires a great deal of thought, experience, and commitment. It is much easier to learn high-technology, dehumanized medicine, which is the model practiced on wards of academic centers. Cassell (1984), has identified two additional and major issues in the clinical education of students: (a) A sophisticated concern with pathophysiology taught in medical school and the unexamined reliance on patterns of tests to substantiate the defects, leading to its "cookbook," but not an integrated treatment of the patient. (b) A generation of teachers with clinical experience under their belts who have the responsibility, but not the authority, to care for patients which the house officer has preempted.

What, then, can be done? It follows from the above that to focus exclusively on pathophysiology in the critically ill patient is to acquire an immediate bias which most students never relinquish. Thus, the wards of university hospitals do not provide the best experience that would acquaint students with the illnesses for which most patients seek help. If students were initially exposed to a wide range of illnesses (not only disease), they would also be forced to acknowledge the preeminent role of social and behavioral factors in their etiology.

This exposure would impel the student to learn to gather data, not only about symptoms and signs of illness and disease, but about sick perons living in their social, familial, and work environments. They should also be enjoined to learn to analyze their data, assess its reliability, explicate the process by which they reached diagnostic decisions, and learn to use laboratory data only as validating criteria and not as their main diagnostic tools. Above all, they should systematically learn specific skills in recognizing the cognitive, emotional, and personal responses of their patients, and learn to analyze the illness and disease. Such specific skills should be taught and continuously reiterated in the manner outlined by Engel (1983).

I. Characteristics of the Symptom
   A. How often or how continuous is it during the day or night?
   B. When does it occur during the day, etc.—associated with what? Time course (meals, at work, at home, exercise, etc.)
   C. The nature of the symptom
      Describe symptom how? (e.g., Pain: sharp, dull, continuous, intermittent; as a simile, metaphor, etc.)
   D. What vital function, if any, does it interfere with?
II. Antecedent Factors
   A. Are there prodromal symptoms (aura, rapid heartbeat, dry mouth, etc.)?
      1. Nature
      2. Duration
   B. Availability of relief
   C. Nature of medication
      1. Name of drug
      2. Amount taken
      3. When taken
   D. Under what circumstances or conditions do these antecedent symptoms occur?
III. Contingent Factors
   A. Social context of symptoms (alone, with others)
   B. Behavior during episode
      1. Stopped activity, etc.
      2. Sought help
      3. Tried to relieve it
   C. Behavior after episode
      1. Continued activity
      2. Reported it, hid it, etc.
   D. Behavior associated with symptom (appropriate, inappropriate)
   E. Behaviors—actions, emotions, cognitions associated with symptom (fear, shame, self-blame, etc.)
   F. Responses of others to symptom

The teacher should at all times make explicit the relevance of this information for the diagnosis and care of the patient. The teaching of an integrated medicine is today honored only in the breach, in part because the entire training of young students and physicians takes place in an atmosphere of crisis, emergency, and impending death in tertiary-care hospitals.

Rather, students should first be taught medicine in ambulatory care settings and emergency rooms. There they would acquaint themselves with the range of misery, distress, injury, and disease that is most commonly seen. In short, they must first learn what the content of medicine is, what doctors do, and how patients do or do not function, without first determining to what specialist they can "punt" the patient. The student should then follow his or her patient from the ambulatory setting to the inpatient or outpatient unit in which the patient is next cared for. Students should initially have an extensive rather than intensive experience, paying particular attention to every aspect of the patient's functioning and care.

Students should have experiences in prenatal and well-baby clinics, in weight-reduction clinics, and so forth. They should also be exposed to methods of changing behaviors and bad habits and modifying symptoms by behavioral and psychosocial means.

A more intensive clinical experience with the hospitalized patient might occur in the fourth year, at no time neglecting the patient-oriented approach, which hopefully the student will have acquired. This learning must, however, at all times be reinforced by a broad approach to each patient that emphasizes the relevance of the context in which the patient became sick: the nature of the disease(s) and how it is (they are) affecting the vital biological functions of the patient; the manner in which the patient is coping with his or her disease; and whether the capacity to cope is impaired by altered language, cognition, mood, or feeling states; an understanding of the present state of patients in terms of their personal histories and background; how all of this information is best used to care for patients and treat their diseases; and a careful weighing of the effects and benefits (or not) of medications.

Such a revised curriculum will require much thought and reorganization of training, re-education of faculties, and a much greater emphasis on the aim and process of medical education in the face of a long tradition, inertia, and strong resistance to change.

REFERENCES

Association of American Medical Colleges. (1984). Physicians for the twenty-first century. *Journal of Medical Education, 59,* 1-208.

Cassell, E. J. (1984). Practice versus theory in academic medicine: The conflict between house officers and attending physicians. *Bulletin of the New York Academy of Medicine, 60,* 297-308.

Chin, D., Hopkins, D., Melman, K., & Holman, H. R. (1985). The relation of faculty academic activity to financing sources in a department of medicine. *New England Journal of Medicine, 312,* 1029-1034.

Committee on Medical Education. (1984). Symposium on the training of tomorrow's physicians: How well are we meeting society's expectations? *Bulletin of the New York Academy of Medicine, 60,* 219-310.

Eichna, L. W. (1983). A medical school curriculum for the 1980s. *New England Journal of Medicine, 308,* 18-21.

Engel, B. T. (1983). Fecal incontinence and encopresis: A psychophysiological analysis. In R. Hoelzl & W. E. Whitehead (Eds.), *Psychophysiology of the gastrointestinal tract* (pp. 301-310). New York: Plenum.

Institute of Medicine. (1983). *Medical education and societal needs: A planning report for the health professions.* Washington, DC: National Academy Press.

Josiah Macy, Jr., Foundation. (1980). *Graduate medical education present and prospective: Call for action.* New York: Josiah Macy, Jr., Foundation.

Lloyd, G. (1983). Medicine without signs. *British Medical Journal, 287,* 539-542.

Patient's reasons for visiting physicians: National ambulatory care survey—United States, 1977-1978. Data from National Health Survey, Series 13, No. 56. Hyattsville, MD: DHHS Publication No. (PHS) 82-1717, U.S.-DHHS, NCHS.

Seldin, D. W. (1981). Presidential Address. *Transactions of the Assoc. of Am. Phys., xclv:* lxxv-lxxxvi.

Shapiro, M. F., & Charrow, R. P. (1985). Scientific misconduct in investigational drug trials. *New England Journal of Medicine, 312,* 731-736.

Sierles, F., Hendrick, I., & Circle, S. (1980). Cheating in medical school. *Journal of Medical Educaion, 55,* 124-125.

Swanson, A. G. (1984). The medical school student and the faculty forest. *Bulletin of the New York Academy of Medicine, 60,* 290-296.

9
TRAINING OF FAMILY PHYSICIANS IN BEHAVIORAL MEDICINE

Hiram B. Curry
Department of Family Medicine
Medical University of South Carolina

Physicians in ancient times must have helped their patients. Patients sought their care, they were appreciative, they returned. This was the pattern for at least 8,000 years of recorded history. Everyone thought medical care was excellent until the Flexner Report came out in 1910.

The Flexner Report pointed out the difference between the best-prepared and the poorest-prepared physicians of the 1910 era. It brought about a great improvement in the scientific training of physicians. I would not presume to comment further, except to say that I do not believe Flexner intended for physicians to lessen their understanding of patients and their behavior.

I attended medical school from 1946 to 1950. My training was scientific. The good physician was praised in general terms if the subject came up, but no one had a responsibility to help us become good physicians. It was as if we were to become good physicians unconsciously, unknowingly, by osmosis, through occasional contact with good physicians. And we were exposed to worthy models on the wards and in the clinics.

I know that the members of this Academy are in favor of behavioral education for all health professionals. I believe you have a special interest in medical students. I am in complete agreement with the GPEP Report. You are as familiar with this important report as I am.

Now the question is, how do we "emphasize the acquisition and development of skills, values, and attitudes by students, at least to the same extent that they do their acquisition of knowledge?" Do we talk about the characteristics of good health professionals in the lecture hall? Perhaps a few lectures will do some good, but the real payoff will come when they see residents and senior students modeling the values and attitudes we associate with excellent patient care. Students spend much less time with faculty members.

We embraced a strategy in Charleston whereby we focus our attention on our residency program. Our residents work in the hospital. They work with and teach students. Students come to the Family Medicine Center for electives. Here they work with our faculty and residents, whose actions and behaviors are louder than their words. Many comments by many students cause me to believe that our strategy is working.

I propose to tell you why I changed my career in order to experiment in the area of medical education, to produce a new kind of family physician. Then I wish to discuss the curriculum for these trainees, excluding training in the medical sciences which I will not describe. I want to mention how the behavioral sciences material is presented, by whom, and how learning in this area is evaluated. Finally, I wish to comment on the change in the person of the young doctor which must occur if he is to become a physician capable of giving truly, wholistic and optimal care.

When I taught neurology in the 1960s, I would ask students to make a symptomatic diagnosis, then an anatomic diagnosis, next a pathophysiologic diagnosis, and finally an etiological diagnosis. Most of the time, making an etiological diagnosis for a "simple" tension headache stumped the students, and stumped me. I realized that I didn't know enough about people and their life styles and stresses to make an etiological diagnosis. I could run the tracts, review the anatomy and physiology of the nerve-muscle endplate; but that wouldn't help the patient. Earlier I had felt anger when general practitioners and internists referred tension-headache patients to me—a waste of my time. I changed my attitude. Someone needed to learn to help these patients. And there were many of them.

Perhaps a patient that I saw October 3, 1984, will demonstrate several points I wish to make.

Mrs. G., a 58-year-old, right-handed, white housewife has had severe headaches since age 15. She recalls seeing a doctor once during high school. She was reassured that they were not serious. She took aspirin and BCs. BCs are a well-known headache powder, more popular 30 years ago than now. The headaches have occurred about five days out of each week for 43 years. She has always been a hard worker. Only when her headache was very bad and long-lasting would she go to bed or not attend to her usual duties.

There was generalized head discomfort which started any time of day. The headache usually began in the back of her head and neck. Only with long-lasting headaches and after medication would she become nauseated and vomit. She had never experienced any prodromata.

She married at 19. Her husband was a mortician in the Air Force. They lived on many bases, including several in Europe. They had two daughters who are now college graduates, married, and have one and two children.

Mrs. G. has been seen by many physicians of several specialties. She has had scores of tests: skull x-rays, EEGs, even a pneumoencephalogram, arteriograms, and three CT scans—all normal.

9. TRAINING OF FAMILY PHYSICIANS   187

She has followed various diets and avoided certain foods. She worked with a psychologist to learn relaxation therapy. Later she worked with another to learn biofeedback. These techniques were helpful, but only for a brief period.

Recently she was seen several times by a university neurologist. He was worried by the frequency of her severe headaches and the number of visits to emergency rooms, where she was usually given injections of Demerol and Phenergan. He knew I had a special interest in headaches and asked me to see her. No family member had severe headaches or migraine. Her general physical and neurological examinations were normal.

As a general practitioner in the 1950s, what would I have done for such a patient? I believe I would have examined her carefully. I would have classified this as a muscle-contraction headache. Then I would have reassured her and given her non-narcotic analgesics. When I became frustrated after many visits, I would have referred her to an internist or a neurologist.

As an internist in the early 1960s, how would I have managed her? I would have done the same as when a GP and made the same diagnosis. I would have excluded a chromaffin-type tumor, and I might have considered hypoglycemia as a possible trigger. Maybe I would have used various diets to exclude an allergy or an offending food.

As a neurologist later in the 1960s, I could have done little better. I would have made the same diagnosis. I would have been more confident of my ability to exclude structural disease, but that would not have helped the patient.

Circumstances developed in 1970 that gave me the opportunity to experiment in medical education, to design a program that would (a) provide training in the medical sciences appropriate for primary care, and (b) include relevant topics in the behavioral sciences to help the young medical doctor understand people, their coping behaviors, responses to stress, effects of life styles, etc. (i.e., a behavioral sciences curriculum appropriate for primary care).

Earlier the Medical University of South Carolina had asked me to propose a plan that would produce a primary-care doctor who would be a competent patient-care physician, could be as proud of his work as other specialists, and the MUSC would be proud to claim. I shall spare you a long story, and only say that I was given the opportunity to implement that proposal which was for a new major department in the School of Medicine. Thus the blueprint for my future effort did not come from the American Academy of Family Physicians or any organization. I did take care that the residency exceeded the requirements for a fully approved residency in family medicine.

An early question was, who will teach how to understand people? I had in mind two or three general practitioners who more or less modeled the qualities I had in mind. But more than this was needed. We needed to look at these qualities, analyze them, and decide the kind of learning experiences that would produce the new type of physician we had in mind. After two or three years, we learned that psychologists were more helpful for that task than psychiatrists. I must give much of the credit for our success to Dr. Alan Johnson, who helped identify and characterize these desirable traits in our early faculty. Once described and given a name, then we could talk about these traits and work to develop them in our program.

In the early years, we determined that a family physician had to assume personal responsibility for his actions (or inactions), values, style, attitude, and the advice he offered. The legal decisions pertaining to abortion at that time focused attention on this issue. This led me to invite Mr. Bert Keller, an ordained minister with a degree in ethics, to join the Department. Over the years, he has had an important influence in having residents identify what they believe as persons and remain faithful to that as physicians.

Now I wish to describe the personnel we found effective in producing the physician we had in mind. In addition to our family physicians, there was Dr. Alan Johnson with his training in Jungian psychology. Another psychologist had emphasized child rearing and the marital relationship in his training. An experienced social worker joined us early. A young psychiatrist who had a special interest in the family joined us—we could depend on him to teach the proper role for psychotropic drugs. The first head of our Division of Behavioral Sciences was an experienced family physician who had had extra training in psychiatry, and he had a special interest in stress and life-style problems.

I will now summarize the content of the behavioral sciences component of our curriculum:

(1) the family, including the life cycle of the family
(2) the community and its meaning
(3) the resident's self-awareness and understanding of himself or herself
(4) ethics and value systems
(5) professional role and function
(6) psychotherapies and counseling skills

In these six areas, there were 38 objectives (Johnson et al., 1977).

The process of teaching the behavioral sciences is important. The first month in this residency program is an orientation to family medicine. At least half of this month is devoted to behavioral topics or activities. In the second and third years, there is a one-month rotation which focuses on applying behavioral sciences information and techniques in family medicine. Many topics are discussed in depth: depression, obesity, school phobias, recurrent headaches, and many more.

In the first month, each new resident is observed by a family physician and a behavioral scientist as he interviews, examines, and advises an adult. The same is repeated for a child. The two faculty members may spend hours with the resident discussing his work and reviewing the videotape of these encounters.

During the initial monitoring and for subsequent taping sessions, deficiences are noted and a plan agreed upon to correct these by a stated date. Clinical monitoring can be initiated at any time by any faculty member or resident.

The behavioral sciences content is taught in several different formats, including encounter groups, role playing, lectures, and videotaping interviews with group analysis of the encounter. There is pre- and post-evaluation for certain courses. It is very difficult to determine the number of hours devoted to behavioral science training because it is often a part of the discussion of patients having structural diseases. We estimate between 15% and 20% of our curriculum is devoted to this area. Some may object to the amount of time invested in such training, but we believe that the time is wisely spent.

Early in the development of our program, the resident's self-awareness and understanding of himself or herself was recognized as being of great importance. We recognized that the person of the family physician is his or her primary diagnostic and therapeutic tool. This means that the values and attitudes of the resident are perhaps as important as medical knowledge and technical skills in addressing primary-care problems. Charisma or a pleasing personality certainly does not compensate for ignorance in the area of medical science. Likewise, specialized technical competence in an unreflective person can be frightening in health care.

It then seemed important to have the resident examine his or her values, attitudes, and behavior as he or she interacted with patients on a daily basis. For example, the resident was asked to reflect on whether he or she was "parenting" or "playing with" the patient, chastising or complimenting the patient, and why. An observer utilizing the audiovisual monitor might share his or her observations also. This can lead the resident to gain new insights and allow him or her to respond to a patient's behavior in a more productive fashion.

The postulate that the person of the family physician is the primary diagnostic and therapeutic tool says what the resident does not know and experience in himself/herself he/she will find difficult, if not impossible, to identify in the patient. The corollary to this statement is that what the resident has been able to find in himself/herself, but not accept, he/she will find impossible to tolerate and care for in the patient. Practically, this means that our behavioral sciences training must help the resident grow personally if he/she is to be able to grow professionally to help patients and their families. To facilitate this personal growth, we developed a program in personal counseling that encourages each resident (and spouse, if they choose) to reflect on his/her own life and feelings and especially on areas that concern him/her. Some graduates have said that this program has meant a great deal to them.

Several years ago, a Balint-trained physician joined our faculty. Two groups were established. These meetings are very similar to those held at the Tavistock Clinic in London in the 1950s. A resident presents a troublesome patient or an unsatisfactory encounter. Often the resident's peers point out a feature of the resident's behavior or attitude to which the resident is blind. This is a powerful way to bring about change—to have those you work with and trust point out your flaws. A trusting relationship is a prerequisite for this process to work. The group leader acts as a catalyst as the group does its work. After a patient is discussed in this setting, the resident often changes to a new and more effective tack in dealing with the patient.

The Balint experience has another application. The resident begins to understand the significance of his or her relationship with his or her peers and patients. He/she learns how others see and perceive him/her. This is an important insight for functioning well in groups, be it a future group practice or serving on a committee in one's community. The young doctor begins to appreciate the underlying dynamics of the doctor-patient relationship, the relationships within the patient's family, and even within the doctor's own family.

In this program, the resident learns that he/she can appropriately use his/her past experiences to relate to his/her patient. He/she is comfortable to abandon the sterile distant professional facade and utilize his/her personhood or genuine self for building a one-on-one relationship with the person of the patient. There is a difference in this kind of a relationship and the usual doctor-patient relationship. A one-on-one personal relationship will tolerate heavy usage for weighty emotional matters. It also embodies trust, and compliance is much improved.

The bottom line for this type of behavioral preparation of the person of the family physician is that he/she grows to recognize and accept himself/herself as an imperfect, error-making, and inconsistent person. It is one thing to intellectually accept this statement. It is another to incorporate it into one's daily life and work. Acknowledging that all patients are imperfect, error-making, and inconsistent comes easily. When two people build a relationship on this basis, it is realistic. And it works very well for the doctor and for the patient.

The physician is no longer to be trained simply as a medical technician who manipulates physiological and biochemical processes. Rather, the physician is to be educated as an individual whose whole personality is to be the "instrument" through which he/she works as a physician to promote growth and to help restore persons to a state of wholeness or wellness. It is, therefore, essential that the behavioral sciences curriculum be structured to include learning experiences in which the physician can gain a greater awareness of himself/herself, his/her interpersonal style, and his/her professional role.

Until three years ago, the second- and third-year residents had a one-month behavioral sciences rotation in the Family Medicine Center. During the early years, we said repeatedly that we wished that the residents would become a new type of physician, having balanced abilities in the medical and behavioral sciences. We depended largely on the behavioral scientists for the behavioral component. The time came about four years ago when our family physicians were actually teaching as well as modeling the synthesis of the medical and behavioral sciences. We had been waiting for this to happen. The rotation name was changed to the family medicine rotation, and our family physicians now take a leadership role in it. At one time the Behavioral Sciences Division had seven positions. Now there are four and one-half: psychiatrist, one and one-half psychologists, ethicist, and social worker.

After that description of our residency program, let me return to Mrs. G. Have I learned yet how to help such patients? I know that I must learn more about the person, Mrs. G., who has had these thousands of headaches.

The nurse commented that Mrs. G came almost an hour before her appointment. I mentioned this to Mrs. G and learned that her mother had insisted that everything be done on time or, better, be done *ahead* of time. And what were the consequences if not done on time? "She would crawl my back."

I asked her to tell me about her mother. There was a highly significant hesitation. Then she related that her mother had been a 13-year-old, full-blooded Cherokee Indian. "What is the earliest memory of your mother?" "She and her sister, who couldn't have a child, arguing because the aunt wanted me to live with her. 'God gave me this young'n' to raise, and I'll do it.' " The patient did not recall ever hearing her mother say that she loved her. In fact, she could recall the opposite. She was repeatedly told that she was trash and worthless. She had three stepfathers before she was 12 years old. All of them died violent deaths.

Mrs. G reported that at age the age of 17, she stole money from her mother's purse to buy a Greyhound bus ticket to Los Angeles. Tears came to her eyes. In Los Angeles, she enjoyed life more and had fewer headaches than before. Her mother found her and forced her to return. She finished high school. She began dating an Air Force private. At his first mention of marriage, she said "yes"(she accepted his proposal), although she says she really did not love him.

I asked her if she had ever told the story of her childhood to anyone. She said "No." She said doctors asked if family members had headaches, but not about how she grew up. I asked if she had told her husband. She had not, and they have been married 39 years. "He's from a good family. He would not understand. I'd be ashamed to tell him how I grew up."

Then I asked if any doctor had ever told her that she needed to talk about her problems. Yes, one doctor had told her that she should talk to herself in the mirror. She did not change her facial expression, so I asked if that helped. "Maybe a little, but it didn't last."

Then I asked if any doctor had suggested that she should talk to a psychiatrist or psychologist. Yes, one did, but she didn't think she was crazy, so she didn't go back to him.

Then I asked Mrs. G if she would say after me "I am a good person." She said "I am _____," but could not say the last three words.

What would be your management plan for Mrs. G? She and her husband live on an enlisted man's military retirement income. They are proud people who wish to pay their way. Does anyone wish to take on this patient?

Because I thought her self-image was poor, I again asked her to say that she was a good person. She said she was *not* a good person. She had told me that she attended every function at her Southern Baptist Church. I told her that I knew the Scripture that troubled her (". . . 'Why do you call me good? No one is good but God alone.' ", Luke 18: 19). I mentioned that I, too, am a Christian. I pointed out that I had not asked her to say that she was perfect. When I listed the worthwhile things she had done and was doing, and affirmed that I thought she was indeed a good person, she finally said it, "I am a good person," and smiled.

I thanked her for telling me about her childhood, for trusting me. I was not ashamed to mention that I had a strict father, that I could understand to a degree her feelings about her childhood. Knowing the potential effectiveness of the wounded healer, I mentioned that I used to have severe headaches. Here I was using my person, my self, to strengthen our relationship so that I could help her.

I believed that she needed to ventilate feelings locked within her memory since childhood but to whom? This process might need to be continued for years. "Do you have a good friend?" "Yes, I have one that I would be comfortable to tell anything to." I then suggested that this church friend and the patient meet at least twice a week to talk about the details of her childhood. "Muster up your courage and talk." She said that she would.

And I had to help her improve her self image. "Every time you think of your headaches or yourself or pass a mirror, say to yourself 'I am a good person, and God loves me.' " She said she would do it.

I stressed that there was no medicine for her problem—that only *she* could help herself, by talking; and I believed that she could and would overcome her headache problem. I recommended only aspirin or Tylenol for partial relief of her headache saying this was the only safe medicine. I told her that stronger medicines were addictive and potentially harmful and would cause her to feel bad even after the headache was over.

When should I see this patient again? Would she do as I suggested to please me or would she do these things to help herself? I decided to make no subsequent appointment. I had spent one hour and fifteen minutes with her.

Two weeks later I called her at home. She was very surprised and pleased that I called. I did so to prove that I valued her as a person, I respected her as a good person, and I was interested in her and her headache problem. And since there was no money involved in my calling, she could not think my reasons were otherwise.

I was absolutely delighted when she said that she had met with her friend as suggested and both were enjoying getting to know each other better. She also said that she was saying "I am a good person" and "God loves me." And she told me that she had not had a headache since we met—unbelievable, but true.

I called again after another three weeks. The report was as favorable as the first one, and again in three or four weeks the report was the same.

About three months after seeing Mrs. G, I decided to share her story with the family medicine residents and faculty at a noon conference. I am not sure everyone believed the story completely. At the end of five months, with monthly calls and no return of headaches, I asked Mrs. G if she would be willing to come for a noon conference. She quickly said she would. On mentioning her friend, she volunteered to bring her too.

I was very pleased when she arrived on time but not ahead of schedule. The noon meeting was in the style of a Phil Donahue program with the audience asking Mrs. G and her friend any and as many questions as they wished. The conference went overtime. She told them that she had not had any more headaches.

I called her recently (June 4, 1985). She had one mild headache two weeks ago while preparing grades for the kindergarten children. She did not see a physician.

I have chosen my most dramatic success story to illustrate why and how we emphasize the behavioral sciences in the education of family physicians. Not only do I recognize that the person of the family physician is his or her primary diagnostic and therapeutic tool, my person is the tool I use most in helping patients like Mrs. G. I use what I have learned and what I have experienced in my medical training and in my entire life to help such patients. Being a part of this Department of Family Medicine has helped me to become the physician I have always wished to be. And I believe its faculty and programs will help each young medical doctor realize his or her dream to become a physician.

I have also learned that the person is the most powerful tool of the teacher. My person is my best tool as a teacher. That which I have not learned and experienced as a person, I have difficulty in teaching. I continue to learn and to have new experiences. I hope to become a good teacher.

REFERENCE

Johnson, A. H., Fisher, J. V., Guy, L. J., Keith, J. A., Keller, A. H., & Sherer, L. M. (1977). Developing behavioral science for a family practice residency. *The Journal of Family Practice*, *4*(2), 319.

10
TEACHING BEHAVIORAL CONCEPTS IN CARDIOVASCULAR DISEASE WITH REMARKS ON CHALLENGES TO MEDICAL EDUCATION

Alvin P. Shapiro
University of Pittsburgh School of Medicine

A review of what has been written and said on the topic of medical education and its problems reveals material that is often painfully repetitive. One runs the gamut of literature ranging from dire predictions of disaster to sweeping generalizations of hope for the future. In conferences, panel reports, and individual papers from the AMA, the AAMC, and various foundations, the crises of medical education have been belabored, it seems in 5-year cycles, by many who are more erudite than I. For instance, you heard earlier in this symposium from Dr. Smith that the Flexner report was a failure and from Dr. Geiger that medical education is reductionist and mechanistic and we should abandon the teaching hospitals and return to the community hospitals. These opinions attack basic premises in medical education and I cannot possibly agree with them because, if carried to their inevitable conclusions, we would return to a medical education in which scholarship is secondary to technical training.

Despite all the criticisms, there seems to have been little substantive change in medical education. Perhaps because we are living in the midst of perceived change, the landmarks which indicate that a true need for change in medical education has evolved are hard to find. To be sure, from my present-day perspective, I can recognize that the major redirections, as Dr. Smith so clearly noted, which occurred following the Flexner report, redefined the relations of medical schools to universities and led to the joint development of basic science and clinical teaching. What is unclear to me is whether the current arguments that the Flexner model has failed, and that medical education must develop a more humanistic, a more compassionate, and a better-rounded physician with a greater awareness of the socioeconomics of medicine, the impact of disease on behavior or behavior on disease, and the problems of "medi-business" do indeed represent new revelations, requiring a new point of departure.

Kenneth Warren (1984) has discussed this in a recent article by pointing out that, to a considerable extent, changes that are being recommended or even being made are done on the basis of a number of mirages which are repeatedly expressed in both the lay and the professional literatures. For instance, he discusses the question of the preparation of our medical students during their premedical programs. Premedical education has been criticized as lacking sufficient input from courses in the humanities, a situation which arises because students perceive that medical school admission is so difficult that they must concentrate on the biological and chemical sciences and neglect the humanities and social sciences. Yet, as Warren points out, the data clearly show that it is not as difficult as it seems to get into medical school because although only one of 20 may get into a particular school, 50% of applicants overall are being admitted, with the data on low acceptance rates obviously distorted by the average of 10 applications per student. Moreover, recent data from the AAMC have demonstrated that acceptance rates are not appreciably affected by whether the student has majored in English, philosophy, or foreign languages or in biology, chemistry, or physics. In fact, the highest perentage acceptance (67%) was in students who majored in music!

And yet, this mirage has now reached the proportion of the proverbial story of the Emperor's new clothes, and recently the Dean of the Johns Hopkins Medical School announced that Hopkins will no longer require MCAT examinations because "they make students concentrate too much on the sciences, and we are interested in well-rounded students." However, in defending his position in an interview which was given to a reporter on National Public Radio, he stated that Hopkins will not ignore the sciences but will look more carefully at grades in courses in the sciences in college, instead of at the MCATs only—something we have always done in admissions policy.

But I would hesitate to abandon the MCATs since they generally show a correlation with college grades at the better universities and also provide a better uniformity among universities. He then further pointed out, in answer to the reporter's questions, that "No, the decision does not mean that it will be more likely that a student who did poorly in sciences would find it easier to get into medical school." In other words, we are planning to take away a symbol, but not change our practice of evaluating performance in the sciences which, in any case, is a good practice.

A student's major field of undergraduate education does not necessarily determine his or her avocational attributes. Until someone demonstrates that a student of the sciences cannot be just as capable of compassion and humanity as a colleague who has not disciplined himself or herself to achieving academic excellence in this area, I will continue to believe that students who are able to think quantitatively and to know biological principles can also be aware of the beauty of a Chagall painting, the profound insights of Tolstoy and Shakespeare, and, yes, even the batting averages of his/her favorite major league ballplayer. Moreover, I believe that a thorough knowledge of the biological and quantitative sciences makes it easier to be a physician and is just as important as the basis for learning how to care for a patient as is an understanding of musical scales to becoming a violinist or of the physics of the stresses and strains of various materials in learning to be an engineer and build bridges.

One other point about premedical education is worthy of note. Dr. Geiger and others have pointed out that much of what is taught in baccalaureate programs, particularly in sciences, is not pertinent to medical practice and could be eliminated and that, accordingly, the duration of premedical education could be shortened. Why, for instance, asks Dr. Geiger, should pre-med students in organic chemistry be required to learn about petroleum chemistry? I would reply that the premedical education, which is pertinent to medical school education, is in fact only a small part of the overall experience of the student in a 4-year undergraduate program. The latter should be an experience unto itself, and the more it can encompass in terms of a liberal arts education, the more it achieves the goal of providing the physician with the same opportunities as the future lawyer, the business executive, and even the engineer to become a broadly educated person. To be sure, the "scholastic ideal" may not always be achieved for any of the above, but I would think it inappropriate and defeatist for us to sacrifice the undergraduate program to the faster production of physicians.

My thesis, therefore, is that we are not in an educational crisis with regard to how we prepare our premedical students or what we teach them in medical school. Although we have different facts to teach now than we had 30 years ago, the fundamental goal is still the same—namely that of providing quality teaching, providing role models, and providing an atmosphere of inquiry and curiosity by research from which, hopefully, will emerge the medical student who will maintain habits of learning and attitudes of compassion throughout his/her medical career. To be sure, there are practical problems which do, at times, achieve crisis levels, such as the financing of medical schools, the financing of students, and the changes created by new methods of health care funding in the hospitals which serve as our educational laboratories. But these are operational considerations, which we share with all of society, and they should not make us wish to change our educational mission and goal. In brief, we must take the bright, curious, and highly intelligent group of students who come to us with an avowed basic interest in "helping people by applying scientific knowledge" (I have heard this statement so many times from premedical students being interviewed for admission to medical school that I now believe it) and create in him/her an attitude of lifelong striving for excellence along with learning habits which will make them continue to acquire knowledge and be excited about performing in this profession.

To illustrate that this is not new, consider the following conclusion from the report by the Commission on Medical Education to the AAMC in 1932, the same report which Dr. Smith quoted to emphasize concerns about rigidity and standardization in curriculum.

> The medical course cannot produce a physician. It can only provide the opportunities for a student to secure an elementary knowledge of the medical sciences and their application to health problems, a training in the methods and spirit of scientific inquiry, and the inspiration and point of view which come from association with those who are devoting themselves to education, research, and practice. Medicine must be learned by the student, for only a fraction of it can be taught by the faculty. The latter makes the essential contributions of guidance, inspiration, and leadership in learning. The student and the teacher, not the curriculum, are the crucial elements in the educational program. (Rappleye, 1932)

How does one go about achieving such goals with particular attention to my topic, the teaching of behavioral medicine in internal medicine in general and in cardiovascular disease in particular?

One can look at this from the point of view of an old Talmudic comment: "When you do not know where you are going, it makes no difference which road you take." But I would prefer to follow Lincoln's advice, from his "House Divided" speech in 1858: "If we could first know *where* we are, and *wither* we are tending, we could better judge *what* to do and *how* to do it." Therefore, I shall speak to the *who*, the *where*, the *what*, and the *how* of such teaching: (a) *Who* should teach behavioral and psychosomatic concepts; should this be done primarily by psychiatrists and behavioral scientists or by internists and cardiologists or a combination of same? (b) *Where* should the material be taught; on the medical wards or in psychiatric units and at which time of the curriculum? (c) *What* should one teach in terms of content; what specific body of behavioral theory and management should be included? (a) *How* should it be taught; on rounds, in conferences, in group sessions, etc.?

I should preface my remarks on teaching by a few words about terminology. I will speak of the material which should be taught as "behavioral medicine" because that is the catchword of today, and it is name of our Academy. I must confess, and with apologies to some of my colleagues, that this term to me is not any different from what I called "psychosomatic medicine" in my youth in Cincinnati when Gene Ferris, Milt Rosenbaum, John Romano, George Engel, and Arthur Mirsky were conducting a grand experiment under the sponsorship of the Commonwealth Fund in training students and fellows in psychosomatic concepts ranging from research to therapy in conditions such as hypertension, peptic ulcer, syncope, and so forth. The field has been called "comprehensive medicine," "somatic-psychic medicine,"and "holistic medicine" and has been included more recently under the rubrics of "family medicine" and "general medicine." In fact, even then and still now one can include under this heading anything that affects man and his emotions, including the care of the indigent, funding of medical services, and Selye's adaptation syndrome. The field is a continuum which ranges from Hippocrates to Cannon, from Pavlov to Neal Miller, from Flanders Dunbar's descriptions of the coronary-prone personality to present Type A and B classifications, and from Franz Alexander's specificity theories to current concepts in hypertension concerning whether hostile and withdrawn attitudes are causes or consequences of hypertensive disease. So, I will use "behavioral medicine" as the catchword, but I cannot accept a dichotomy between it and what has gone before.

The first question is *Who* should teach behavioral aspects of cardiovascular disease? I will say that at all levels of medical education, those who are teaching the physiology, the pharmacology, and the biochemistry of the cardiovascular system as well as the clinical care of cardiac patients should introduce into their material those established facts as well as the appropriate speculations about behavioral influences. Increasingly, I think this is done in neurophysiology and neurosciences courses even in first-year medicine in which concepts presented by Schneiderman in this volume are discussed. But it has not caught on as well in the teaching of cardiovascular physiology where reactivity to behavioral stimuli should be an important part of the material presented and in biochemistry where the effects of behavioral stimuli on hormonal changes and on lipid risk factors should at least be introduced. More and more this teaching can come from psychologists trained in behavioral medicine. Although in the past their education has largely been lacking in physiology, now many coming from a research orientation are increasingly adept at understanding and teaching cardiovascular psychophysiology. Our institution started a behavioral cardiovascular training program several years ago, and its purpose is to train psychology "postdoctorates"(Ph.D.) in cardiovascular research methodology and to train M.D. internists, psychiatrists, and pediatricians in the use of quantitative behavioral research techniques. We are hoping to develop individuals from these programs, who in the future can participate in teaching the sciences basic to medicine.

In the clinical years, a body of knowledge about risk factors in the development of cardiovascular disease is available which has many psychological implications. It is best introduced by the clinical faculty who are teaching the "Introduction to Medicine" in the second-year courses, and at our school we try to do this with varying degrees of success. It depends almost entirely on the interests of the individual who is teaching a given block of the course. I devote at least one lecture, of the three or four which I give each year on hypertension, to the behavioral aspects of the disease because this is one of my interests, and my colleagues in epidemiology who teach about risk factors in coronary heart disease talk about the personality aspects of the individual as a risk factor, as well as about smoking, cholesterol, diabetes, and so forth. I think every effort should be made within each block of such "Introduction to Medicine" courses, whether it be gastroenterology, endocrinology, infectious disease, etc., to introduce what is known and what is speculated about with regard to behavioral factors with the same emphasis as we do in teaching the "harder" facts. Such courses are only an introduction to clinical medicine but set the pattern for further study. That we do not do more of it is a reflection of the problem of getting certain materials into a curriculum when planning is left to individual entrepreneurs, a problem which I will discuss further later in this essay.

It is during clinical teaching on the wards in the third and fourth years that the best opportunity is present for teaching of behavioral concepts. There is a regrettable tendency on the part of many present-day "rounders" to move away from the bedside and discuss lab findings on the chart and history as obtained secondhand from the house staff and students rather than as supplemented by the attending physician going to the bedside. I have been aghast in recent years at being told by students and young house staff that I am one of their better "rounders" for no other reason than that I go to the bedside, talk to the patient, and do a physical examination at that time. I don't expect kudos for this activity because it is the way I was trained, and I regret that it is disappearing. Dr. Jack Myers at our institution, who was Professor and Chairman of the Department of Medicine for many years and who now has put his encylopedic factual knowledge onto a computer and is in the forefront of computer use for facilitating diagnosis, has nevertheless made the point that the most important data he puts into his computer are those obtained at the bedside (Myers, 1984). The data base derived from a discerning history and a careful physical examination is still, and will ever be, the data which his computer needs to call up other information and start the analytic process.

In the course of this bedside experience, one then has the opportunity to observe the emotional state of the patient; to talk to him; to find out about his family, his fears, and their impact on his illness; and to lead from this to discussion of how such data impact on the specific illness. My late mentor, Arthur Mirsky, has said that the disease state is the outcome of a chain of relevant events which encompass the three Ps of predisposition, precipitation, and perpetuation; students must be encouraged during bedside teaching experiences to recognize this chain of events and not just to think about causality in a one-dimensional fashion. I find that students are extraordinarily perceptive of such connections and easily respond to encouragement to explore these links. We do not, as some have feared, drill this empathy out of them by teaching them biochemical facts and molecular events, but we do not always provide the role models among teachers who encourage them to speak of their feelings and observations about behavioral matters. Let me provide several examples.

Years ago in Cincinnati, Chambers and Reiser (1953) studied 25 consecutive patients who came into the hospital with acute pulmonary edema. These were people with organic heart disease, but in 76% of the patients, the precipitating event was not eating too much salt or running up a flight of stairs but a profound emotional event occurring within the previous few days—information elicited by talking to the patient, with one's stethoscope removed from one's ears.

Many times during my rounding activities on a patient who has recently incurred a myocardial infarction, the simple question, "What were you doing during the day before the pain developed?" provides incidents, often elicited by the students, such as the illness of a family member, an impending break-up with a loved one, a job crisis, etc. An example of one dramatic incident was a man who was our orchestra's assistant conductor and who was scheduled for his first venture in leading the local orchestra himself the next day, in the presence of scouts from a prestigious orchestra who were looking for a new conductor. He developed chest pain while sitting in the barber chair the afternoon before the concert. When he was brought to the emergency room, an EKG revealed a newly developed inferior infarct. When he was informed of this, he said, "Oh no, it can't happen today; I've got too much to do," at which point he promptly went into ventricular fibrillation. Incidents such as these are impressive and not altogether anecdotal and make believers in behavioral impact on disease, of students and even cardiologists. In brief, I think it is the role of the internist to teach behavioral connections in cardiovascular disease to his/her students in cardiology and the role of the psychiatrist and psychologist to supplement them both in formal lectures and conferences as well as to teach some of the behavioral techniques which can be utilized in management of cardiovascular patients. Both groups of faculty should provide impetus and encouragement to obtaining quantitative research data.

I think my remarks have already covered *where* one should teach the behavioral material. It should be taught wherever the opportunity presents but, more formally, teaching on the medical wards by internists and by consultation-liaison psychiatrists on specific patients is crucial. Basic material can be given in the second year and even in the first year, but the major efforts are in the clinical years.

What should be the content of our teaching in the behavioral aspects of cardiovascular disease?

1. We should cover *cardiovascular reactivity*, specifically as it relates to the sympathetic nervous system and neurohormonal release, as well as the intrinsic factors in the heart, blood vessels, and the brain-periphery connections which influence response. There is a vast body of evidence, in this area. This includes information about variability of cardiovascular response to drugs and the comparison of their pharmacologic effects and their placebo effects.

2. We should discuss *behavioral and personality considerations which constitute risk factors*, with specific attention to Type A and all its problematic assumptions and the various deviations from the "classical" which are coming into vogue at the present time. These are risk factors which should be taught, just as we teach about cholesterol, and so forth. In addition, there is an increasing interest in disease effects on behavior which should be introduced.

3. We should teach about *adjustment* to cardiovascular illness. Heart disease produces profound changes in one's life style. The ultimate of this now, in which

we have had increasing experience at our institution, is the profound quality-of-life change experienced by people who survive cardiac transplantation. This topic will lead to further discussion of the ethics of such heroic procedures, again a subject for discussion on rounds as well as for special sessions which now are held regularly in many medical schools and hospitals. Quality-of-life issues, as well as specific ways to handle the disabilities of cardiac illness both by the patient and his or her family, can be taught by the experienced internist with the help of the psychiatrist and social workers who now regularly work on most medical units. Students and house staff are extremely receptive to these approaches. I am often impressed by the concerns which they express about plans for people when they leave the hospital, and not just for the traditional reason of getting that patient off their ward. (The latter is, of course, the well-known "Gomer" syndrome—for those of you who are uneducated in house staff parlance, "Gomer" is an acronym for "get out of my emergency room.")

4. We should teach about *behavioral methods for treatment* and as primary and secondary preventive measures. Specific techniques are perhaps too specialized for the average internist or even psychiatrist to teach; but their potential can be discussed and the facilities available in the community can be explored. In this area, behavioral scientists can play a large role.

5. We cannot easily teach *compassion*, but we can encourage it in our students, and we can set examples, as Dr. Curry so well described in his discussion. We can point out that it is not always necessary to like a patient in order to care for him; a mature physician adapts his approach to the patient. We must not set a dichotomy between brisk, efficient competence and compassion, because "compassion" without "competence" is "care-less." My grandmother was a most compassionate woman, but she was unskilled in applying medical care, and her much-praised chicken soup does not replace the prompt recognition of pneumonia and its treatment with penicillin.

Finally, *how* should behavioral medicine be taught? I think I have covered this question in my earlier remarks—namely that behavioral medicine in cardiovascular disease should be taught primarily in patient-oriented sessions, as in "old-fashioned ward rounds." There is a place, however, for conferences; behavioral concepts should occasionally grace grand rounds and should be regularly part of consultation-liaison conferences held on the medical units. The latter have tended, in recent years, to become somewhat more didactic than I think they were in the past when we presented individual patients and discussed individual problems. The art of interviewing a patient in a group session seems to be slowly disappearing. I think that is because of a misplaced consideration on the part of some that it is an invasion of privacy of the patient to have him talk to you with a group of students present. I did this for many years, and I usually found that patients were open in their comments and enjoyed talking to the group. Of course, it requires some technique, and the avoidance of topics which one realizes are too sensitive to discuss in an open session; but this is a matter of experience and tact, and I would hate to see it disappear for the wrong reasons.

Most importantly, throughout all behavioral teaching must run the theme of the research which is going on in one's own laboratory, in the institution, and in the behavioral sciences at large. We should introduce into the discussions the work which has been done, with the proper literary references, and the work which needs to be done. We should encourage students to think about the unsolved problems and invite some of them to become involved in our laboratories. The latter takes time and the former produces the risk of making one known as the person who always talks about his/her own research. However, when research data are intelligently and properly presented with the proper mix of clinical input, they prepare the student to contribute to the future of behavioral medicine. A medical school's mission is not complete unless it encourages and is involved in investigation; and investigation is not complete unless it is talked about, presented, and set forth for comment and criticism. New ideas often stem from clinical observations, which, when they are brought back to the laboratory, become the most exciting parts of ecucation. Research need not only be at the bench but case-oriented research, epidemiologic investigations, acute studies of the effects of stress, etc., are only a few of the areas which lend themselves to student involvement.

Over the years I have used many methods to try to teach behavioral medicine at the three universities with which I have been associated. In the halcyon days in Cincinnati, we ran weekly psychosomatic conferences which were case presentations and discussions. We developed a Psychosomatic Clinic as part of the outpatient medicine clinic, which in current parlance would be a general medicine clinic. We required junior students on the ward to write up at least one case report during their service on medicine, which went into depth in the emotional aspects of the patient's disease, and this was reviewed, criticized, and discussed with junior and sometimes senior faculty people. And we developed a research ward jointly staffed by psychiatric and medical residents in which "interesting psychosomatic cases" were hospitalized, treated, evaluated, and became the subjects of research projects.

When I went to Dallas as an assistant professor, I started a course called the "Art of Medicine" in the first year which consisted of a case presentation in which I would try to emphasize the emotional as well as the physical aspects of the individual's disease. It was hard work, requiring hours of preparation for each weekly session, and I felt it to be unrewarding and discontinued it after about a year. To my surprise, even years later I have had former students come up to me, and in spite of anything else I have done, they remember me for those sessions. We conducted occasional psychosomatic conferences, and now and again we spoke at grand rounds about specific diseases. There was really little of a Department of Psychiatry in Dallas at the time, and I worked almost entirely out of Internal Medicine. At the same time, I carried on an active research program on stress as it related to hypertension and a variety of other diseases, such as peptic ulcer.

In Pittsburgh, I came to join Arthur Mirsky and Jack Myers with the hope of setting up a medical–psychiatric unit such as we had had at Cincinnati, but, for a variety of reasons it did not work out. Nevertheless, I continued weekly psychosomatic conferences on the medical wards for 20 years and then participated when several of my trainees successively took them over. These were primarily done with the students with a modest and occasionally an enthusiastic input from the house staff, and from these students or house staff members came a few fellows who went on to do productive work in the area. We required students to write up cases as we had done in Cincinnati, and occasionally we again did grand rounds. We gave a few lectures in the first year of psychiatry on psychophysiology, and when I was in the Dean's Office, we began to bring in psychiatrists and social workers as major teachers of history-taking. Many of these programs were started with great enthusiasm. The problem was that after a few years one's enthusiasm waned, but, in some instances, sufficient people were trained to take over these tasks.

At present, I find that much of what we attempted to teach at that time has been spread around among departments. I am continually pleased at our heart-transplant conferences to hear our excellent cardiac surgeons discuss at length the emotional aspects of their patients and the role that these factors play in their suitability for and the success of their surgery. There is active investigation of emotional aspects of disease in thyroid patients and a comprehensive program in the care of young diabetics at our institution. In the epidemiologic studies on the care of hypertensives which are going on in our Graduate School of Public Health, a considerable investment is being made to look at the behavioral consequences of labeling and of pharmacologic therapy. I think that the present-day medical student is, in many ways, more sophisticated, appreciative and demanding of behavioral input than were my colleagues. Although he or she is bombarded with a great many facts, and this is used as an excuse not to bombard him or her with more, I am impressed by the capacity these young people have for information when it is properly formulated in its presentation to them. We sometimes forget that we cannot cram into the heads of our students in four years the accumulated knowledge and perspective that we have taken 30 years to gather, but we can provide the information from research and from example to stimulate them to continue their curiosity through their next 30 years.

I should make a few remarks about the problems of getting behavioral material, or *any* material for that matter, into the curriculum of a medical school from the perspective of one who was a former Dean of Academic Affairs, responsible for the curriculum, and then later was vice-chairman of the Department of Medicine, responsible for the teaching programs in that department. To get anything formally incorporated into a medical school curriculum is a formidable task. It actually has two phases—the first is to get the allotted time to put a given course or new approach into the curriculum, and the second is the control of the content of that course and its evaluation once it is in the curriculum.

The major roadblock in introducing new courses into the curriculum is that of *departmental autonomy*. The departments all want their alloted time, they do not want their turf trodden upon, and unless there is a strong Curriculum Committee chaired by someone with direct authority from the Dean (something which I fear is vanishing from some medical schools), the committee will have little authority as compared to the respective departmental chairmen. The department chairman, himself, once he has been alloted time and in turn re-allots it to the subsections within his department, has relatively little influence on what those particular subsections teach. It is difficult for him to exert his influence on what they present unless he undertakes the impossible task of attending all lectures by every member of his department and offering detailed criticism to them.

Second, there is not a good plan to *evaluate changes in the curriculum*. The criteria used for analyses of the impact of the program change are sometimes misguided, as demonstrated by the events which took place at our medical school in the 1970s (Shapiro, Schuck, Schultz, & Barnhill, 1974). Elimination of the laboratory portions of several of the basic science courses in freshman and sophomore years and subsequent substitution of a completely elective senior year led to a prompt drop in scores on National Boards, Parts I and II, over the next few years. This was, of course, blamed by the faculty on the curricular changes, particularly since MCAT scores in successive classes were continually rising during this time. The same sequence was noted at other schools with resultant retreat to the older curriculum. We persisted in maintaining the changes, and over the next few years, scores gradually returned to previous levels. There obviously could be a number of explanations, for these events, but it seems likely that perturbation per se was as likely the cause of the effect as were differences in content of the curriculum. Moreover, National Board exams were never intended as a means to evaluate changes in curriculum, and it is inappropriate to use them in this fashion. In any case, this lack of proper ways to evaluate the consequences of changes in medical education, leads to resistance to and fear of change.

Third, when changes are contemplated, there is often *a lack of facilities and the funding* necessary to pursue them, both hardware and software. If we decided to make computers available for all of our students, where would we get the monies? Some schools are rich; most of us cannot afford it.

Fourth, there is a *lack of impact from educators trained in course design and evaluation*. This is becoming even worse in medical schools today as funding problems have dried up what investments many schools made in hiring such people in the medical schools. Most medical faculty not only have a dearth of interest in educational techniques but actually an antipathy to it. Many do not understand the concept of devising a course by using educational objectives and developing techniques to test attainment of these objectives. We did some of it at our school while I was in the Dean's Office, but it was not popular; and as one powerful basic science chairman said to me, "Al, you've done a good job in improving our organization; now don't screw it up by asking us to do ridiculous things like defining objectives." In addition, rapidly changing personnel on curriculum committees will assure that continuity of evaluation is *not* maintained when new programs are developed.

Fifth, there is the problem of *evaluating student opinion concerning corruculum*. We can rationalize by saying that it is more important that one pleases the faculty because they are "here forever," whereas students are "gone tomorrow." However, student input can be quite valuable, and it should be listened to with great care. Students have good insights, and they want to be heard. They are as realistic as the rest of us in that they do not necessarily expect all things to change to their satisfaction, and they know that there is no nirvana in which you can be given a discrete amount of material which will allow you to pass your exams, leaving all the rest of your time to "creative learning," which may include sleeping and skiing. Students are willing to accept much of what we throw at them, but they must be listened to as the intelligent, thinking people that they are, and their evaluations of courses and of professors can be of great help.

Sixth, I think that there is a *lack of understanding*, on the part of many of our faculty, *of modern-day concepts of knowledge transmittance*. In other words, we are slow to learn the uses of new techniques. We are slow in using computers for storing knowledge; we tend to mix up process and facts and don't always understand what people like Jack Myers are trying to do by putting the facts into the computer as a textbook and using that as a source for then developing the thinking processes in diagnosis and management.

Finally, there is the "nitty-gritty" problem of *scheduling of students* to provide a continual flow through the various medical school stations (departments), so that all are "touched" by each student and that the faculty is not always out of town when the teachers are scheduled to give lectures. I struggled with the former when I was an academic dean, and we finally worked out a linear programming system which is equivalent to that used in warehouses to make sure that every box gets through every station to get the proper stamp on it as it passes through the warehouse.

May I conclude as I started by saying that I see no crisis in medical education when it comes to the type of students entering and the material we have to teach them. We have practical problems of facilities and funding which are sometimes at a crisis level, but the process of bringing bright students into a medical school, helping them to have fun while learning, and teaching them how to pursue knowledge for the rest of their lives is unchanged. We cannot expect that in four years the student will accumulate the knowledge and experience that we have accumulated over a lifetime, but we can at least develop in him and her the patterns which will encourage a lifetime of *curiosity, competence*, and *compassion*. And, in this respect, research is an important part of the curriculum because without this as the background, all progress stops, and there is little need to continue to be excited about further learning.

Role models are vital, and we must help the student of medicine to find those which he needs. We must not get into the trap which to some extent psychiatry has gotten into, as expressed several years ago by John Romano, who commented that one of the reasons that students were having difficulty selecting psychiatry as a career choice was that

> When the student comes to these (psychiatric) floors, unlike the other clinical services, he find that most of the staff are not in uniform. He finds them in open shirts, loose gypsy blouses, hip-hugging jeans, wooden shoes, Indian beads, and an abundance of hair. There are nurses, nurse assistants, nurse clinicians, assistant clinicians, psychiatric technicians, social workers, social workers' assistants, mental health aides, program coordinators, psychology students, primary therapists, mental health information service clerks, junior psychiatric faculty, senior faculty (not many of these), full-time (less of these), part-time (often in a hurry), sometime, onetime, and characteristically, most of them never on time. —Small wonder the medical student asks, "Who is the psychiatrist and what does he do?" (Romano, 1980, pp. 109-110)

Whom should he model in his career? Hopefully, he will model himself after those physicians who not only teach him scientific medicine, but also perform well at the bedside, do research, stimulate his thinking, and provide examples in their manners with patients.

ACKNOWLEDGMENT

Preparation of this chapter was supported by NHLBI Cardiovascular Behavioral Medicine Research Training Grant #HL07560.

REFERENCES

Chambers, W. N., & Reiser, M. F. (1953). Emotional stress in the precipitation of congestive heart failure. *Psychosomatic Medicine, 15*, 38–60.

Myers, J. D. (1985). Educating future physicians: Something old, something new: In J. V. Warren & G. L. Trzebiatowski (Eds.), Medical education for the 21st century. Columbus, OH: Ohio State University College of Medicine.

Rappleye, W. C. (Director). (1932). *Medical education: Final report of the Commission on Medical Education*. New York: Association of American Medical Colleges Commission on Medical Education.

Roman, O. J. (1980). On the teaching of psychiatry to medical students: Does it have to get worse before it gets better? *Psychosomatic Medicine, 42* (Suppl.), 103–111.

Shapiro, A. P., Schuck, R. F., Schultz, S. G., & Barnhill, B. N. (1974). The impact of curricular change on performance on National Board Examinations. *Journal of Medical Education, 49*, 1113–1118.

Warren, K. S. (1984). The humanities in medical education. *Annals of Internal Medicine, 101*, 697–701.

AUTHOR INDEX

A

Ader, R., 32, *45*, 50–51, *53*, 54–56, 60, *63*
Adkins, J.R., 16, *22*
Agras, W.S., 87, 93, 96, 97, 99–101, 103, 104, *108*, *109*, *110*
Agrawal, R.C., 96, *108*
Ainslie, G.W., 15, *18*
Alderman, E.A., 89, *108*
Alexander, A.B., 114, 115, 129, 132, 134, 140, 143, *153*, *156*
Alexander, F., 127, *155*, 199
Alexander, K.R., 164, *173*
Allen, M.T., 4, *20*
Allen, R.A., 93, 96, 97, 99, 104, *108*, *110*
Altman, J., 48, 49, *65*
Altszuler, N., 170, *171*
Ams, P.A., 89, *109*
Anderson, D.E., 2–3, 4, 7, *18*
Astley, C.A., 8, 9, 15, *22*
Astley, C.H., 9, *22*
Austen, K.F., 124, *155*
Ayllon, T., 72, *86*
Azrin, N., 72, *86*

B

Backial, M., 139, 142, 145, 151, *154*
Baker, L., 166, *171*, *172*
Bali, L.R., 7, *18*, 91, 100, 101, *108*
Bandura, A., 150, *153*
Barber, J.H., 3, *18*
Barcai, A., 166, *171*
Barker, G.F., 4, *20*
Barlow, D.H., 90, *108*
Barnett, P.M., 70, *86*
Barnhill, B.N., 205, *207*
Baum, D., 132, 136, 138, 139, 147, *153*
Beaudry, J., 16, *21*
Becker, H.C., 28, *45*
Beecher, H.K., 47, 48, *63*, *64*
Beidel, D.C., 97, *109*
Bell, I.R., 6, *18*
Bell, T.D., 118, *156*
Benson, H., 3, 7, *18*, 89, 91, 100–102, 104, *108*, *109*, *110*
Benson, J., 89, *110*
Bergman, J.S., 6, *18*
Bertelson, A.D., 159, *171*
Better, W.E., 4, *18*
Birch, J., 112, *157*
Bisariya, B.N., 96, *108*
Blainey, A.D., 121, *155*
Blanchard, E.B., 6, *18*, *23*, 90, *108*
Blount, W.P., 67, 72, 84, *86*
Bolin, J.F., 121, *155*
Bonner, J.R., 112, 113, *154*
Bose, S., 96, *108*
Bouchard, M.A., 16, *18*
Bovbjerg, D., 50–51, 55, 60, *63*

209

Bradley, C., 166, 167, *171*
Brady, J.P., 91, 98, 100, 103, *109*, 132
Brady, J.V., 2-3, 5, 17, *18*, *19*, 49, *64*
Branscomb, B.V., 117, *154*
Brauer, A.P., 93, 100, 101, 104, *108*
Brett, L.P., 35, 36, *46*
Brickman, A., 17, *18*
Brierley, H., 88, *109*
Brody, H., *63*
Buck, V.M., 118, *156*
Budzynski, T.H., 167, *172*
Bunch, W.H., 70, *86*
Burchfield, S.R., 26, 28, 44, *46*
Burns, K.L., 139, 142, 143, 145, 151, *154*, *156*

C

Cannon, W.B., 161, *171*n, 199
Capponi, R., 161, *171*
Cardozo, C., 9, *19*
Carey, V., 121, *158*
Carpenter, C.B., 50, *65*
Carter, W.R., 166, *171*
Casey, R., 138, *158*
Casey, T.P., 47, 51, *63*
Cassell, E.J., 181, *183*
Chai, H., 114, 117, 118, 129, 132, 134, 139, 140-43, 147, *153*, *154*, *155*, *156*
Chambers, W.N., 200, *207*
Charrow, R.P., 175, *184*
Chase, G., 51, *65*
Cherksey, B., 170, *171*
Cherniack, L., 126, *154*
Cherniack, R.M., 126, *154*
Chesney, M.A., 17, *20*
Chin, D., 175, *183*
Christian, W.P., 135, 136, 139, 147, *155*
Circle, S., 175, *184*
Clancy, R.L., 51, *64*
Clark, G.A., 38, 39, *46*
Clark, L.S., 3, *18*
Clark, T.J.H., 111, 117, 118, 130, *154*
Clarke, W.L., 166, *171*
Clemens, W.J., 17, *18*
Cluss, P.A., 139, *154*
Cochrane, C., 169, *172*
Coe, C.L., 26, 43, *45*
Cohen, A.S., 90, *108*
Cohen, D.H., 1, 8, 9, *18*

Cohen, M., 91, 98, 100, 103, *109*
Cohen, N., 50-51, *53*, 54, 55, 60, *63*
Cohn, M., 55, *64*
Collins, D.K., 82, 85, *86*
Cooley, R.L., 118, *156*
Coover, G.D., 31, 43, *45*
Corbit, J.D., 42, *46*
Corby, J.C., 89, *108*
Corey, E.J., 124, *155*
Corley, K.C., 3, *18*
Cottier, C., 7, *20*, 90, 98, 100-102, 106, *108*
Cowdery, J.S., 51, *65*
Cox, D.J., 166, *171*
Coyle, S., 36, *46*
Creer, P.P., 149, *155*
Creer, T.L., 9, 111, 113-22, 128-30, 132-36, 138-52, *153*, *154*, *155*, *156*, *157*, *158*
Cripps, A.W., 51, *64*
Crits-Christoph, P., 87, 91, 93, 98, 100, 103, 105, *109*, *110*
Cropp, G.J.A., 143, 145, 151, 152, *153*, *155*, *156*
Crowther, J.H., 105, *108*
Cruz, P.T., 162, *172*
Cullen, J.W., 49, *65*
Cuskey, W., 138, *158*
Cuthbert, B., 92, 102, *108*

D

Dahlem, N.W., 115, 144, *156*
Dahms, T.E., 121, *155*
Danker-Brown, P., 114, 129, 132, 134, 140, *156*
Datey, K.K., 17, *18*, 96, *108*
Dauth, G., 9, *23*
Davidson, D.M., 89, *108*
Davidson, J.M., *172*
Davidson, M.B., 159, 160, 166, *171*
Davidson, R.J., 6, *18*, 90, *108*
Davies, R.J., 121, *155*
Davis, A.L., 137, *155*
Davis, H., 59, *63*
Davis, M.H., 114, 129, 132, 134, 140, *156*
DeBoer, K.F., 167, *173*
Deckert, T., 168, *172*
DeGood, D.E., 166, *171*
Delamater, A.M., 159, *171*
DeLeo, J., 89, *110*

Desjardins, C., 29, 30, *45*
Deutsch, R., 48, *64*
De Vellis, R., 150, *158*
Devito, J.L., 9, *22*
DiCara, L.B., 5, *19*
Dietiker, K.E., 142–43, *157*
Dikshit, N., 96, *108*
Di Nardo, P.A., 90, *108*
Dirks, J.F., 115, 144, *156*
Dirks, R., 137, *158*
Dixon, F.J., 51, *64, 65*
Donegan, N.H., 38, 39, *46*
Donjan, M., 40, *45*
Downs, D., 9, *19*
Drazen, J.M., 124, *155*
Driscoll, P.A., 13, *20*
Drummond, D.S., 67, *86*
Dubey, D.R., 146, *157*
Dunbar, F., 199
Dunbar, J.M., 97, *108*
Duncan, H.J., 59, *64*
Dworkin, B.R., 5, *21*, 60, *65*, 85, *86*

E

Eagleston, J.R., 91, *110*
Edmonson, A.S., 67, *86*
Eichna, L.W., 175, *184*
Eikelboom, R., 28, *45*, 49, 55, 60, *64*
Ellenberger, H., 8, 10, 11, *19, 21, 22*
Ellis, E.F., 124, *156*
Elster, A.J., 8, *22*
Eney, R.D., 138, *155*
Engel, B.T., 7, 15–17, *18, 19, 20, 21*, 99, 105, 106, *108*, 182, *184*
Engel, G., 198
Epstein, L.H., 139, *154*
Ernst, F.A., 7, *19*
Erskine, M.S., 41, *46*
Esterly, J., 51, *65*
Evans, F.J., 48, *64*
Evans, F.M., 165, *172*

F

Falliers, C.J., 132, *154*
Farquhar, J.W., 93, 100, 101, 104, *108, 109, 110*
Farr, R.S., 123, 125–26, *158*

Farrell, L., 59, *64*
Faust, R., 137, *155*
Feinberg, G., 124, *155*
Feinglos, M.N., 159, 160, 162, 164, 165, 167–69, *171, 172, 173*
Feldman, J., 6, *22*
Feldstein, M.A., 5, *22*
Ferguson, D.G., 48
Ferris, G., 198
Fertiziger, A.P., 49, *65*
Findley, J.D., 5, *19*
Fine, T.H., 90, *109*
Fireman, P., 139, *154*
Fischer, T.J., 123, *155*
Fisher, E.B., Jr., 159, *171*
Fisher, J.V., 188, *193*
Fisher, L., 104, *109*
Fitzgerald, J., 137, *158*
Flaherty, C.F., 28, *45*
Flannery, G.R., 50, *66*
Fletcher, C.M., 112, *155*
Flood, J.F., 51, *65*
Floyer, J., 111
Forester, W.E., 100, 101, *110*
Forsyth, R.P., 2, 3, *19*
Fortmann, S.P., 104, *109*
Fowler, J.E., 167, *172*
Fox-Kenning, C., 47, *66*
Francis, J., 8, *19*
French, T.M., 127, *155*
Friday, G., 139, *154*
Friedman, B., 82, 85, *86*
Friedman, H., 105, 106, *108*
Friedman, R., 3, *19*
Frysinger, R.C., 11, *20*
Fujimoto, K., 169, *172*
Furedy, J.J., 17, *21*

G

Gaarder, K.R., 99, 105, 106, *108*
Gadow, K.D., 47, 48, *64*
Gaebelein, C.J., 3, 6, *21*
Gallagher, M., 10, 11, *20*
Gallimore, R., 47, *66*
Galosy, R.A., 6, *21*
Galvis, S.A., 139, *154*
Gamsu, D.S., 167, *171*
Gantt, W.H., 48, 49, 60, *64, 65*
Gartside, P.S., 123, *155*

Geiger, 197
Gelfand, M.C., 51, 65
Gellman, M., 10, 11, 19, 22
Gentile, C.G., 8, 11–15, 19, 20, 21
Gershon, E., 6, 22
Gerstenfeld, D.A., 165, 173
Gibbs, C.M., 59, 64
Gill, A., 89, 109
Gilliam, W.J., 5, 19
Glasgow, M.S., 99, 105, 106, 108
Glasgow, R.E., 137, 155
Gleidman, L.H., 48, 64
Glover, A., 48, 64
Golden, T., 9, 21–22
Goldman, L., 43, 45
Goldstein, D.S., 5, 17, 19
Goldstein, E.O., 138, 155
Goldstein, I.B., 87, 93, 99, 104, 105, 109, 110
Goldstein, R., 144, 155
Goleman, D.J., 90, 108
Gonzalez, C.A., 35, 36, 46
Gonder-Frederick, L.A., 166, 171
Gorczynski, R.M., 51, 55, 64
Gormenzano, I., 59, 64
Gormezano, I., 9, 21
Gortmaker, S.L., 121, 155
Graham, J.M., 29, 30, 45
Green, L.W., 144, 155
Green, N., 51, 63
Greer, S., 87, 93, 98, 105, 110, 140
Griffin, M., 124, 155
Grignolo, A., 3, 4, 19, 21
Groshen, S., 167, 172
Grota, L.J., 51, 53
Guilfoile, T.D., 123, 155
Guillemin, R., 55, 64
Gunnar, M.R., 35, 36, 46
Gurr, J., 67, 86
Guy, L.J., 188, 193

H

Hackel, D.B., 162, 172
Hager, J.L., 6, 22
Hahn, B.H., 51, 64
Hall, P., 28, 45
Halter, J.B., 170, 172
Hamburg, S., 166, 172
Hamilton, R.B., 10, 11, 19, 20, 22

Hamilton, T.R., 51, 64
Haque, N., 166, 171
Harada, M., 170, 172
Harano, Y., 170, 172
Hardick, H., 137, 158
Hardin, J.A., 51, 65
Harm, D.L., 115, 116, 118, 120, 121, 141, 142, 147, 151, 154, 155, 156, 158
Harris, A.H., 5, 19, 22, 49, 64
Harris, D.B., 150, 157
Harver, A., 142, 156
Haselton, J.R., 8, 10, 11, 19, 20, 21
Hastedt, P., 167, 168, 171
Hayashi, T., 48, 64
Haynes, M.R., 6, 18
Haynes, R.B., 138, 156
Hedberg, B., 16, 21
Hendler, R., 166, 172
Hendrick, I., 175, 184
Hennessy, J.W., 33–35, 39, 40, 45, 46
Herd, J.A., 3, 18, 19
Hernandez, L.L., 8, 19
Herrnstein, R.J., 48, 49, 57, 64
Hershkoff, H., 143, 153
Heybach, J.P., 31, 45
Hicks, J.D., 51, 65
Higgins, G., 10, 11, 22
Hinde, R.A., 41, 45
Hindi-Alexander, M., 145, 151, 152, 155, 156
Hinkle, L.E., Jr., 165, 172
Hippocrates, 199
Hoard, J.L., 3, 21
Hochstadt, N., 140, 156
Hodes, R., 92, 102, 108
Hoelscher, T.J., 97, 109
Hoffer, J.L., 3, 21
Hoffman, A., 114, 129, 132, 134, 140, 156
Hoffman, J.W., 89, 109
Hohimer, A.R., 8, 9, 15, 22
Holman, H.R., 175, 183
Holroyd, K.A., 150, 158
Hopkins, D., 175, 183
Horlick, L., 93, 100, 101, 104, 108
Horne, N., 103, 108
Howard, J.L., 6, 21
Huang, S.W., 161, 172
Hubbard, J.W., 4, 20
Hughes, J.C., 25, 39, 45
Hunt, E.P., 151, 158
Hurwitz, H.M.B., 59, 63

Husband, M.G., 51, *64*
Huston, D.P., 51, *65*
Hutton, R.A., 28, *45*, 164, *173*

I

Ingels, N.B., 89, *108*
Ishizawka, K., 123, *156*
Ishizawka, T., 123, *156*
Iwai, J., 3, *19*

J

Jachuck, S., 88, *109*
Jachuck, S.J., 88, *109*
Jackson, M.A., 124, *155*
Jacob, R.G., 17, *20*, 87, 93, 97, 104, 105, *109*
Jacobs, F.H., 121, *155*
James, J.I.P., 78, *86*
Jarrell, T.W., 8, 11–15, *19*, *20*, *21*
Javonic, L., 167, *172*
Jensen, R.A., 39, *45*
Jevning, R., 89, *109*, 166, *172*
Johnson, A.H., 188, *193*
Johnson, H.J., 6, *18*
Johnson, K., 167, *172*
Jones, L.G., 3, *19*
Jones, N.F., 115, 144, *156*
Jones, R.S., 116, *156*
Jordan, D., 10, *20*
Joseph, J.A., 15, 16, *19*, *20*
Julius, S., 7, *20*, 90, 98, 100–102, 106, *108*

K

Kadlec, G.J., 138, *158*
Kaestner, E., *46*
Kaliner, M., 124, 125, 127, *156*
Kane, W.J., 67, *86*
Kapp, B.S., 10, 11, 13, *20*, *22*
Karibo, J.M., 138, *158*
Karlman, P., 70, *86*
Kashiwagi, A., 170, *172*
Katkin, E.S., 7, *20*
Katz, R.M., 113, 137, *158*
Kaufman, M.P., 11, *20*
Kawada, M.E., 161, *171*

Kaye, R., 166, *171*
Kearns, G.L., 4, 123, *155*
Keiser, R.P., 68, *86*
Keith, J.A., 188, *193*
Kelleher, R.T., 3, *18*, *19*
Keller, A.H., 188, *193*
Kennedy, M., 51, 55, *64*
Kesarwala, H.H., 123, *155*
Khalid, M.E.M., 10, *20*
Kimball, W.H., 85, *86*
Kimble, G.A., 59, *64*
King, M., 51, *64*
Kinsman, R.A., 115, 137, 144, *156*, *158*
Kirkley, B.G., 159, *171*
Kirmil-Gray, K., 145, *158*
Klemchuck, H.M., 7, *18*
Klemchuk, H., 104, *108*
Klerman, G.L., 62, *65*
Klosko, J.S., 90, *108*
Klosterhalfen, S., 51, *64*
Klosterhalfen, W., 51, *64*
Knapp, P.H., 126, *156*
Knight, G., 167, *171*
Knotts, L., 51, *64*
Knowles, J.B., 48, *64*
Koepke, J.P., 4, *19*, *108*, *109*
Kojima, H., 170, *172*
Kolp, L.A., 36, *46*
Konorski, J., 38, 39, *45*
Kopell, B.S., 89, *108*
Kordenat, R.R., 7, *19*
Koski, G.B., 138, *158*
Kotses, H., 115, 141, 142, 147, 151, 153, 154, *155*, *156*, *158*
Kraemer, H.C., 87, 93, 99, 104, *108*, *109*
Krantz, D.S., 96, *109*
Krieger, D.T., 25, 39, *45*
Kristeller, J., 92, 102, *108*
Kristt, D.A., 7, *20*
Kron, R.E., 91, 98, 100, 103, *109*
Kuhn, C.M., 162, 169, *172*, *173*
Kulkosky, P.J., 28, *46*, 163, *173*
Kurland, A.A., 48, *64*
Kusnecov, A.W., 51, *64*

L

Labelle, J., 16, *18*
Lal, H., 48–49, *65*
Lammers, C.A., 167, *172*

Landberg, L.L., 89, *109*
Landis, B., 167, *172*
Landis, E., 167, *172*
Lando, H., 137, *156*
Lang, P.J., 6, *20*
Lang, W.J., 48, *64*
Langer, A.W., 3, *21*
Lasagna, L., 48, *64*
Latham, S.B., 59, *64*
Laughlin, K.D., 104, *109*
Lavond, D.G., 38–39, *46*
Lawler, J.E., 3, 4, 6, *20*, *21*
Lawler, K.A., 3, *20*
Lawry J.A., 26, *46*
Lazarus, A.A., 105, *109*
LeBlanc, W., 10, *19*
Lebovitz, H.E., 162, 168, *171*, *172*
Lehman, D.H., 51, *64*
Leigh, D., 115, *156*
Leitch, A.G., 124, *155*
Leung, P., 118, 139, 142, 145, 151, *154*, *156*
Levine, J., 28, *45*
Levine, S., 26, 33–37, 39–43, *45*, *46*
Levy, L., 91, 98, 100, 103, *109*
Lewis, S.B., 166, *172*
Liberman, R., 47, *64*
Lichstein, K.L., 97, *109*
Lichtenstein, E., 137, *156*
Light, K.C., 3, *21*, *108*, *109*
Lincoln, J.S., 38, 39, *46*
Linde, J., 168, *172*
Linden, W., 90, *109*
Lisina, M.I., 7, *21*
Liskowsky, D.R., 10, 11, *19*, *22*
Livingston, E.G., 162, 164, *173*
Lloyd, G., 176, *184*
Locurto, C.M., 59, *64*
Long, A.J., 92, 102, *108*
Loren, M.L., 118, *156*
Lowenthal, D.T., 51, *65*
Luborsky, L., 87, 91, 93, 98, 100, 103, 105, *109*, *110*
Lukas, S.E., 5, *22*
Lulla, S.H., 140, *156*
Lynch, J.J., 49, *65*
Lyon, R., 142–43, *157*

M

Mackintosh, N.J., 27, *45*, 59, *65*
Macrae, S., 51, 55, *64*
Madden, J., 38, 39, *46*
Magnusson, E., 16, *21*
Maheshwari, R., 96, *108*
Makinodan, T., 51, *65*
Makous, W., 28, *45*, 164, *173*
Malcuit, G., 16, *21*
Mamounas, L.A., 38, 39, *46*
Manning, A.A., 9, *21–22*
Manning, J., 3, *21*
Manuck, S.B., 96, *109*
Margolis, A., 42, 43, *46*
Marion, R.J., 115, 116, 118, 120, 121, 139, 142, 143, 145, 147, 149, 151, 152, *154*, *155*, *156*
Marlatt, C.A., 91, *109*
Marmot, M.G., 89, *110*
Marques, J.K., 91, *109*
Martin, P.L., 3, *21*
Martinez, J.L., Jr., 39, *45*
Marzetta, B.R., 7, *18*, 104, *108*
Mason, J.W., 25, *45*
Mathe, A.A., 126, *156*
Mauck, H.P., 3, *18*
Mauk, M.D., 38, 39, *46*
McCabe, P.M., 8, 11–15, *19*, *20*, *21*
McCormick, D.A., 38–39, *46*
McCormick, M.C., 138, *158*
McCubbin, J.A., 3, *21*, 162, 164, 165, *173*
McDaniels, S.M., 51, *65*
McFadden, E.R., Jr., 111, 117, 121–25, *155*, *156*
McGaugh, J.L., 39, *45*
McGee, D.J., 165, *173*
McGrady, A.V., 90, *109*
McLesky, C.H., 166, *172*
McNall, C.D., 10, *20*
Melman, K., 175, *183*
Melnechuk, T., 55, *64*
Messing, R.B., 39, *45*
Meyer, M.P., 150, *157*
Middleton, E., 124, *156*
Mikat, E.M., 162, *172*
Miklich, D.R., 114, 126, 129, 132, 134, 139, 140, 142, 143, 145, 151, *153*, *154*, *156*
Milburn, P., *46*
Miller, K.A., 138, *156*
Miller, N.E., 5, *19*, *21*, 49, 60, *65*, 85, 86, 167, *172*, 199
Minuchin, S., 166, *172*

Mirsky, A., 198, 200, 204
Mitchell, E.A., 153, *157*
Moe, J.H., 67, 72, 84, *86*
Molk, L., 140, *155*
Moomaw, C.J., 123, *155*
Morris, A.D., 51, *65*
Morris, J.T., 67, *86*
Morse, W.H., 3, *18, 19*
Moses, J.L., 167, *171*
Mosteller, F., 48, *64*
Mowrer, O.H., 26, 38, 39, 44, *45*
Munoz, A., 121, *158*
Murphy, R.H., Jr., 121, *157*
Murray, E.H., 7, *20*
Myers, J., 200, 204, 206, *207*

N

Naliboff, B.D., 167, *172*
Nau, E., 142–43, *157*
Nelson, E., 93, 100, 101, 104, *108, 110*
Newcomb, R.W., 117, *154*
Ng, M., 51, *64*
Nisho, Y., 170, *172*
Noble, M.E., 7, *22*
North, W.R.S., 7, *21*
Numan, R., 48–49, *65*

O

O'Brien, F., 72, *86*
Obrist, P.A., 3–6, 8, 16, 17, *18, 19, 20, 21, 23, 108, 109*
O'Halloran, J.P., 89, *109*
Ohashi, K., 48, *64*
O'Leary, S.G., 146, *157*
Oliver, M.F., 87, *110*
Ordentlich, M., 137, *155*
Overmier, J.B., 26, *46*

P

Pagano, R.R., 91, *109*
Pain, M.C.F., 141, *157*
Parcel, G.S., 150, *157*
Parker, S.R., 144, *155*
Patel, C., 7, 17, *21*, 89, 104, 106, *110*
Patterson, J.M., 37, *46*

Pavlov, I.P., 40, 41, *46*, 199
Pearlman, D.S., 112–14, 118, 119, 122, 123, *157*
Pepys, J., 121, *155*
Perez-Reyes, M., 17, *21*
Perski, A., 17, *21*
Peter, J.M., 100–102, *110*
Peters, R.K., 91, 100–102, *110*
Peterson, C.M., 167, *172*
Petrie, A., 48, *65*
Petrik, G.K., 11, *20*
Picon, L., 161, *172*
Piers, E.V., 150, *157*
Pihl, R.O., 48, 49, *65*
Pirkle, H., 89, *109*
Plout, S.M., 161, *172*
Poling, A.D., 47, *64*
Pollard, S.J., 138, *158*
Ponseti, I.V., 82, 85, *86*
Porte, D., Jr., 164, 170, *172, 173*
Porter, D., 91, *110*
Porter, R., 112, *157*
Portha, B., 161, *172*
Powell, D.A., 8, *19*
Pride, N.B., 112, *155*
Purcell, K., 127, 128, 132, *154, 157*

R

Rachelefsky, G.S., 113, *158*
Rachelefsky, O., 137, *158*
Raczynski, J.M., 85, *86*
Raeburn, J.M., 102, *110*
Randall, D.C., 1, 8, 9, *18*
Rapp, P.R., 10, 11, *22*
Rappleye, W.C., 198, *207*
Raveche, E.S., 51, *65*
Ray, W.J., 85, *86*
Reddy, C., 49, *65*
Redgate, E.S., 166, *171*
Reed, C.E., 119, 121–26, 153, *156, 157*
Rees, J., 113, *157*
Reeves, J.L., 17, *21*
Reich, P., 50, *65*
Reiser, M.F., 200, *207*
Renne, C.M., 114–18, 128–30, 132, 134–36, 139–43, 147, 152, *155, 156, 157*
Rescorla, R.A., 26, 39, *46*
Revusky, S., 40, *46*
Reynolds, R.V.C., 152, *156*

Rigter, H., 39, 45
Riley, D.M., 17, 21
Rizza, R.A., 160, 173
Roberts, B.W., 100, 101, 110
Robertson, P.R., 170, 172
Roffman, M., 49, 65
Rogala, E.J., 67, 86
Roger, T., 85, 86
Rogers, M.P., 50, 65
Roll, D., 72, 86
Romano, J., 198, 207
Romanski, L.M., 12–14, 19, 20
Rose, B.J., 14, 20
Rose, R.M., 91, 109
Rosenbaum, L., 167, 172
Rosenbaum, M., 198
Rosenthal, T.L., 97, 109
Rosman, B., 166, 172
Rosner, B., 121, 158
Rosner, B.A., 7, 18, 104, 108
Ross, P., 48, 64
Ross, R.S., 5, 17, 19
Ross, S., 48, 49, 65
Rotter, J.B., 150, 157
Roudier, M., 161, 172
Rounsaville, B.J., 62, 65
Rowan, G.A., 28, 45
Rubin, H., 72, 86
Rubinfeld, A.R., 141, 157
Ruch-Ross, H., 121, 155
Russell, P.J., 51, 65

S

Sackett, D.L., 138, 156
Sakaguchi, T., 169, 172
Sakula, A., 111, 157
Salanova, C., 84, 86
Sandman, C.A., 7, 19
Sandman, M.S., 7, 19
Santiago, J.V., 160, 173
Sato, K., 51, 65
Savchenko, V.A., 164, 172
Schachter, S., 139, 157
Schade, D.S., 160, 173
Schaub, R.G., 4, 20
Schiffer, C.G., 151, 158
Schlosberg, H., 48, 65
Schneider, J.A., 93, 96, 97, 99, 104, 108, 110

Schneiderman, N., 1, 8–15, 17, 18, 19, 20, 21–22, 23, 199
Schnitzer, S.B., 48, 49, 65
Schuck, R.F., 205, 207
Schuler, R., 28, 45
Schull, J., 42, 46
Schultz, S.G., 205, 207
Schwaber, J.S., 10, 11, 13, 20, 22
Schwartz, G., 47, 66
Schwartz, G.E., 5, 6, 16, 18, 22, 90, 108
Scott, D., 166, 171
Scott, R.W., 6, 18
Scovern, A.W., 159, 160, 173
Seeburg, K.N., 167, 173
Seer, P., 87, 93, 102, 105, 110
Seldin, D.W., 175, 181, 184
Sevastikoglou, J.A., 70, 86
Shanks, E.M., 6, 21
Shanks-Teller, E., 3, 21
Shapiro, A.K., 47, 65
Shapiro, A.P., 97, 109, 205, 207
Shapiro, D., 5, 6, 16, 17, 21, 22, 87, 93, 99, 104, 105, 109, 110, 166, 173
Shapiro, K., 90, 98, 100–102, 106, 108
Shapiro, M.F., 175, 184
Sharp, G.C., 51, 65
Shattock, R.J., 17, 18
Shearn, D.W., 4, 22
Shepard, J., 140, 156
Sherer, L.M., 188, 193
Sherrard, D.J., 104, 109
Sherwin, R.S., 166, 172
Shiel, F.O., 3, 18
Shigeta, Y., 170, 172
Shogren, R.E., 164, 173
Shufflebarger, H.L., 68, 86
Sideroff, S., 8, 22
Siegel, S., 28, 42, 46, 49, 65, 113, 137, 158, 164, 173
Sierles, F., 175, 184
Simons, R., 92, 102, 108
Singer, G., 50, 66
Sirota, A.D., 6, 16, 22
Sivyer, M., 51, 64
Skinner, B.J., 48, 65
Skyler, J.S., 160, 173
Slavin, R.G., 121, 155
Sly, R.M., 117, 137, 158
Smith, A.C., 9, 21
Smith, G.R., 51, 65
Smith, J.C., 90, 110

Smith, M., 28, *45*
Smith, M.C., 9, *21*
Smith, N., 48–49, *65*
Smith, O.A., 8, 9, 15, *22*
Smith, S.B., 121, *158*
Smithson, K.W., 3, *21*
Smotherman, W.P., 33–36, 40, 42, 43, *45*, *46*
Snyder, C., 7, *22*
Solomon, H., 5, *22*
Solomon, R.L., 26, 39, 42, *46*
Southam, M.A., 93, 100, *108*
Spector, S.L., 123, 125–26, 137, *158*
Speizer, F.E., 121, *158*
Spence, K.W., 59, *65*
Spiro, H.M., 47, *65*
Spyer, K.M., 10, *20*
Stanley, W.C., 48, *65*
Stanton, M.E., 26, 37, 43, *45*, *46*
Steinberg, A.D., 51, *65*
Steinbrook, G.L., 89, *109*
Stephenson, R.B., 8, 9, 15, *22*
Steptoe, A., 115, *158*
Stern, J.M., 41, *46*
Stern, M., 6, *22*
Stevens, J.B., 111, *156*
Stewart, J., 28, *45*, 49, 55, 60, *64*
Stone, R.A., 89, *110*
Straatmeyer, A.J., 167, *172*
Strom, T.B., 50, *65*
Sublett, J.L., 138, *158*
Surwit, R.S., 6, *22*, 159, 160, 162, 164–69, *171*, *172*, *173*
Surwit, R.W., 5, 6, *22*
Sussman, K.E., 165–66, *173*
Sutton, B.R., 31, *45*
Suzuki, M., 170, *172*
Swanson, A.G., 181, *184*
Szakmary, G.A., *46*

T

Tager, I.B., 121, *158*
Takadoro, S., 48, *64*
Talal, N., 51, *65*
Tan, S.T., 90, *109*
Taplin, P.S., 139, 141, 142, 145, 151, *154*, *158*
Taub, H.A., 105, 106, *108*
Taurog, J.D., 51, *65*

Taylor, C.B., 89, 93, 96, 97, 99–101, 103, 104, *108*, *110*
Taylor, D.W., 138, *156*
Taylor, G., 161, *172*
Taylor C.B., *108*
Teich, A., 11, 12, 15, *19*
Teitelbaum, H.A., 48, 49, *64*, *65*
Telch, M.J., 91, *110*
Terrace, H.S., 59, *64*
Terry, D.J., 89, *110*
Thananopavaran, C., 99, 104, *109*
Theofilopoulos, A.N., 51, *65*
Thompson, R.F., 38–39, *46*
Thoresen, C.E., 91, *110*, 145, *158*
Tinker, T.R., 142, *158*
Titus, C.C., 165–66, *173*
Tobin, D.L., 150, *158*
Tosheff, J., 2, *18*
Townley, R.G., 119, 121–23, 125, 126, *157*
Tunved, J., 16, *21*
Turkkan, J.S., 5, *19*, *22*
Turner, J.L., 47, *66*
Tursky, B., 5, 6, *22*, 47, *66*
Twentyman, C.T., 6, *20*

U

Ui, M., 169, *172*
Ullman, S., 139, 142, 145, 151, *154*
Underwood, M.D., 10, *20*
Uzwiak, A.J., 28, *45*

V

Vandenbergh, R.L., 165–66, 167, *172*, *173*
VanDercar, D.H., 5, 9, 12, 15, *19*, *21–22*
Varela, C., 161, *171*
Vargas, L., 161, *171*
Vasselli, J.R., *46*
Vaughan, G.D., 166, *173*
Vermilyea, B.B., 90, *108*
Vitiello, M.V., *46*
Voelker, S., 28, *45*
Von Pelsinger, J.M., 48, *64*

W

Waddell, M.T., 90, *108*

Wadden, T.A., 87, 91, 93, 97, 98, 105, *110*
Wagner, A.R., 42, *46*
Walker, D.K., 121, *155*
Wallace, R.K., 89, *110*
Wallach, J.H., 10, 11, *19*, 22
Wallston, B.S., 150, *158*
Wallston, K.A., 150, *158*
Walsh, R.N., 89, 90, *109*, *110*
Walton, T.R., 89, *108*
Ward, J.D., 167, *171*
Wareheim, B.A., 161, *172*
Warren, K., 196, *207*
Wayner, E.A., 50, *66*
Webb, R.A., 8, *21*
Weinberg, E., 140, *155*
Weinberg, J., 35, 36, *46*
Weinberger, N.M., 14, 22
Weinstein, A.G., 138, *158*
Weiss, J.H., 128, 150, *157*, *158*
Weiss, J.W., 124, *155*
Weiss, S.T., 121, *158*
Weiss, T., 91, 98, 100, 103, *109*
Weissman, M., 62, *65*
Weissmann, G., 124, *158*
Wells, D.T., 6, 22
White, L., 47, 48, *66*
Whitehorn, D., 10, *20*
Wickers, F.C., 70, *86*
Wickramasekera, I., 48, *66*
Wigal, J.K., 150, *158*
Wigal, J.L., 142, *158*
Wikler, A., 48, *66*

Williams, J.L., 16, 22
Williams, M.H., Jr., 112, 115, 117, 124, 140, *158*
Williams, R.B., 5, 6, 22
Willis, P.W., *108*, *109*
Wilson, A.F., 89, *109*, *110*, 166, *172*
Wilson, C.B., 51, *64*
Winant, J.G., Jr., 123, *155*
Winchester, M.A., 89, *108*
Winder, J.A., 116, 117, 144, 149-52, *155*, *158*
Woerner, M., 90, *109*
Wolf, S., 48, *66*, 165, *172*
Wolpe, J., 140, *158*
Wood, D.M., 8, 17, *21*, *23*
Wood, P.R., 28, 138, *158*
Woodruff, R.E., 166, *172*
Woods, S.C., 26, 28, 44, *45*, *46*, 47, 163, 164, *173*

Y

Yehle, A., 9, *19*, *21–22*, *23*
Yingling, J.E., 3, 7, *18*
Young, J.B., 89, *109*
Young, L.D., 6, *18*, *23*

Z

Zarcone, V.P., Jr., 89, *108*

SUBJECT INDEX

A

Absenteeism, 91
Abstinence, 137
Adipose tissue, 161
Adjustment, 201
Adrenal cortex, 161
Adrenocortical steroids, 32, 51
Adrenomedullary system, 161
Allergy, 118, 122
Amygdala-vagal bradycardiac pathway, 13
Anaphylaxis, 124
Anticipation, 3, 16
Antihypertensive medications, 87
Anxiety, 20, 179
Approach-avoidance conflict, 34
Aspirin, 123
Associative learning, 2
Asthma, 120, 121, 133, 137, 149
Asthma diaries, 150
Asthma interventions, 127
Asthma precipitants, 120, 136
Atrophine methylnitrate, 7
Attitudes, 147, 150, 181, 185, 197
Auditory cortex, 13
Autoimmune disease, 49
Automated postural feedback, 67–86
Autonomic arousal, 89
Autonomic nervous system, 160

B

B lymphocyctes, 51
Behavior modification, 183
Behavioral deficits, 135, 138–139, 141–144
Behavioral excesses, 135, 136–137, 139–141
Behavioral intervention strategies, 127
Behavioral risk factors, 201
Behavioral techniques, 135
Behavioral treatment of hypertension, 7–15
Beta-adrenerg blockade, 125, 166
Biofeedback, 2, 5, 7, 16, 90, 105
Blood pressure, 5–6, 87, 93, 100
Brochospasm, 125
Bronchi, 113
Bronchial asthma, 111–158
Bronchitis, 112
Bronchoconstriction, 112

C

Carbohydrate metabolism, 160
Cardiovascular disease, 195
Cardiovascular reactivity, 17, 201
Cardiovascular regulation, 1–17
Cardiovascular response modification, 15–17
Catecholamines, 170
Central nervous system, 88
Chemotherapy, 55

219

Cigarette use, 121
Classical conditioning, 8–15
Compliance, 68, 96, 132, 138, 189
Conditioned emotional response, 9
Conflict, 35
Control, 92, 117
Control procedures, 130
Coping, 88, 181
Corticoids, 32
Corticosterone, 51
Corticothalamic pathway, 14
Cortisol, 38, 161 (see also adrenocortical steroids)
Counseling skills, 188
Cyclophosphamide, 49, 51, 57

D

D-amphetamine, 49
Dehydration, 159
Dependence, 57
Depression, 91, 179, 188
Desquamation, 125
Diet, 3, 161
Doctor-patient relationship, 189
Dorsal vagal nucleus, 10
Drug administration, 48
Drug withdrawal, 49, 55
Dying patients, 181

E

Ejection fraction, 89
Emg biofeedback, 167
Emotion arousal, 38, 90, 122
Emphysema, 130
Endocrine abnormalities, 162
Endocrine response, 25–46
Environment, 25, 114, 163
Epinephrine, 101 (see also catecholamines, endocrine response)
Epinephrine bitartrate, 162
Ethics, 188
Euglycemic, 162
Exercise, 17, 121
Exhaustion, 179
Experimenter-subject interaction, 92

F

Family physician training, 185–194

Family relationships, 152
Family therapy, 166
Fatigue, 159
Fear, 37, 39
Fear conditioning, 38
Furosemide-stimulated renin activity, 89

G

Glucose control in diabetes mellitus, 159–173
Glucose intolerance, 162
Glucose levels, 166
Glucose metabolism, 165
Glycochemoglobin, 167
Grief, 181
Growth hormone, 25

H

Habituation, 41
Headache, 179, 185, 188
Health education, 90
Hemaglutinating antibody titers, 50
Histamine, 125
Hospital overuse, 140
Hyperadrenocorticism, 162
Hyperglycemia, 28, 159
Hyperinsulinemia, 162
Hyperosmolar coma, 159
Hypertension, 87–111
Hypnosis, 105
Hypoglycemia, 28
Hypogonadotrophism, 162
Hypometabolic state, 89
Hypothalamic pituitary adrenocortical, 161
Hypothalamus, 10
Hypothermia, 49

I

IgE, 123
Immunosuppression, 49
Immunology of asthma, 123
Immunologic reactivity, 49
Infections, 122
Information processing, 146
Instrumental learning therapy, 72
Insulin, 28

K

Ketoacidosis, 159

L

Latent inhibition, 41
Lateral preoptic region, 11
Laughing, 122
Leukotrienes, 124
Lifestyle, 188
Lithium chloride, 33
Locus-of-control, 150
Luteinizing hormone, 29–30

M

Medial forebrain bundle, 11
Medical education, 195–207
Medical monitoring, 138
Medical school curriculum, 175–207
Medication, 182
Medication scores, 152
Medication use, 143
Meditation, 87
Memory, 88
Morphine, 49
Mucosal edema, 125

N

Neuromuscular pathways, 125
Neuropathy, 159
Noise stress, 166
Norepinephrine, 89 (see also catecholamines)
Nucleus ambiguus, 10

O

Obesity, 162, 188
Oligosynaptic bradycardia pathway, 11
Operant conditioning, 2, 4–7
Opponent process theory, 42

P

Pancreatic islets of Langerhans, 160
Panic, 117, 139
Parabrachial nucleus, 11
Parental behavior, 117
Patient-oriented theory of disease, 176
Pavlovian conditioning, 25–46
Perception, 90, 117
Performance, 3, 148
Personality, 199, 201
Pharmacotherapy, 56
Pituitary-adrenal system, 25, 43 (see also adrenal cortex, adrenocortical steriods, cortisol)
Pituitary-gonadal axis, 28
Placebo, 47–66, 101
Plasma dopamine-beta-hydroxylase activity, 89
Professional role, 188, 190
Prostaglandins, 124
Proteinuria, 52
Psychological intervention strategies, 127
Psychosomatic disease, 119
Psychotherapy, 91, 188
Pulmonary function, 151
Punishment, 75

Q

Quality-of-life, 202

R

Reciprocal inhibition, 115
Rehabilitation, 134
Relaxation training, 7, 87–111, 143, 166
Renin, 90
Retinopathy, 159
Reward, 75
Rhinitis, 118
Role models, 197, 207

S

Saccharin, 33
School absenteeism, 151
School data, 151
School phobias, 188
Scoliosis, 67–86
Scopolamine hydrobromide, 49

Second-order conditioning, 40
Self-concept measures, 150
Self-control, 135
Self-efficacy, 150
Self-instruction, 146
Self-management, 131, 135, 138, 142, 144, 145, 152
Self-monitoring, 135, 146
Sensory preconditioning, 40
Sex differences, 35
Sexual interest, 88
Side effects, 60, 101
Smoking, 130
Social affiliation, 37, 91
Social drinkers, 91
Social factors, 38
Spirometer, 142
Spontaneous remission, 118
Steptozotocin, 161
Stress, 163, 165, 166
Stroke volume, 89
Superior olivary nucleus, 13
Sympathetic discharge, 160
Sympathetic nervous system, 88
Sympathetic tone, 89
Symptom characteristics, 182
Systematic desensitization, 140
Systemic lupus erythematosus, 51

T

T lymphocyctes, 51
Tantalum myocardial markers, 89
Testosterone, 25
Theophylline, 130, 138
Tolbutamide, 164
Trachea, 113

V

Vagal reflexes, 125

W

Weight gain, 179
Weight loss, 159
Work performance, 91